ADHD AND THE NATURE
OF SELF-CONTROL

ADHD
AND THE NATURE
OF SELF-CONTROL

Russell A. Barkley, PhD

THE GUILFORD PRESS
New York London

Library of Congress Cataloging-in-Publication Data

Barkley, Russell A., 1949–
    ADHD and the nature of self-control / Russell A. Barkley.
      p. cm.
    Includes bibliographical references and index.
    ISBN 1-57230-250-X
    1. Attention-deficit hyperactivity disorder–Etiology. 2. Self-
control. 3. Inhibition.   I. Title.
RJ506.H9B368 1997
616.85′89071—dc21   97-25931
                                             CIP

For my sons, Ken and Steve

15.61

The end of summer hits a person my age with special force. . . . Over the years, the turning of the seasons has become an irrefutable image of the life cycle itself. Your youth is precious to me, in part as compensation for the loss of my own. . . . The end of summer lays bare the law of time. My life ends, and so will yours. Time itself will end. . . . Young as you are, you know this. . . . At a certain point you had accumulated enough past to imagine a future. The arc of experience revealed itself to you. You sensed your own beginning, which prepared you then to think of your mother's end and mine—which is a way of thinking of your own. This was the beginning of the end of your childhood, when looking backward forced you to look ahead. Before that, the lack of a larger frame within which to interpret occurrences left you at the mercy of a dislocated present, a condition of absolute immediacy. Young children take such a state for granted. We call it pure innocence. What you were innocent of was time. . . . The awareness of mortality, and only that, enables us to see fully our real place in the universe, and the name for our place is time. Once we see this, everything changes. The sadness in the death of living things does not go away, but it takes on a silent and equal partner, which is the feeling of acceptance. That is the definition of happiness—when we mortal beings accept ourselves as such. The two-dollar word for this change is "transcendence," and what we have transcended, in accepting time, is time itself.

From "A Chill in the Air," by James Carroll, *The Boston Globe Magazine* (September 1, 1996, pp. 16–21)

99935

Preface

THIS BOOK REPRESENTS an unabashed and unapologetic attempt to construct a wholesale theory of attention-deficit/hyperactivity disorder (ADHD). It is the culmination of nearly 5 years of work toward this end, ranging from the nearly continuous critical conceptual thinking that has almost obsessed me since my discovery of this model 4 years ago, to the literature searches and the subsequent reading and rereading of several hundred scientific papers. It also involved multiple discussions with my close friends and colleagues about the fruits of these labors and their implications for understanding self-control and ADHD. Throughout, I maintained a running diary of various free-associated thoughts from these enterprises so that no new perspective, idea, hypothesis, or implication of this model for ADHD would escape my memory. The substantial scientific literature I read spans that of child psychopathology on the cognitive deficits associated with ADHD, theories of and empirical research into the executive functions of the prefrontal cortex in neuropsychology, empirical research on the development of self-regulation in children as reflected in the developmental psychological literature, and readings outside of these disciplines (e.g., evolutionary biology). I then made several attempts to develop rudimentary forms of this theory and set them to paper. However, each attempt, though more adequate than the last, seemed imperfect to me. I had the nagging sense that only a book could cover so much material in any persuasive way. I have no doubt, however, that this text will prove imperfect as well, given time.

Out of this extended conceptual analysis, I have attempted to synthesize a theory of executive functions and their critical role in human self-regulation. I have then extended this theoretical model to an understanding of ADHD. My original goal was the construction of a scientific theory of ADHD. But along the way I had, of necessity, to construct a theory of self-regulation for at least two reasons. First and foremost, any theory of a child psychopathological condition such as ADHD will ultimately have to be linked to larger theories of the nature of normal developmental psychological processes and the neuropsychological processes that comprise them. Pathological states are variations from normal states. An understanding of the development of those normal psychological functions, therefore, can provide substantial insight into the development of the psychopathological condition. In short, the literature about a psychological disorder and that about its normal developmental counterpart must be bridged at some point in theory construction. Second, a model of self-regulation was required because evidence has been growing within the literature on ADHD that it is not a disorder of attention, but rather one of behavioral inhibition and self-regulation. The model, then, had to become a model of executive neuropsychological functions as well because it became clear that these functions are the self-directed actions that permit self-control. Consequently, any theory of ADHD is, of necessity, a theory of executive functions and self-regulation.

My conclusion that ADHD involves delays in the development of inhibition and self-regulation is not new or original. George Still made this point in what appears to be the first scientific clinical treatise on the disorder, published in 1902. Virginia Douglas has been the more recent proponent of a similar view since the late 1980s, along with myself and, more recently, Bruce Pennington and Martha Denckla. What distinguishes my attempt here from these others is my effort to (1) specify the nature of self-regulation, (2) show how the executive functions are involved in it, (3) articulate the basic number and nature of these functions, (4) demonstrate their critical dependence on behavioral inhibition, (5) argue that the purpose of executive functioning and self-regulation is to increase the control of behavior by time and hypotheses the individual constructs about the future, and (6) specify that the ultimate utility function of all this activity is the net maximization of long-term consequences for the benefit of the individual relative to just those consequences in the immediate context or short-term.

Out of such a theory comes a richer and deeper understanding of the nature of human self-regulation and of ADHD, as well as a number of new and testable hypotheses about the nature of ADHD that have not previously been predicted to be associated with this disorder by any prior theory of it. While too numerous to list exhaustively here, some of these predictions will be mentioned briefly in order to illustrate the point. The rest are scattered throughout the text, and, in particular, can be found in Chapter 9.

For instance, to my knowledge this is the first theoretical model of ADHD to predict that the disorder (1) disrupts the capacity for working or representational memory and the power of covertly sensing, or, more accurately, resensing, information to oneself; (2) creates a delay in the internalization of speech during development and the self-control dependent upon this rather miraculous developmental process; (3) impairs the development of the psychological sense of time, hindsight, and forethought and, particularly, the employment of those senses in the regulation of one's own behavior relative to time and the future; (4) disrupts not only the power to internally represent information but also the capacity to reconstitute that information in the service of goal-directed behavioral creativity and the cross-temporal organization of behavior; (5) diminishes the capacity for private, covert emoting and motivating to oneself that is critical to objectivity, perspicacity, intentionality, and the motivational support of behavior as it is driven toward the future; (6) impairs the capacity to imitate or replicate the complex behavioral sequences of others; (7) results in more externalized or public than internalized or covert "thinking" behavior than is typical of normal individuals; and (8) interferes with the goal-directed persistence, volition, and free will of the individual.

Indeed, this is the only theory to my knowledge that even makes a critical distinction between two forms of sustained attention. One is context-dependent and contingency-shaped (externally controlled). The other is rule-governed, goal-directed, and internally guided and motivated. It is the latter, not the former, that is impaired by ADHD. This explains the apparent inattention of those with ADHD and why it fluctuates so much as a function of the task and context. So long as the environment provides the ongoing reinforcement needed to sustain responding, those with ADHD will have no difficulties in doing so. It is when minimal or no reinforcement is available and behavior must be created, organized, and self-sustained toward a future goal that those with ADHD will be found to be impersistent or "inattentive."

While other researchers have certainly noted some of these deficits in their findings on ADHD, they were not testing predictions from a theoretical model of ADHD. Nor could they account for such results within any extant viewpoint of this disorder. Instead, they were largely engaged in descriptive or exploratory research about the disorder, laudable in its own right, using relatively novel approaches to measurement for research on ADHD.

The theory of ADHD espoused here is also the only one of which I am aware that asserts that the very process by which various forms of behavior become internalized is delayed in those with the disorder. This means that the multiple forms of thought or "cognition" that regulate behavior and that depend upon such internalization to create them will also be delayed in this disorder. The implications for clinical practice from such a radical shift of perspective on this disorder are numerous and profound, as I attempt to show in the last chapter of this book, and so, I believe, are the implications of this model for society's perspective on self-control more generally.

Based on this new theory of ADHD, I make the point repeatedly throughout this text that understanding the nature of self-control, the process of developmental internalization of behavior, and the process of directing behavior toward the future are absolutely critical to achieving a more complete understanding of the nature of the cognitive and social impairments created by ADHD and to treating those with this disorder. Equally crucial are the concepts of time, timing, and timeliness that are inherent in self-regulation and future-oriented behavior. In this volume I will eventually argue that humans have evolved an instinct for self-regulation so as to bring behavior under the control of time and the probable futures that lay before them. I liken this developmental instinct to the human instinct for language that, upon stimulation by a linguistic community, displays a rapid developmental acquisition in the child during neurological maturation. The capacity for language is not a cultural product, though its contents clearly are so. The same it seems to me is true of self-control as well, as the evidence presented here appears to make plain. ADHD results in a delay in this socially critical neuropsychological instinct that results in a pervasive impact on the day-to-day adaptive functioning of individuals having this disorder. As a consequence, ADHD is not a disorder of attention—it is a developmental disorder of inhibition, self-control, and time.

To make my case, I have structured this book as a lawyer might present evidence at a trial, laying out the evidence for each assumption I wish to make and building my case toward the final verdict that ADHD is a developmental disorder of self-regulation that impairs the capacity to direct behavior toward time and the future. First, I give a brief summary of research on the nature of ADHD and a discussion of current criteria used in its diagnosis as these forms of information may impact the construction of a theory of the disorder (Chapter 1). I then discuss what is known about the biological factors that appear to cause or at least to contribute to this disorder and the implications such findings have for any attempts at developing a theory of ADHD (Chapter 2). That chapter concludes that ADHD must be viewed as a neuropsychological disorder having a substantial biological, and largely genetic, contribution to its expression and that a theory of ADHD therefore will need to be neuropsychological in nature and must include constructs that have a substantial heritability to them. In Chapter 3, I specifically define those terms that will prove critical to developing a theory of ADHD as a disorder of inhibition that disrupts the executive functions and so impairs self-regulation. Subsequently, I marshal the substantial evidence that supports the conclusion that ADHD is a disorder of behavioral inhibition (Chapter 4). With this key assumption in place as a foundation, I move to a discussion of past models of the executive functions, all of which incorporate inhibition as a necessary precursor to them and protector of them (Chapter 5). From these earlier models, four executive functions apart from behavioral inhibition can be extracted. Further evidence for the existence of these functions is then presented in Chapter 6. Having established the likelihood that such executive functions exist and are separable, though clearly inter-active in their performance, I then set about combining them into a hybrid model of executive functions and self-regulation in Chapter 7. The following chapter highlights some of the developmental findings on these executive functions and their probable developmental staging during maturation (Chapter 8). I then proceed to one of the major purposes of this text, the extrapolation of this model to a theory of ADHD (Chapter 9). In Chapter 10, I review the literature on the cognitive and neuropsychological deficits documented in prior research as associated with ADHD, examining it for its consistency with the predictions of the theoretical model. The general consistency of the evidence with the predictions is most reassuring but not always confirmatory of the predictions, owing in large part to an absence of research on these various predictions. Even so, what evidence does exist does not seem to me to contradict the theory in most of its predictions about ADHD. Finally, in Chapter 11, I discuss what I believe are the major implications of this model for the clinical understanding and diagnosis of ADHD as well as for the assessment and treatment of the disorder.

An author often has many hopes for the eventual outcome of a project such as this. For me, I can honestly say that the achievement of its completion has, in large measure, met those hopes and justified the extensive amount of work I was called upon to put into it. Seeing it done and out the door is its own reward. The specter of this project has haunted me for many months. Its siren's call to undertake it has been like a compulsion that has plagued my very being for almost 5 years. Now that my pen has gleaned this matter from my teeming brain, I can take some satisfaction simply from its publication. But if in some small way this book improves the way in which scientists, clinicians, and the general public view ADHD, if by some small measure it further dignifies this condition as a legitimate developmental disorder, or if it serves to remove even a shade of the aura of negative moral aspersions often cast upon those with the disorder by others naive to this condition, then it will have been well worth the many months of time and toil in its preparation.

Acknowledgments

AS WILL BECOME EVIDENT in Chapter 5, I owe a substantial debt to Jacob Bronowski, the late British scientist, mathematician, poet, and lifelong student of human evolution. This debt stems from several sources. The lesser of these was Bronowski's book and television program of popular science on *The Ascent of Man,* which appeared in December 1976. His enthusiasm for the study of man, language, and mind and their evolution was contagious to this then-young student with a love of evolutionary biology who was proceeding into the field of psychology. As I moved into that field and eventually into its specialty of clinical neuropsychology, Bronowski's work infused my early training with his excitement about science and the process of discovery. As a fledgling behavioral scientist at the time with a seemingly unquenchable curiosity, I was most impressed by the passion and insight Bronowski brought to his subjects. Bronowski conceived of science as a form of play. Undoubtedly, it is play that is more highly ritualized and codified than the play of children, but it is no less exciting in its exercise and joyful in the products of discovery it yields. In earlier years, my first mentor in psychology, Donald Routh, nicely demonstrated these points to me—that psychological science is play, that such play could be fun and exciting, and that the discoveries it revealed were never-ending. Now, some 25 years since our initial chance meeting, I see that Don still epitomizes these principles that Bronowski made about science-as-play and that both of them are still correct in their assessments of science as a means of creativity and discovery.

More to the point of this book, however, I owe Dr. Bronowski an even more profound debt for his having written and published the paper "Animal and Human Languages." This paper first served as a speech to honor Roman Jakobson in 1967, and was later republished in 1977 by MIT Press as a posthumous collection of Bronowski's essays, titled *A Sense of the Future*. It was my chance selection of that book at the Boston Museum of Science on a visit there with my children in the spring of 1992 that, in hindsight, proved fateful to this theory and this book. And it was my reading of his essay shortly thereafter on a plane flight to Atlanta, Georgia, that led to one of those rare moments of "eureka!" in the career of a scientist. For it is in that moment that a major problem with which one has been grappling and that seems apparently unsolvable is resolved in a flash of insight, a scientific epiphany.

As I discuss in Chapter 5, Bronowski's views on the unique properties of human language relative to the languages of other animals, as presented in his essay, provided the conceptual framework and theoretical foundation I needed to achieve a better understanding of the nature of ADHD. Prior to this discovery, findings in the literature on cognitive deficits seen in ADHD seemed to me like so much flotsam and jetsam on the vast ocean of research on the disorder. By putting Bronowski's model together with that literature on ADHD, I was able to conceive instantly of a new conceptual paradigm from which to understand that literature. Just as importantly, from that paradigm I was able to generate nearly instantly numerous exciting and testable hypothesis about additional cognitive deficits that might be associated with the disorder. Over time, as I delved into relevant aspects of the literatures of child psychopathology, neuropsychology, developmental psychology, and evolutionary biology with more thoroughness in pursuit of evidence for or against this model, I was able to appreciate that Bronowski's concepts could be extended from language to the larger domain of human behavior. That framework provided a rudimentary template on which to better conceive of the nature of the executive functions as discussed in neuropsychology and the development of self-regulation as it has been studied in developmental psychology. Ironically, this event of scientific serendipity for me served to illustrate beautifully several of the lessons Bronowski repeatedly put forth in his popular writings on science—chance does favor prepared minds, necessity is the mother of invention, science and art share common processes of creativity and discovery, and new discoveries often arise by reading or exploring outside of one's chosen scientific discipline. My debt to Bronowski, then, is limitless, and I acknowledge it humbly, respectfully, and most appreciatively here. Without his formidable insights into the unique characteristics of human language, I would still be searching for the clues to a theory of ADHD.

There are others deserving of acknowledgment for their assistance with this project. Among them are my close friends and colleagues

Charles Cunningham, Michael Gordon, and Eric Mash for their tolerance of my initial mania around the discovery of this new theory, my fits and starts at attempting to mold it to an understanding of ADHD, and my repeated impositions on them to listen and comment on my ideas as I tried to forge those ideas into a useful theoretical model of ADHD. Better friends than these would be difficult to find. I am sure I often appeared to them as would a love-struck teenager in the throes of a romantic infatuation who attempts to convince his pals of the matchless beauty of his lover. Chuck and Eric witnessed fully my excitement and tolerated well my incessant chatter about Bronowski's ideas for understanding ADHD as we wined and dined our way through the 1993 meeting of the International Society for Research in Child and Adolescent Psychopathology, with the incomparable beauty of Santa Fe, New Mexico, as a backdrop. Thank you, my good friends, for your patience with me in these matters of the theoretical heart.

I must also express appreciation to Megan Gunnar, PhD, Associate Editor of the *Psychological Bulletin*, and the anonymous reviewers she employed in the repeated reviews of my recent theoretical paper on which this book is based (see Barkley, 1997). The challenges that all of them raised to my ideas in their series of reviews and critiques of that paper, which spanned nearly 2 years, forced me ever deeper into the psychological literature to justify my positions, pushed me to be more self-critical than I would have otherwise been, and encouraged me to be far clearer about this theory and its constructs than I would have been had it not been for their feedback. Those collegial and constructive reviews were most helpful and encouraging, and I thank all of those reviewers here for their assistance in that project, which served to inspire the present one.

And I must surely thank my friends Seymour Weingarten and Robert Matloff of The Guilford Press for their willingness, once again, to support me during the preparation of another book, particularly one on a theory, of all things, that hardly rings of bestseller status and market share. Over the 17 years of their steadfast support of my career as a psychologist and writer, they, often more than I, have seen the hidden worth in my ideas for books and have gambled to publish them when others might not have taken the chance. A more congenial, honest, supportive, and dedicated publishing company could not be found. I am also most appreciative of Rochelle Serwator for her initial editing of the manuscript. In the midst of any publishing house toil the yeomen of the publisher's trade, the production editors, who make me appear in print as far more scholarly, pithy, witty, and intelligent than I actually am in person. In this case, much gratitude is owed to Anna Brackett and her associates for shepherding this book through the publication process, while correcting the errors of my grammatical ways and reigning in my penchant for the dramatic. I am also very appreciative of Bonnie Murphy and Pat Barkley for kindly assisting me with the preparation of the references and with the editing and retyping of the manuscript in the course of this project. Gratitude is also owed to Beth H. Maynard Mellor, illustrator/computer artist extraordinaire, for skillfully rendering the figures that appear in Chapters 2, 7, and 9 from my feeble drawings of them.

During the preparation of this book, I was also financially supported, in part, by grants from the National Institute of Mental Health (MH45714, MH41583) and the National Institute for Child Health and Human Development (HD28171). The contents of this book, however, are solely my responsibility and do not necessarily represent the official views of these institutes. I was also financially supported during this time by funds from the Department of Psychiatry, University of Massachusetts Medical Center. The Chairman of that Department, Paul Appelbaum, MD, and the Chancellor of the University Medical School, Aaron Lazare, MD, have both been very supportive of my scholarly endeavors at a time when managed health care is making heavy demands on psychiatry departments for fiscal frugality. For all of this financial support, I am most grateful.

Contents

ADHD AND THE NATURE
OF SELF-CONTROL

CHAPTER 1

———•———

The Nature of Attention-Deficit/ Hyperactivity Disorder

IT IS COMMONPLACE for children, especially young preschool children, to be active, energetic, and exuberant and to flit from one activity to another as they explore their environment and its novelties. They are also notorious for getting bored easily with tasks that lack intrinsic appeal for them. Acting without much forethought and responding on impulse to events that occur around them, their emotional reactions to these events often readily apparent, are typical characteristics of young children. If opportunities arise that offer young children the promise of immediate reward or gratification, then their indulgence in these activities is to be expected, rather than the restraint of self-control that would be demanded of someone older. To be a child is to be less accountable than an adult for controlling one's impulses. But when children persistently display levels of activity that are far in excess of their age group, when they are unable to sustain their attention, interest, or persistence as well as their peers with regard to their activities, longer-term goals, or the tasks assigned to them by others, or when their impulse control and self-regulation lag far behind expectations for their developmental level, they are no longer simply expressing the *joie de vivre* that characterizes childhood. They are,

This chapter is adapted from Barkley (1996). Copyright 1996 by The Guilford Press. Adapted by permission.

instead, highly likely to experience a number of problems in their social, cognitive, academic, familial, and emotional domains of development and adjustment, and they are at great risk for falling substantially behind other children in their ability to meet the demands increasingly placed upon them for daily adaptive functioning.

Such demands will include the need to become more personally organized and self-sufficient; more reflective, objective, and measured in their consideration of events and their choice of actions; and more responsible and self-caring. They also will need to become more planful and concerned about the future, more independent from but thoughtful of others, and better able to adhere to progressively more numerous and complex social rules. They will be expected increasingly to turn away from the pleasures and seductions of the moment, and even engage in self-deprivation, so as to concentrate their attention on maximizing future gains, incrementally more distant in time, through various acts of deferred gratification. Further, the social pressure to organize their own behavior ever more toward time and the future, and ever less to the immediate context, will prove unrelenting.

Highly active, inattentive, and impulsive youngsters will find themselves far less able than their peers to cope successfully with these developmental progressions toward self-regulation, time, and the future. They will often experience the harsh judgments, punishments, moral denigration, and social rejection and ostracism reserved for those society views as reckless, impulsive, lazy, unmotivated, selfish, thoughtless, immature, and irresponsible. For society holds widespread and deeply seated beliefs about the nature of self-control and moral conduct. Its members are quick to morally judge those who may fall short of the mark and behave in less than responsible fashion. Such impulsive children may both fascinate and repel us, causing us consternation about why they cannot seem to control their own behavior, follow through on what they are told to do, and pay attention to getting ready for the future, and simultaneously shocking our sensibilities with their often heedless risk taking, disregard for others, devil-may-care attitudes, and hell-bent, seemingly self-destructive ways. As a result, these children have captured public interest and commentary for at least 130 years, and scientific interest for nearly 100 of these. While the diagnostic labels for children manifesting such disturbances in attention and impulse control have changed numerous times over this century, the actual nature of the condition has changed little, if at all, from descriptions of it at the turn of the century (Still, 1902). The triad of inattentive, impulsive, and hyperactive behavior problems may constitute one of the most well-studied childhood disorders of our time. Yet these children remain an enigma to Western societies, which are struggling to accept the notion that these children may have a developmental disability of chiefly biological origins when nothing apparently seems physically or outwardly to be wrong with them.

Children who are excessively active, are unable to sustain their attention, and are deficient in their impulse control to a degree that is deviant for their developmental level are now given the clinical diagnosis of attention-deficit/hyperactivity disorder (ADHD; American Psychiatric Association, 1994). Their problematic behavioral characteristics are thought to arise early, often before age 7 years, and to be persistent over development in many cases. Approximately 3–7% of school-age children are believed to have this disorder, with most estimates erring toward the higher end of this range (Szatmari, 1992). As has been well documented elsewhere, such children are at risk for a variety of negative outcomes across childhood and into adolescence and adulthood (Barkley, 1990, 1996; Hinshaw, 1994; Weiss & Hechtman, 1993). It is not the purpose of this text to discuss these aspects of ADHD. My purpose, instead, is to provide an overview of the nature of this disorder, briefly consider its history, describe its diagnosis, and briefly summarize the known potential causes, to the extent that this information may pertain to my attempt to construct a scientific theory of ADHD. Some of the critical issues related to these topics will be raised along the way, but only insofar as they may be relevant to my goal of developing a theory of ADHD and what constitutes the essence of this disorder. Given the thousands of scientific papers on this disorder, an overview of these various topics, indeed, is all that space here can afford.

This overview is necessary as a prelude to the introduction of a new theoretical model of ADHD that will be developed in later chapters. That model will provide a more parsimonious accounting of the many features of the disorder while pointing to numerous promising directions for future research. By the end of this book, I hope the reader will have gained not only a deeper appreciation of the developmental significance of this disorder and the seriousness with which it should be taken, but also a richer understanding of the nature of human self-control and how it comes to be disrupted in those with ADHD. Perhaps then it will become clearer why continuing to refer to this disorder as simply an attention deficit may be a gross understatement of what has become increasingly evident in contemporary research: ADHD represents a developmental disorder of behavioral inhibition that interferes with self-regulation and the organization of behavior toward the future. The implications of such a theoretical model of ADHD are numerous and important and will be explored in separate chapters later in this text. Even more important, however, may be the implications of this model for the manner in which society may have to alter its views on the nature of human self-control and how it judges others who are deficient in this psychological faculty, through no fault of their own or their upbringing.

A BRIEF HISTORY OF ADHD

Literary references to individuals having serious problems with inattention, hyperactivity, and poor impulse control have been with us for some time. Shakespeare made reference to a malady of attention in one of his characters in *King Henry VIII*. A later description specifically of a hyperactive child can be found in the poem "Fidgety Phil," published by the German physician Heinrich Hoffman in the mid-1800s (see Stewart, 1970). William James (1890), in his *Principles of Psychology*, also described a normal variant of character that he called the "explosive will," which resembles the characteristics that today might be attributed to having ADHD: "There is a normal type of character, for example, in which impulses seem to discharge so promptly into movements that inhibitions get no time to arise. These are the 'dare-devil' and 'mercurial' temperaments, overflowing with animation, and fizzling with talk . . . " (p. 800).

Yet serious clinical interest in children with this constellation of symptoms seems to have first occurred in three lectures, subsequently published, before the Royal Academy of Physicians by the English physician George Still (1902). Still described a group of 20 children in his clinical practice whom he defined as having a deficit in "volitional inhibition" (p. 1008) or a "defect in moral control" (p. 1009) over their own behavior. Aggressive, passionate, lawless, inattentive, impulsive, and overactive were descriptions he applied to these children, many of whom today would be diagnosed not only as ADHD but also as having oppositional defiant disorder (ODD) or even conduct disorder (CD) (see Hinshaw & Anderson, 1996). Still's observations were quite astute, describing many of the associated features of ADHD that would come to be corroborated in research more than 50–90 years later: (1) an overrepresentation of males (the ratio of 3:1 in Still's sample applies today as well); (2) an aggregation of alcoholism, criminal conduct, and depression among the biological relatives; (3) a familial predisposition to the disorder, implying heredity to be at work in some cases; and (4) the possibility of the disorder also arising from acquired injury to the nervous system.

Initial interest in children with similar characteristics seems to have arisen in North America around the time of the great encephalitis epidemics of 1917–1918. Children surviving these brain infections were noted to have many behavioral problems similar to those comprising contemporary ADHD (Ebaugh, 1923; Hohman, 1922; Stryker, 1925). These cases and others known to have arisen from birth trauma, head injury, toxin exposure, and infections (see Barkley, 1990) gave rise to the concept of a brain-injured child syndrome (Strauss & Lehtinen, 1947), often associated with mental retardation, that would eventually come to be applied to children manifesting these same behavioral features but without evidence of brain damage or retardation (Dolphin & Cruickshank, 1951; Strauss & Kephart, 1955). The concept of a brain-injured child syndrome in the absence of evidence of brain injury would later evolve into the diagnostic term "minimal brain damage," and later, into that of "minimal brain dysfunction" (MBD). Such changes in terms were in part due to challenges raised by critics concerning the dearth of evidence of brain injury in many of these cases (see Kessler, 1980, for a more detailed history of MBD).

At this same time (the 1950s and 1960s), others became interested in the more specific behaviors of hyperactivity and poor impulse control, labeling the condition as "hyperkinetic impulse disorder" and attributing it to cortical overstimulation due to poor thalamic filtering of stimuli entering the brain (Knobel, Wolman, & Mason, 1959; Laufer, Denhoff, & Solomons, 1957). These and other papers marked a shift in diagnostic terminology away from the obvious conclusion that such symptoms indicated brain damage or dysfunction and toward a more descriptive view of the disorder. These changes in perspective gave rise to the diagnostic term "hyperactive child syndrome" (Burks, 1960; Chess, 1960), which was said to be typified by daily motor movement far in excess of that seen in normal children of the same age. Nevertheless, a belief continued among clinicians and researchers of this era that the condition had some sort of neurological origin. Yet the larger influence of psychoanalytic thought held sway over child psychiatry, and along with it the belief that children's mental disorders necessarily arose as a reaction to various environmental factors, particularly early events in the family life of the child. Therefore, when the second edition of the *Diagnostic and Statistical Manual of Mental Disorders* (DSM-II; American Psychiatric Association, 1968) was created, all childhood disorders were described as "reactions," and hyperactive child syndrome became "hyperkinetic reaction of childhood." It was defined simply (and completely) as follows: "This disorder is characterized by overactivity, restlessness, distractibility, and short attention span, especially in young children; the behavior usually diminishes in adolescence. If this behavior is caused by organic brain damage, it should be diagnosed under the appropriate non-psychotic organic brain syndrome" (p. 50).

Important in this definition was the inclusion of problems with attention and distractibility along with those of hyperactivity/restlessness already being emphasized in the existing research literature of the time. Another important distinction was the assertion that the condition seemed developmentally benign, diminishing as it did at adolescence. Also, the recognition that the disorder was *not* caused by brain damage seemed to follow a similar argument made somewhat earlier by the prominent child psychiatrist Stella Chess (1960), and created the beginnings of the major conceptual rift between professionals in North America and those in Europe that continues to some extent to the present. European clinical professionals continued to view hyperkinesis as a relatively rare condition of extreme overactivity often associated with mental retardation or evidence of organic brain damage. This discrepancy in conceptualizations seems to be abating as of this writing, at least between scientists on both continents (cf., e.g., Barkley, 1990, with Sandberg, 1996, or Taylor, 1986) and, more recently, in diagnostic criteria (see the DSM-IV criteria presented later in this chapter). Nevertheless, the manner in which clinicians and educators on both continents view the disorder continues to be quite at odds; in North America, hyperactive–impulsive children are labeled as having ADHD, which is viewed as a developmental disorder having substantial biological origins. In Europe, by contrast, these same children are viewed as having conduct problem or disorder because of their often hostile, defiant, and belligerent nature. There it is viewed as a behavioral disturbance believed to originate largely in poor parental management of children, family dysfunction and social disadvantage, and in some cases poor diet.

By the 1970s, research was appearing that emphasized the importance of problems with sustained attention and impulse control in addition to hyperactivity in understanding the nature of the disorder (Douglas, 1972). Douglas (1983) would eventually come to theorize that the disorder was comprised of four major deficits, these being in (1) the investment, organization, and maintenance of attention and effort; (2) the ability to inhibit impulsive behavior; (3) the ability to modulate arousal levels to meet situational demands; and (4) an unusually strong inclination to seek immediate reinforcement. Significant in retrospect but apparently unnoticed at the time was the observation by Douglas, akin to that of Still some 70 years earlier, that the disorder was associated with significant problems in moral development. The repeated mention of this association throughout the history of ADHD, as will be shown later, is not merely coincidental.

Douglas's seminal paper, along with the numerous studies of attention, impulsiveness, and other cognitive sequelae of this disorder that followed (see Douglas, 1983, and Douglas & Peters, 1978, for reviews), eventually led to retitling the disorder as "attention-deficit disorder" (ADD) in 1980, when the third revision of the DSM appeared (DSM-III; American Psychiatric Association, 1980). No longer was the disorder viewed as simply a behavioral reaction of childhood. Instead, the cognitive and developmental nature of the disorder was emphasized and more explicit criteria for defining and diagnosing the condition were now provided. Specifically, symptom lists and cutoff scores were recommended for each of the three major symptoms to assist with identification of the condition.

Equally as significant, historically, as the renaming of the condition was the distinction in DSM-III between two types of ADD: with hyperactivity and without it. Little research existed at the time on the latter subtype that would have supported such a distinction being made in an official and increasingly prestigious diagnostic taxonomy. Yet, in hindsight, this bald assertion led to further valuable research on the differences between these two forms of ADD that otherwise would never have taken place. That research may have been fortuitous, as will be shown later, for it may be leading to the conclusion that ADD without hyperactivity is actually a disorder of attention that is separate and distinct from ADD with hyperactivity, in which the nature of the attention deficit may be qualitatively different (Barkley, DuPaul, & McMurray, 1990; Goodyear & Hynd, 1992; Lahey & Carlson, 1992).

Nevertheless, within a few years of the creation of the label ADD, concern arose that problems with hyperactivity and impulse control were features critically important to differentiating the disorder from other conditions and to predicting later developmental risks (Barkley, 1990; Weiss & Hechtman, 1993), and that therefore these symptoms warranted a place in the name for the condition. Perhaps as a result, in 1987, the disorder was renamed as attention-deficit/hyperactivity disorder (ADHD) in DSM-III-R (American Psychiatric Association, 1987). A single list of items incorporating all three symptoms and a single threshold for the number of symptoms needed for diagnosis were specified. Also important here was the placement of the condition of ADD without hyperactivity, now named undifferentiated attention deficit disorder, in a section of the manual separate from ADHD, with the specification that insufficient research existed to guide in the construction of diagnostic criteria for it at that time.

During the 1980s, reports began to appear that challenged the notion that ADHD was primarily a disturbance in attention, instead focusing upon problems with motivation generally, and an insensitivity to response consequences specifically (Barkley, 1989; Glow & Glow, 1979; Haenlein & Caul, 1987). Research was demonstrating that children with ADHD did not respond in the same way to alterations in contingencies of reinforcement or punishment as did normal children. Under conditions of continuous reward, the performances of children with ADHD were often indistinguishable from those of normal children on various laboratory tasks, but when reinforcement patterns shifted to partial reward or to extinction (no reward) conditions, children with ADHD showed significant declines in their performance (Douglas & Parry, 1983, 1994; Parry & Douglas, 1983). It was also becoming evident to me that deficits in the manner in which rules and instructions governed behavior existed in these children (Barkley, 1981, 1989, 1990). When rules specifying behavior were given that were in conflict with the prevailing immediate consequences in the setting that were available for other, competing forms of action, the rules did not control behavior in children with ADHD as well as they did in normal children. Thus, I hypothesized that the class of human behavior initiated and sustained by rules (and language), called *rule-governed* behavior by behavior analysts (Hayes, 1987; Skinner, 1953), may be impaired in those with ADHD.

Over the next decade, researchers employing information-processing paradigms to study ADHD had a difficult time demonstrating that the problems these children had with attending to tasks were actually attentional in nature. Instead, problems with response inhibition and motor system control were more reliably demonstrated and appeared to be specific to this disorder (Barkley, Grodzinsky, & DuPaul, 1992; Pennington & Ozonoff, 1996; Schachar & Logan, 1990; Sergeant, 1988; Sergeant & Scholten, 1985a; Sergeant & van der Meere, 1989, 1990). Researchers were also finding that the problems with hyperactivity and impulsivity were not separate symptoms but formed a single dimension of behavior (Achenbach & Edelbrock, 1983; Goyette, Conners, & Ulrich, 1978; Lahey et al., 1988), which I previously described as *disinhibition* (Barkley, 1990). The symptoms of hyperactivity and impulsivity seemed to be both a single and signal problem for the disorder. All of this research led to the creation of two separate lists of items and thresholds for ADHD when DSM-IV diagnostic criteria were published (American Psychiatric Association, 1994); one list was for inattention and another for hyperactive–impulsive behavior. Unlike its predecessor, DSM-III-R, the establishment of the inattention list once again permitted the diagnosis of a subtype of ADHD to be granted that consisted principally of problems with attention without problems with hyperactive–impulsive behavior (ADHD–predominantly inattentive type). DSM-IV also permitted, for the first time, the distinction of a subtype of ADHD that consisted chiefly of hyperactive–impulsive behavior without significant inattention (ADHD–predominantly hyperactive–impulsive type). Children having significant problems from both item lists were designated ADHD–combined type. The specific criteria from DSM-IV are set forth and discussed in more detail in the section "Diagnostic Criteria for ADHD," later in this chapter.

In conclusion, as of this writing, debate continues over the core deficit(s) in ADHD, but increasing weight is being given to the problem of behavioral inhibition as somehow being central to at least two subtypes of the disorder (Barkley, 1997; Pennington & Ozonoff, 1996; Quay, 1988a, 1988b). The nature of the problems with sustaining attention demonstrated by these children remains controversial, but apparently will need to be explained by deficiencies within the anterior or motor control systems of the brain rather than in the more posterior sensory or information-processing systems themselves. Likewise, controversy continues to swirl around the place of that subtype composed primarily of inattention within the larger condition of ADHD. Many, though by no means all, researchers seem to be coming to view it as probably a deficit in focused or selective attention and speed of information processing that may have distinctive features from the other two types of ADHD and may be more akin to internalizing rather than to externalizing disorders (Barkley, 1990; Barkley et al., 1992; Goodyear & Hynd, 1992; Hinshaw, 1994; Lahey & Carlson, 1992). Consequently, the theoretical model to be developed in Chapters 2 and 3 does not address this type of attention disorder. Instead, the model applies primarily to those children having hyperactive–impulsive symptoms, whether inattention has yet arisen in those children or not. It will become evident why this is so in Chapter 9. There, a critical distinction will be made between different types of inattention and why one of them is so dependent on inhibition and self-regulation.

CORE SYMPTOMS OF ADHD

As discussed above, ADHD is generally viewed at this time as comprising two major symptoms: (1) inattention and (2) hyperactive–impulsive behavior (or disinhibition) (American Psychiatric Association, 1994).

Inattention

The problem with attention is witnessed in the child's inability to sustain attention or responding to tasks or play activities as long as others of the same age, and to follow through on rules and instructions as well as others. It is also seen in the child being more disorganized, distracted, and forgetful than others of the same age. Parents and teachers frequently complain that these children do not seem to listen as well as they should for their age, cannot concentrate, are easily distracted, fail to finish assignments, daydream, and change activities more often than others, typically without completing them if such completion was necessary (Barkley, DuPaul, & McMurray, 1990). Research employing objective measures of these attributes corroborate their presence in ADHD in that such children are often recorded as being more "off-task" and less likely to complete as much work as normal children. They are also observed to look away more from the activities they are requested to do (including television), and to persist less in correctly performing boring activities, such as continuous performance tasks (Barkley & Ullman, 1975; Ceci & Tishman, 1984; Luk, 1985; Milich & Lorch, 1994). ADHD children have also been noted to be slower to return to an activity once interrupted and even less likely to return to it at all than normal children (Schachar, Tannock, & Logan, 1993). These inattentive behaviors have also been noted to distinguish ADHD children from those with learning disabilities (Barkley, DuPaul, & McMurray, 1990) or other psychiatric disorders (Oosterlaan & Sergeant, 1996a, 1996b; Werry, Elkind, & Reeves, 1987). Yet objective research does not find children with ADHD to be generally more distracted by extraneous events occurring during their task performance, although they may be so distracted if the irrelevant stimuli are embedded within the task itself (Campbell, Douglas, & Morganstern, 1971; Cohen, Weiss, & Minde, 1972; Rosenthal & Allen, 1980; Steinkamp, 1980).

Hyperactive–Impulsive Behavior (Disinhibition)

The problems with disinhibition noted in children with ADHD are manifest in difficulties with fidgetiness, staying seated when required, moving about, running, and climbing more than other children, playing noisily, talking excessively, interrupting others' activities, and being less able than others to wait in line or take turns in games (American Psychiatric Association, 1994). Parents and teachers describe them as acting as if driven by a motor, incessantly in motion, always on the go, and unable to wait for events to occur. Research objectively documents them to be more active than other children (Barkley & Cunningham, 1979b; Barkley & Ullman, 1975; Luk, 1985; Porrino et al., 1983; Teicher, Ito, Glod, & Barber, 1996; Zentall, 1985), to be less mature in controlling motor overflow movements (Denckla & Rudel,

1978), to have considerable difficulties with stopping an ongoing behavior (Milich, Hartung, Matrin, & Haigler, 1994; Schachar, Tannock, & Logan, 1993) to talk more than others (Barkley, Cunningham, & Karlsson, 1983), to interrupt others' conversations (Malone & Swanson, 1993), to be less able to resist immediate temptations and delay gratification (Anderson, Hinshaw, & Simmel, 1994; Campbell, Szumowski, Ewing, Gluck, & Breaux, 1982; Rapport, Tucker, DuPaul, Merlo, & Stoner, 1986), and to respond too quickly and too often when they are required to wait and watch for events to happen, as is often seen in impulsive errors on continuous performance tests (Corkum & Siegel, 1993). Although less frequently examined, differences in activity and impulsiveness have been found between children with ADHD and those with learning disabilities (Barkley, DuPaul, & McMurray, 1990) and other psychiatric disorders (Halperin, Matier, Bedi, Sharma, & Newcorn, 1992; Oosterlaan & Sergeant, 1996a, 1996b; Roberts, 1990; Werry et al., 1987).

Interestingly, recent research shows that the problems with disinhibition arise first (at 3–4 years of age), with those related to inattention emerging later in the developmental course of ADHD (at 5–7 years), often by entry into formal schooling. The type of attention problems characterizing the predominantly inattentive subtype of ADHD may arise even later than this, by the early to middle elementary school grades or even later (Applegate et al., in press; Hart, Lahey, Loeber, Applegate, & Frick, 1996; Loeber, Green, Lahey, Christ, & Frick, 1992). Whereas the symptoms of disinhibition in DSM item lists seem to decline with age, those of inattention remain relatively stable during the elementary grades (Hart et al., 1995). Yet even the inattentive symptoms decline by adolescence (Fischer, Barkley, Fletcher, & Smallish, 1990) and, indeed, apparently throughout life (Murphy & Barkley, 1996b). Why inattention arises later than the disinhibitory symptoms and does not decline over development at the same time as the latter do remains an enigma that I attempt to address in this book.

SITUATIONAL AND CONTEXTUAL FACTORS

The symptoms comprising ADHD are greatly affected in their level of severity by a variety of situational and contextual factors. Any credible theory of ADHD will have to provide an explanation for such fluctuations in the presence and severity of symptoms. Why, for instance, can ADHD children play videogames for prolonged periods of time, even for hours, yet not sustain their attention to schoolwork, academic homework, or chores for more than a few minutes? Why is their impulsiveness and sustained attention on laboratory tasks, such as continuous performance tests (CPTs), improved when an adult merely sits in the room with them, compared with when the adult is not present? And why is their work productivity and task performance so variable over time relative to normal peers?

Douglas (1972) commented on the greater variability of task performances made by ADHD compared to control children. Many others since then have found that when the ADHD child must perform multiple trials within a task assessing attention and impulse control, the range of scores around their own mean performance is frequently greater than in normal children (see Douglas, 1983). The finding is sufficiently common in measures of reaction time (Chee, Logan, Schachar, Lindsay, & Wachsmuth, 1989; Zahn, Krusei, & Rapoport, 1991) to have led several developers of CPTs to recommend that variability in this measure serve as one indicator for the presence of the disorder in clinical patients (Conners, 1995; Greenburg & Waldman, 1992).

A number of other factors have been noted to influence the ability of children with ADHD to sustain their attention to task performance, control their impulses to act, regulate their activity level, and produce work consistently. These include: (1) Time of day or fatigue (Porrino et al., 1983; Zagar & Bowers, 1983); (2) increasing task complexity, such that organizational strategies are required (Douglas, 1983); (3) extent of restraint demanded for the context (Barkley & Ullman, 1975; Luk, 1985); (4) level of stimulation within the setting (Zentall, 1985); (5) schedule of immediate consequences associated with the task (Barkley & Sivage, 1980; Douglas & Parry, 1983, 1994); and (6) absence of adult supervision during task performance (Draeger, Prior, & Sanson, 1986; Gomez & Sanson, 1994b).

Besides the aforementioned factors, which chiefly apply to task performance, variability has also been documented across more macroscopic settings. For instance, using a rating scale of 16 different contexts within the home (the Home Situations Questionnaire), it has been shown that children with ADHD are most problematic in their behavior when persistence in work-related tasks is required (e.g., chores, homework, etc.) or where behavioral restraint is necessary, especially in settings involving public scrutiny (e.g., in church, in restaurants, when a parent is on the phone, etc.) (Altepeter & Breen, 1992; Barkley & Edelbrock, 1987; DuPaul & Barkley, 1992). Such children are least likely to pose behavioral management problems during free play, when little self-control is required. Although they will be more disruptive when their fathers are at home than during free play, children with ADHD are still rated as much less problematic when the father is at home than in most other contexts. Fluctuations in the severity of ADHD symptoms have also been documented across a variety of school contexts (Barkley & Edelbrock, 1987; DuPaul & Barkley, 1992). In this case, contexts involving task-directed persistence are the most problematic, with significantly lesser degrees of problems posed by contexts involving an absence of supervision (i.e., at lunch, in hallways, at recess, etc.), and even fewer problems being posed during special events (i.e., field trips, assemblies, etc.) (Altepeter & Breen, 1992).

Current views of ADHD as an attention deficit are simply unable to account for such findings regarding the fluctuation of symptoms across settings and the variability of behavior over time. One advantage of the model of ADHD to be developed in subsequent chapters is that it can provide a reasonable explanation for these findings in addition to predicting new research directions that should prove fruitful to pursue.

ASSOCIATED COGNITIVE IMPAIRMENTS

Although ADHD is defined by the presence of the two major symptom dimensions of inattention and disinhibition, research finds that such children often demonstrate deficiencies in many other cognitive or mental abilities. Among these, the most reliably demonstrated are difficulties with (1) motor coordination and sequencing (Barkley, 1997; Barkley, Fischer, Edelbrock, & Smallish, 1990; Breen, 1989; Carte, Nigg, & Hinshaw, 1996; Denckla & Rudel, 1978; Mariani & Barkley, 1997); (2) digit span and mental computation (Anastopoulos, Spistor, & Maher, 1994; Mariani & Barkley, 1997; Zentall & Smith, 1993); (3) planning and anticipation (Barkley, Grodzinsky, & DuPaul, 1992; Douglas, 1983; Grodzinsky & Diamond, 1992); (4) verbal fluency and confrontational communication (Grodzinsky & Diamond, 1992; Zentall, 1988); (5) effort allocation (Douglas, 1983; Sergeant & van der Meere, 1993; Voelker, Carter, Sprague, Gdowski, & Lachar, 1989); (6) applying organizational strategies in tasks (Hamlett, Pellegrini, & Conners, 1987; Voelker et al., 1989; Zentall, 1988); (7) the internalization of self-directed speech (Berk & Potts, 1991; Copeland, 1979); (8) adhering to restrictive instructions (Barkley, 1985; Danforth, Barkley, & Stokes, 1992; Roberts, 1990; Routh & Schroeder, 1976); and (9) self-regulation of emotional arousal (Barkley, 1997; Cole, Zahn-Waxler, & Smith, 1994; Douglas, 1983; Hinshaw, Buhrmeister, & Heller, 1989). Several studies have also demonstrated what both Still (1902) and Douglas (1972) noted anecdotally years ago—ADHD may be associated with less mature or diminished moral reasoning (Hinshaw, Herbsman, Melnick, Nigg, & Simmel, 1993; Nucci & Herman, 1982; Simmel & Hinshaw, 1993).

The commonality among most or all of these seemingly distinct abilities is that most have been considered to fall within the domain of *executive functions* in the field of neuropsychology (Denckla, 1994; Torgesen, 1994) or *metacognition* in developmental psychology (Flavell, 1970; Torgesen, 1994; Welsh & Pennington, 1988), and all have been considered to be mediated by the frontal cortex, particularly the prefrontal lobes (Fuster, 1989, 1995; Stuss & Benson, 1986). This is an important point, as evidence (to be discussed in the next chapter) is increasingly mounting that ADHD originates from problems in the development or functioning of these brain regions.

DIAGNOSTIC CRITERIA FOR ADHD

The most recent diagnostic criteria for ADHD as defined in DSM-IV (American Psychiatric Association, 1994) are set forth in Table 1.1. They stipulate that individuals have had their symptoms of ADHD for at least 6 months, that the degree of these symptoms is developmentally deviant, and that the symptoms have developed by 7 years of age. From the inattention item list, six of nine items must be endorsed as developmentally inappropriate. From the hyperactive–impulsive item list, six of nine items must be endorsed as deviant. Depending upon whether criteria are met for either or both symptom lists will determine the subtype of ADHD that is to be diagnosed: predominantly inattentive (ADHD-I), predominantly hyperactive–impulsive (ADHD-HI), and combined type (ADHD-C).

These diagnostic criteria are some of the most rigorous and most empirically derived criteria ever available in the history of clinical diagnosis for this disorder. They were derived from a committee of some of the leading experts in the field, a literature review of ADHD, an informal survey of rating scales assessing the behavioral dimensions related to ADHD and the particular items they contained, and statistical analyses of the results of a field trial of the items using 380 children from 10 different sites in North America (Lahey et al., 1994).

Despite being an improvement over prior sets of DSM diagnostic criteria, some problems and critical issues still remain. These have been discussed in more detail elsewhere (Barkley, 1996), but a few will be mentioned here as they may apply to understanding the nature of ADHD or developing a theoretical model of it. For one thing, as discussed earlier, *it is not clear that ADHD-I, the predominantly inattentive*

TABLE 1.1. DSM-IV Criteria for ADHD

A. Either (1) or (2):

(1) six (or more) of the following symptoms of **inattention** have persisted for at least six months to a degree that is maladaptive and inconsistent with developmental level:

Inattention
(a) often fails to give close attention to details or makes careless mistakes in schoolwork, work, or other activities
(b) often has difficulty sustaining attention in tasks or play activities
(c) often does not seem to listen when spoken to directly
(d) often does not follow through on instructions and fails to finish schoolwork, chores, or duties in the workplace (not due to oppositional behavior or failure to understand instructions)
(e) often has difficulty organizing tasks and activities
(f) often avoids, dislikes, or is reluctant to engage in tasks that require sustained mental effort (such as schoolwork or homework)
(g) often loses things necessary for tasks or activities (e.g., toys, school assignments, pencils, books, or tools)
(h) is often easily distracted by extraneous stimuli
(i) is often forgetful in daily activities

(2) six (or more) of the following symptoms of **hyperactivity–impulsivity** have persisted for at least 6 months to a degree that is maladaptive and inconsistent with developmental level:

Hyperactivity
(a) often fidgets with hands or feet or squirms in seat
(b) often leaves seat in classroom or in other situations in which remaining seated is expected
(c) often runs about or climbs excessively in situations in which it is inappropriate (in adolescents or adults, may be limited to subjective feelings of restlessness)
(d) often has difficulty playing or engaging in leisure activities quietly
(e) is often "on the go" or often acts as if "driven by a motor"
(f) often talks excessively

Impulsivity
(g) often blurts out answers before the questions have been completed
(h) often has difficulty awaiting turn
(i) often interrupts or intrudes on others (e.g., butts into conversations or games)

B. Some hyperactive–impulsive or inattentive symptoms that caused impairment were present before age 7 years.

C. Some impairment from the symptoms is present in two or more settings (e.g., at school [or work] and at home).

(cont.)

TABLE 1.1 (cont.)

D. There must be clear evidence of clinically significant impairment in social, academic, or occupational functioning.

E. The symptoms do not occur exclusively during the course of a Pervasive Developmental Disorder, Schizophrenia, or other Psychotic Disorder and are not better accounted for by another mental disorder (e.g., Mood Disorder, Anxiety Disorder, Dissociative Disorder, or a Personality Disorder).

Code based on type:
314.01 **Attention-Deficit/Hyperactivity Disorder, Combined Type:** if both Criteria A1 and A2 are met for the past 6 months.
314.00 **Attention-Deficit/Hyperactivity Disorder, Predominantly Inattentive Type:** if Criterion A1 is met but Criterion A2 is not met for the past 6 months.
314.01 **Attention-Deficit/Hyperactivity Disorder, Predominantly Hyperactive–Impulsive Type:** if Criterion A2 is met but Criterion A1 is not met for the past 6 months.

Coding note: For individuals (especially adolescents and adults) who currently have symptoms that no longer meet full criteria, "In Partial Remission" should be specified).

Note. From American Psychiatric Association (1994, pp. 83–85). Copyright 1994 by the American Psychiatric Association. Reprinted by permission.

type of ADHD, is actually a subtype of ADHD, sharing a common attention deficit with the other types. This will be discussed further later. For another, it is also unclear whether ADHD-HI is really a separate type from ADHD-C or simply an earlier developmental stage of it. The field trial found that ADHD-HI was primarily comprised of preschool-age children, while ADHD-C was primarily comprised of school-age children. As noted earlier, this is what one would expect to find given that research has previously revealed that the hyperactive–impulsive symptoms appear first, followed within a few years by those of inattention. If one is going to require that inattention symptoms be part of the diagnostic criteria, then the age of onset for such symptoms will necessitate that ADHD-C have a later age of onset than ADHD-HI. Thus, it seems that these two types may actually represent separate developmental stages of the same type of ADHD rather than separate subtypes.

By permitting younger children to receive the diagnosis by meeting only the criteria for ADHD-HI, however, DSM-IV now may be capturing more of the preschool children referred to clinics with this behavior pattern who are impaired. Previously, under DSM-III-R, they might have gone undiagnosed for want of sufficient inattention to be eligible for diagnosis. This may be a good thing. Yet this also raises *the issue of whether or not the requirement for significant inattention to diagnose ADHD is even necessary,* given that ADHD-HI children are likely to eventually move into ADHD-C over time. Does the added requirement of significant inattention for the hyperactive–impulsive group add any greater power in predicting additional impairments not already achieved by the hyperactive–impulsive symptoms? Apparently not much, according to the results of the field trial (Lahey et al., 1994). Significant levels of inattention mainly predicted additional problems with completing homework that were not as well predicted by the hyperactive–impulsive behavior. Otherwise, the latter predicted most of the other areas of impairment studied in this field trial. This is consistent with follow-up studies that have found that childhood symptoms of hyperactivity are more strongly predictive of negative adolescent outcomes while those of inattention are much less so, if at all (Fischer, Barkley, Fletcher, & Smallish, 1993; Weiss & Hechtman, 1993). Such findings intimate that it is the hyperactive–impulsive symptom dimension that may be more important in striving to understand the essence or true nature of ADHD, rather than the problems with inattention. But if that is so, why do follow-up studies tend to show that the hyperactive–impulsive symptoms, although often emerging before those of inattention, decline more sharply with age than do those of inattention? Such apparent contradictions in the importance of these dimensions for understanding ADHD need to be addressed and explained by any new theoretical model of the disorder. Suffice it to say here that the present view of ADHD gives no clue to the resolution of such findings.

Another critical issue deserving consideration is *how well the diagnostic thresholds set for the two symptom lists apply to age groups outside of those used in the field trial* (ages 4–16 years, chiefly). If ADHD is a category of pathology, as its title and placement in DSM with other mental disorders imply, then a listing of its pathognomonic symptoms should suffice to define the disorder across the life span. But if the essence of ADHD is that of a psychological trait that is dimensional in nature and varies in degree in the normal population, and if that essence is not one of attention but of some other developmental process, then the approach taken in DSM will fall short. The same symptom lists and diagnostic thresholds for those lists will not apply equally well across development. This is because we recognize that psychological constructs or abilities that are developmental in nature can vary in their manifestations at different developmental stages even though the same underlying mental ability is at work in each such stage.

An analogy should prove instructive of this problem. Mental retardation (MR) is conceptualized as a *developmentally relative* deficiency in general cognitive ability or intelligence—a deficiency defined as such relative to one's peer group and to an individual's stage of development on measures of intelligence and adaptive functioning. Now suppose that instead MR was to be diagnosed like ADHD, using a fixed set of items and fixed diagnostic thresholds developed exclusively on children, such as the following six items: (1) has a vocabulary of 100 words, (2) counts to 10, (3) recognizes and names primary colors, (4) is toilet trained, (5) dresses self, and (6) draws simple geometric designs (i.e., circle, square, diamond, etc.). This might be a useful item set for identifying children as having MR upon entry into school (age 5–6 years), but it would be a terrible set of items for identifying MR in adolescents or adults, failing miserably at diagnosing nearly all individuals having mild to moderate MR at those ages. So, too, would any diagnostic threshold for the number of such items a child had to fail to be identified as having MR relative to other children. The end result of using such a fixed list of items and a fixed cutoff score for them across development would be the illusion that children are recovering from MR with increasing age. In fact, what is happening is that they are simply outgrowing the sensitivity of the fixed-item set and its childhood-based threshold for detecting MR. To continue to identify MR across development, one must employ items that are developmentally appropriate and thresholds that are peer referenced. ADHD, like MR, has come to be viewed as a developmental disorder. Therefore, the same types of adjustments to the diagnostic criteria for ADHD may need to be made as has been done for MR—the use of developmentally sensitive item sets and developmentally referenced thresholds. Notice that the item sets themselves may need to change in order to capture the relative delay in the psychological construct that is the essence of the developmental disorder as children mature. To do otherwise, which is what DSM has done across editions, is to create the same illusion of recovery from the disorder as was shown here with MR.

This is not merely conjectural. The use of DSM criteria developed using only children proves to be increasingly restrictive or severe relative to same-age normal samples when applied to adolescents or adults. For instance, at the adolescent follow-up point in my follow-up study in Milwaukee (Barkley, Fischer, Edelbrock, & Smallish, 1990), the degree of statistical deviance associated with the threshold of 8 out of 14 symptoms (the DSM-III-R criteria in use at that time) was examined. This threshold was found to represent a level equal to 3–4 standard deviations above the normal (control) mean, corresponding to the 99th+ percentile in a normal distribution. This clearly represents a score that will be extraordinarily restrictive of the diagnosis within the teenage or adult population. Likewise, Schaughency and colleagues (Schaughency, McGee, Raja, Feehan, & Silva, 1994) discovered in their study of the prevalence of ADHD symptoms in 15- and 18-year-olds that when DSM-III criteria were used in this population sample, only 0.5% met full criteria for disorder. This could indicate that most children outgrow ADHD by this age, but it could also indicate that the diagnostic criteria are too severe in this age group, as suggested in the Milwaukee study. However, when an empirical definition of ADHD was employed by Schaughency et al. (+1.5 standard deviations on ratings of ADHD symptoms), the prevalence of ADHD was found to be 9–12%, depending upon gender and method of definition.

The young adult outcome phase of the Milwaukee study just recently completed by Mariellen Fischer, PhD, and me illustrates the problem (Barkley, Fischer, Fletcher, & Smallish, 1997). When self-report of DSM criteria was used, the persistence of disorder into adulthood was only 3%. Amazing! This indicates that 97% of ADHD children outgrow their disorder by young adulthood. However, when an empirical (age-referenced) definition was used, again just with self-reported symptoms, the persistence increased ninefold, to 28%. (Lest the reader believe that this would suggest that 72% of ADHD children outgrow the disorder, bear in mind that this analysis was based on self-report of symptoms and that there is reason to believe that ADHD adolescents and adults are more likely to underreport the number of such symptoms they have. When parents were used as the source of information about these young adults, the retention of ADHD into adulthood rose to 58%). Such findings imply that DSM criteria, based on children, pose an increasingly restrictive set of criteria for diagnosis of ADHD in later adolescence and adulthood.

Further underscoring this problem are the findings of Kevin Murphy, PhD, and me (Murphy & Barkley, 1996b) in our study of the prevalence of ADHD symptoms in adults in central Massachusetts. That study found that DSM-IV symptom thresholds were 2–4 standard deviations above the mean for a normal sample of adults. No wonder, then, that earlier follow-up studies seemed to find such a high rate of recovery from the disorder, if DSM criteria served as the basis for diagnosis. The threshold the adult subjects had to meet to get the diagnosis moved further out on the normal distribution, becoming increasingly more extreme the older those subjects became. This results in a situation where only the most severe cases are likely to continue to qualify for the diagnosis in adulthood, even though many ADHD subjects may have retained their identical relative position within the population distribution over development and even though they have impairments. Following the analogy of MR given earlier, this situation is tantamount to requiring an IQ of 70 or less for the diagnosis of MR in children, but then changing it to one of 50 or even 25 for the same diagnosis to be given to the same individual in adulthood.

Further evidence supporting the point that ADHD may need to be defined as a developmentally relative disorder comes from findings that the behavioral items comprising the DSM-IV lists decline significantly in prevalence with age across childhood and adolescence in the normal population (DuPaul et al., 1996, in press). Applying the same threshold across such a declining developmental slope could produce a situation wherein an excessive percentage of young preschool age children (ages 2–3) would be inappropriately diagnosed as ADHD (false positives), while a smaller than expected percentage of adults would meet the criteria (false negatives).

All of this suggests that ADHD is probably the extreme end of a normal psychological trait. That trait probably undergoes developmental elaboration or maturation with increasing age, as do other familiar traits, such as receptive and expressive language ability, intelligence, spatial ability, memory, and even mechanical or motor aptitude. Evaluating that trait at any given developmental stage to determine if a person is developmentally deficient in it (whether he or she is ADHD, in this case) requires an elaborate list of test or diagnostic items that are developmentally referenced and so remain developmentally sensitive to assessing deficiency with age. The range of test items needed to assess verbal intelligence, for instance, across development and into adulthood is lengthy, varied, and increasingly complex or difficult. Any item list that would hope to capture the nature of ADHD across development must be so, too.

Perhaps this accounts for why levels of symptoms of inattention in those with ADHD are more stable across childhood than are levels of symptoms of hyperactive–impulsive behavior, which sharply decline with age (Hart et al., 1995). While this may represent a true developmental decline in the severity of the latter symptoms, and possibly in the severity and prevalence of ADHD itself with maturation, it could also represent an illusory developmental trend. That is, it might be an artifact of the developmental restrictedness of some items (hyperactivity) more than others (inattention) and the minimal sampling of impulsive behavior appropriate for the various developmental periods. Hyperactivity, in other words, is simply that manifestation of the underlying psychological trait that comprises ADHD as it appears in young children. That trait could have very different manifestations at later ages, yet remain the same underlying psychological trait. This would result in precisely what Hart et al. (1995) observed in their study—the list of mainly hyperactive items loses its sensitivity to the disorder with increasing age while the inattention list may remain more developmentally appropriate to detecting the disorder across middle childhood and early adolescence. If the theoretical model to be developed in later chapters is at all accurate, then developmentally sensitive sets of items for disinhibition and its related executive functions will need to be created and tested for use in detecting this disorder so as to more accurately capture its nature. Like MR, ADHD probably represents a developmentally relative deficit, but in this case one of inhibition and the executive functions dependent upon it. As it now stands, ADHD is being defined mainly by one of its earliest developmental manifestations (hyperactivity) and one of its later (school-age) yet secondary sequelae (goal-directed persistence) and only minimally by its central feature (behavioral inhibition and self-regulation).

The requirement of an age of onset for ADHD symptoms (7 years) in the diagnostic criteria has also come under recent challenge from its own field trial (Applegate et al., in press) as well as from other longitudinal studies (McGee, Williams, & Feehan, 1992) and from the practical problems such an age of onset raises for the diagnosis of ADHD in adults (Barkley & Biederman, in press). Such a criterion for age of onset suggests that there is something qualitatively different between those who meet the criterion (early onset) and those who do not (late onset). Some results do suggest that those with an onset before age 6 years may have more severe and persistent conditions and more problems with reading and school performance more generally than those having a later onset (McGee et al., 1992). But these were matters of degree and not of kind in this study, and it was, after all, only a single study, on which no diagnostic dogma should be founded. The DSM-IV field trial also was not able to show any clear discontinuities in degree of ADHD or in the types of impairments it examined between those meeting and not meeting the 7-year age of onset. It remains unclear at this time just how specific an age of onset may need to be established for distinguishing ADHD from other disorders. Meanwhile, Joseph Biederman and I (Barkley & Biederman, in press) have recently recommended that the threshold for onset be broadened to at least 13 years of age, loosely adhered to, in keeping with the view that ADHD has a childhood onset while dispensing with the arbitrary and limiting age threshold of 7 years.

More important to the purposes of this book, specifying so precise an age of onset was not based on any developmental theory of the nature of ADHD or the construct(s) comprising its psychological essence. If

ADHD indeed represents the extreme end of a normal psychological trait and not a category of pathology, then no age of onset should be sharply demarcated in specifying whether a case represents a valid disorder or not. No such precise age of onset criteria are established for other developmental disorders, such as MR, learning disabilities, or language disorders in order for them to be valid disorders, nor should there necessarily be such a criterion for ADHD. All of these other disorders arise in childhood in the vast majority of cases (except those resulting from acquired central nervous system lesions later in life), and are understood to be childhood-onset developmental disorders as such without the need for precision around the age of symptom onset to establish them as valid. The theoretical model to be developed later in this book specifies the psychological construct(s) of which ADHD is likely to be comprised, constructs that are probably developmentally continuous rather than discontinuous.

The diagnostic criteria used to identify individuals as having ADHD, helpful and increasingly empirically based as they have become, should not be taken to be a precise rendering of the nature of the disorder. Instead, they are the result of repeated efforts to more accurately specify the clinical manifestations likely to be seen in the disorder, particularly in elementary school–age children, and to provide some decision-making rules as to how clinicians may reliably identify and diagnose individuals as having the disorder. But in no way do such diagnostic criteria necessarily mean that we have got the nature or essence of the disorder perfectly specified. Such criteria do not provide an adequate scientific theory of ADHD for at least two reasons. First, they do not explain the questions being raised about the disorder (i.e., situational fluctuations, developmental stability or instability of the DSM dimensions over development, developmental sensitivity of symptom lists to disorder across development, deficiencies across various executive cognitive functions, etc.). Second, they do not make new predictions about what else we are likely to find in those with ADHD that has previously been unnoticed and that deserves further investigation. In short, current diagnostic criteria are merely descriptive, not theoretical.

ADHD–PREDOMINANTLY INATTENTIVE TYPE

In 1980, the publication of DSM-III not only changed the name for the disorder from hyperkinetic reaction of childhood to attention deficit disorder, it included a bifurcation of the disorder into two subtypes. One contained the symptoms of inattention, hyperactivity, and impulsivity and was termed "Attention Deficit Disorder with Hyperactivity" (ADD+H), while the other was thought to be comprised of just inattention and impulsivity, and was labeled "Attention Deficit Disorder without Hyperactivity" (ADD-H). The official proclamation of this second subtype was quite unexpected, given that there existed almost no research on such a subtype or its characteristics at that time. Its creation, however, resulted in a number of studies being conducted to investigate its nature and associated features. The result of nearly 17 years of investigation into this subtype suggests the following: (1) the ADD-H subtype actually does represent a condition for which children are referred to clinics for evaluation and treatment; (2) the symptom of impulsiveness is associated more with hyperactivity and not with inattention as was originally set forth in DSM-III; (3) a separate dimension of inattention exists apart from that of hyperactivity–impulsivity, such that a separate group of children having predominantly inattentive symptoms can be identified; (4) the ADD-H subtype is not associated with the other disruptive behavior disorders (ODD, CD) to anywhere near the degree that ADD+H is; and (5) children with ADD-H have distinctly different social problems with peers than do those with ADD+H (Barkley, 1990; Barkley, Grodzinsky, & DuPaul, 1992; Carlson, 1986; Goodyear & Hynd, 1992; Lahey & Carlson, 1992).

Despite the appearance of the ADD-H subtype in DSM-III, the relatively small amount of research on the disorder that existed when DSM-III-R was being prepared resulted in this subtype being relegated to an ill-defined category labeled as Undifferentiated ADD. This was done with the proviso that more research was needed before its rightful place within the DSM generally, and the disruptive behavior disorders specifically, could be better specified. Thus, the ADD-H subtype was not collapsed in with that of ADD+H in DSM-III-R, as some have mistakenly come to believe, nor did DSM-III-R completely ignore the existence of this subtype. The American Psychiatric Association simply stated in DSM-III-R the immature status of the literature on this subtype as it then existed and concluded it was premature to go about inventing new subtypes without more research to guide such an important official endeavor.

By the time DSM-IV was written, much more research was available to support the existence of such a condition, although the question of whether it represented a true subtype of ADHD or an entirely new disorder distinct from ADHD had not been answered. Efforts also were made within the DSM-IV field trial to determine the most appropriate symptom list for the construct of inattention, allowing for this subtype to be better identified. The result was the creation of ADHD–predominantly inattentive type (ADHD–I) within DSM-IV.

Controversy continues over whether this represents a true subtype of ADHD, sharing a common attentional disturbance with ADHD–combined type while being distinguished from it simply by the relative absence of significant hyperactivity–impulsivity. Several recent reviews of this literature have suggested that it is not a true subtype but may actually represent a separate, distinct disorder, probably having a different attentional disturbance than the one present in ADHD–combined type (Barkley, 1990; Barkley, Grodzinsky, & DuPaul, 1992; Goodyear & Hynd, 1992). Another review concluded that evidence for this subtype's existence was at least strong enough to place it within DSM (under ADHD), in order to provide a better definition of it than in DSM-III-R, and to await more research on its course and treatment responsiveness as a means of clarifying its status within this taxonomy of psychopathology (Lahey & Carlson, 1992).

There is no question that statistical (factor) analyses of teacher ratings of these symptoms typically produces a two-factor solution like that created in DSM-IV (inattention, hyperactivity–impulsivity), as these reviews have noted (see also DuPaul et al., in press). These two dimensions often emerge in parent ratings of these symptoms as well, but not always and particularly not when preschool samples of children are studied separately (Achenbach & Edelbrock, 1987). In that age group, a single dimension exists, similar to the older DSM-III-R structure for ADHD, and is often associated with aggressive/oppositional behavior as well. Moreover, some factor analyses of teacher ratings using a somewhat different set of inattention items revealed two dimensions of inattention (disorganized–distractible and sluggish–drowsy), hinting that the cognitive styles of the ADD+H and ADD-H subtypes, in fact, could be different. Factor analyses of direct observations of children's inattentive behavior collected in classrooms, likewise, indicated that the inattention dimension may actually be comprised of two types of inattention, one corresponding to an inattentive–passive form and the other to a problem with persistence and distractibility (Achenbach, 1986).

The latter findings are important if only to remind us that teacher and parent ratings consist of opinions about a child's behavior and represent relatively crude judgments that may overlook or obscure important yet fine-grain distinctions about behavior. This is well demonstrated by neuropsychological research using laboratory measures, which often identifies at least four distinct components of attention (Barkley, 1994a; Mirsky, 1996) and at least two of impulsivity (Gerbing, Ahadi, & Patton, 1987; Milich & Kramer, 1985; Olson, 1989), whereas parent and teacher ratings of these constructs yield a more global, unidimensional list of symptoms for each. Research using clinician ratings has identified a third dimension of behavior labeled as sluggish tempo (Lahey et al., 1988) that is consistent with the research on direct classroom observations that identified two forms of attentional problems, one of which was this passive, sluggish, day-dreamy form of inattention. Thus, we should not assume that the results of factor analyses of parent and teacher ratings of children's behavior accurately reflect the exact nature of these behavior problems or the clinical disorders comprised of them. The items in such rating scales, and indeed in DSM-IV, are relatively global in nature (i.e., difficulty finishing tasks, needs supervision, etc.) and could result from very different disturbances in attention in different children.

This may help to explain why initial research on ADHD-I (or ADD-H) is suggestive of a different attentional disturbance in this group than that found in the combined type (ADHD-C, or ADD+H). The very limited research available to date intimates that ADHD-I children have more problems in the focused or selective component of attention, appear sluggish and less accurate in information processing, and may have memory retrieval problems, while those with ADHD-C have more problems with persistence and, relatedly, working memory as well as inhibition (Barkley, DuPaul, & McMurray, 1990; Barkley, Grodzinsky, & DuPaul, 1992; Goodyear & Hynd, 1992; Lahey & Carlson, 1992; Taylor, Sandberg, Thorley, & Giles, 1991). Both types have significant academic problems (Lamminmaki, Ahonen, Narhi, Lyytinent, & de Barra, 1995). However, the ADHD-I may have more difficulties with math abilities (Morgan, Hynd, Riccio, & Hall, 1996) as well as language delays and reading difficulties (Taylor et al., 1991), although others have not found such learning disabilities to be over-represented in this subtype compared to ADHD-C children (Barkley, DuPaul, & McMurray, 1990). The results of such studies are not sufficiently consistent to conclude unequivocally that these two sub-types have a different attentional disturbance or different patterns of associated cognitive deficits.

Part of the problem with many of the studies, and especially those finding few if any differences in these subtypes, is that most of the measures selected are drawn from the research literature on ADD+H. If uncritically accepted, such research might show that any differences between the two subtypes are merely matters of degree. Yet it is important in research on this issue to choose attentional tasks that represent its distinct components, so as to test for double-dissociation—one subtype may have problems in one component (inhibition and persistence) but not others, while the other subtype may show problems in a different component (focused/selective attention) but not in that of the first subtype. Certainly, the theoretical model of ADHD to be developed in this text applies only to the ADD+H (i.e., ADHD-C and ADHD-HI) subtype because of central problem of disinhibition. The components of the model to be developed in later chapters, however, provide guidelines as to what other cognitive/motor domains may be useful in selecting measures that would distinguish the subtypes ADD+H and ADD-H.

Psychophysiological studies, such as the program of research by Klorman and colleagues (Klorman, 1992; Klorman, Brumaghim, et al., 1988) on evoked responses in ADHD-C, could be very fruitful in helping to distinguish the nature of the subtle distinctions in attention between these subtypes. A pilot study I conducted with Ronald Cohen has revealed that early components of the evoked response may be disturbed in those with ADHD-T, consistent with a problem in the initial processing of sensory information, while those with ADHD-C show a diminished late component of the response at P300 (the electrically positive peak at 300 milliseconds), identical to that found repeatedly by Klorman and colleagues, and suggestive of a problem with resource allocation (response selection and effort), as has been suggested by Sergeant and colleagues (Oosterlaan & Sergeant, 1995; Sergeant & van der Meere, 1990). More recently, a study examining both electroencephalographic (EEG) and evoked response differences between ADHD subtypes suggested that both ADHD-I and ADHD-C may have reduced P300 amplitudes, while the latter has a longer latency to the N100 response (the electrically negative trough at 100 milliseconds), again, implying decreased effort allocation (Kuperman, Johnson, Arndt, Lindgren, & Wolraich, 1996). More research of this type, perhaps using neuroimaging methods such as functional magnetic resonance imaging, may be needed, rather than global symptom ratings by parents and teachers, to sort out the differences in attentional disturbances in these two groups.

Two other areas of functioning that appear to distinguish the subtypes of ADHD are peer relations and the types of emotional disturbances and psychiatric disorders found to be comorbid with them. Research suggests that those with ADHD-I (i.e., ADD-H) may be more anxious, are more likely to have anxiety disorders and perhaps other mood disorders, and are often rated as socially withdrawn, shy, reticent, or apprehensive than those with ADHD-C (i.e., ADD+H). The latter group, in contrast, are typically rated as more aggressive, defiant, and oppositional, are more likely to have oppositional or conduct disorder, and are more often rejected by their peers than those with ADHD-I (Lahey & Carlson, 1992; Morgan et al., 1996; Taylor et al., 1991). The studies of comorbidity and family aggregation of psychiatric disorders by Biederman and colleagues (Biederman,

Faraone, & Lapey, 1992) suggest that those with ADHD-I have far fewer comorbid psychiatric conditions and impairments than those with ADHD-C and that this seems to be so among their biological relatives as well (Barkley, DuPaul, & McMurray, 1990; Taylor et al., 1991), although others have not been able to replicate such differences in family history (Lahey & Carlson, 1992). While more research on these distinctions is needed given the very limited number of studies examining them to date, what little evidence exists points to important differences between these subtypes in their patterns of comorbidity. If replicated in later research, such distinctions would predict very different adolescent outcomes for these subtypes. Findings from follow-up studies have shown that early hyperactive–impulsive behavior is associated with a greater risk for adolescent delinquency, early substance use and abuse, and school suspensions and expulsions, particularly when hyperactive–impulsive behavior is combined with early aggressive or defiant behavior (Barkley, 1990; Biederman, Faraone, et al., 1996; Loeber, 1990; Weiss & Hechtman, 1993). This implies that the ADHD-C (i.e., ADD+H) subtype is probably far more prone to these outcomes than will be the ADHD-I (i.e., ADD-H) subtype when the latter is eventually studied in longitudinal research.

Studies of the prevalence of the subtypes of ADHD are few in number but suggest several important differences between ADD+H and ADD-H (Szatmari, 1992). ADD+H is far more common than is ADD-H, with approximately 85% or more of those having ADHD falling into the ADD+H subtype (i.e., ADHD-HI and ADHD-C) in childhood. In adolescence, however, the ADD-H (ADHD-I) subtype was more common but still less prevalent than the +H subtype. It remains unclear as to whether differences exist in the sex ratios of these two subtypes, though males still seem to predominate in both subtypes relative to females (Szatmari, 1992).

CONCLUSION

The present chapter has attempted to provide an overview of current knowledge about the nature of the principal deficits believed to be associated with ADHD. To date, research has identified two major domains of symptom expression in children having ADHD, these being hyperactive–impulsive behavior and inattentive behavior. Whether both of these are actually separate and primary features of the disorder or whether one is secondary to the other in some way has not been clearly established. The hyperactive–impulsive dimension appears to arise first in development, is associated with a greater diversity of impairments over time, and is more predictive of eventual comorbidity for oppositional defiant disorder and conduct disorder as well as other antisocial acts. Yet this dimension of deficits shows an apparent and significant decrease in severity over the childhood years, in contrast to the apparently greater stability over time of deficits related to the dimension of inattention. The latter appears to arise somewhat later in development, is more predictive of primarily school performance problems and possibly reading difficulties, and is less predictive of later problems with other externalizing disorders and antisocial behavior. Moreover, the dimension of inattention may actually be comprised of two separable types of inattention, one related to poor selective attention, passivity, and sluggish information processing, and the other typified more by difficulties with resistance to distraction and persistence of effort. Such a distinction in forms of attention deficits may help to explain the differences that are emerging in research comparing the ADHD-I (i.e., ADD-H) subtype with the ADHD-HI and ADHD-C subtypes (i.e., ADD+H). The former subtype involves more difficulties with the selective attention component, while the latter subtypes involve greater problems with distractibility and persistence. If findings along these lines continue, they would argue for viewing ADHD-I (i.e., ADD-H) as a separate disorder, rather than as a subtype of ADHD, having little affinity with the other disruptive behavior disorders (ODD, CD). The other two subtypes of ADHD (ADHD-HI and ADHD-C) involve substantial problems with hyperactivity–impulsivity (disinhibition), conjoined with problems of distractibility and impersistence later in development. Thus, ADHD-HI and ADHD-C may not form two subtypes at all but simply represent two different developmental stages of the same disorder. It is this disorder, chiefly characterized by problems with behavioral inhibition, that will be the focus of the remainder of this book and my attempt at theory construction.

CHAPTER 2

---•---

Biological Etiologies
Associated with ADHD

THE PRECISE CAUSES of ADHD are unknown at the present time, if by cause one means the direct, necessary, and sufficient events that immediately precede and directly lead to the creation of this behavior pattern in children. A precise causal chain of events simply has not been unequivocally established as yet for ADHD, nor for any other mental disorder. However, we should not be deterred from considering those factors that appear to be likely candidates in such a chain of causality, those that have been shown to be associated with a significantly increased risk for ADHD in children. They are implicated chiefly by their increased association with the symptoms comprising the disorder. It is among these more indirect forms of causation that one must be content to look for now. Numerous indirect causes of ADHD have been proposed, but evidence for many has been weak or lacking entirely. For that reason, attention will not be given to such factors here, particularly those that are purely social or dietary in nature, even though the general public believes them to be the chief causes of ADHD. Research supporting their role is scant and recent genetic studies, discussed later in this chapter, suggest that those factors contribute little to the disorder. The reader is directed to other reviews for a discussion of unsupported or weakly supported causes of ADHD (Barkley, 1990; Hinshaw, 1994; Ingersoll & Goldstein, 1993; Ross & Ross, 1982; Wolraich, Wilson, & White, 1995).

Not surprisingly, the potentially causative factors associated with ADHD that have received the most research support are biological in nature; that is, they are known to be related to or to have a direct effect on brain development and/or functioning. But, as already noted, the precise causal pathways by which these factors lead to ADHD are simply not known at this time. Far less evidence is available to support any purely psychological or social etiology of ADHD. In the vast majority of cases where such psychosocial risks have been significantly associated with ADHD/hyperactivity—as in child management methods used by parents, parenting stress, marital conflict, or parental psychopathology—more careful analysis of subgroups or later research has shown these risks either to be the result of ADHD in the child (i.e., the effects of the child on his or her parents) or, far more often, to be related to aggression, ODD, or CD in the ADHD child rather than to ADHD itself. Furthermore, genetic studies that will be discussed in detail later in this chapter have shown that environmental factors, such as parental child rearing, combined with all nongenetic sources of neurological impairment account for less than 10–15% of the variance in ADHD symptoms (Goodman & Stevenson, 1989). The strong hereditary influence in ADHD may also contribute to an apparent link between poor child management by a parent and ADHD—a link that may be attributable to the parent's own ADHD (Frick & Jackson, 1993). As Plomin (1995) has noted, even aspects of the home environment once thought to be nongenetic may have genetic contributions to them. For this reason, those few assertions that hyperactivity or ADHD may arise purely from poor child-rearing practices by parents (Silverman & Ragusa, 1992; Willis & Lovaas, 1977) must be viewed with much skepticism until these studies control for the potential presence of ADHD in the parent and its association with that parent's child management ability. Therefore, purely psychosocial factors as causes of ADHD will not receive further attention here.

However, this approach should not be construed as meaning that "biology is destiny." Environmental factors may well shape and mold the nature and severity of an initial biologically created vulnerability toward poor inhibition such that it rises to the level of clinical ADHD. Further, the risk for comorbid disorders such as ODD, CD, anxiety, and depression is largely related to family environmental factors, as previously noted. Given that such comorbid conditions have proven to be the most consistent predictors of later developmental risks and negative outcomes (Fischer et al., 1993; Weiss & Hechtman, 1993), the environment in which the child is raised and schooled may well play a large role in determining outcome, even if it plays much less of a role in primary causation.

NEUROLOGICAL FACTORS

In Still's (1902) first description of ADHD children, he conjectured that the disorder most likely arose out of impairments within the brain as well as hereditary factors. Research on ADHD has provided the greatest evidence for these two potential causes. Throughout the century, investigators have repeatedly noted the similarities between symptoms of ADHD and those produced by *lesions or injuries to the frontal lobes more generally and the prefrontal cortex specifically* (Benton, 1991; Heilman, Voeller, & Nadeau, 1991; P. M. Levin, 1938; Mattes, 1980). Both children and adults suffering injuries to the prefrontal region demonstrate deficits in sustained attention, inhibition, regulation of emotion and motivation, and the capacity to organize behavior across time (Fuster, 1989; Grattan & Eslinger, 1991; Stuss & Benson, 1986).

Numerous other lines of evidence have been suggestive of a neurological origin to the disorder. The early onset of the symptoms in ADHD and their relatively persistent nature over time, their association with other developmental disorders believed to arise from neurological development or impairment (i.e., learning disabilities, language disorders, motor abnormalities, and IQ), their significant relationship to peri- and postnatal adversities (particularly low birth weight and severe prematurity; Breslau et al., 1996; Schothorst & van Engeland, 1996; Szatmari, Saigal, Rosenbaum, & Campbell, 1993), and their relatively dramatic improvement by stimulant medication have served to repeatedly focus research attention on possible causal neurodevelopmental factors. The repeated findings of deficient performances on some neuropsychological tests known to be associated with prefrontal lobe functions, such as inhibition, persistence, planning, working memory, motor control and fluency, and verbal fluency have further supported the view of a neuropsychological origin to ADHD (Barkley, 1990, 1997; Barkley, Grodzinsky, & DuPaul, 1992; Goodyear & Hynd, 1992). The significantly greater risk for the disorder in other family members (see the "Genetic Factors" section, later in this chapter), and the increased risk for ADHD symptoms in children known to have been exposed to toxins (pre- or postnatally) have likewise fueled scientific speculation that biological factors must be involved in this disorder. But is there more direct proof of this connection to brain function and morphology?

It has only been within the past 10–15 years that more direct research findings pertaining to neurological integrity in ADHD have increasingly supported the view of a neurodevelopmental origin to the disorder. Even here, however, far more research is needed before we can be as sanguine about the biological nature of ADHD as we might like to be. Studies using *psychophysiological measures* of central and autonomic nervous system electrical activity, variously measured (electroencephalograms, galvanic skin response, heart rate deceleration, etc.), have been inconsistent in demonstrating group differences between ADHD and control children. But where differences from normal are found, they are consistently in the direction of *diminished arousal or arousability* in those with ADHD (see Ferguson & Pappas, 1979; Hastings & Barkley, 1978; Rosenthal & Allen, 1978; Ross & Ross, 1982, for reviews). Far more consistent have been the results of evoked response measures taken in conjunction with performance of vigilance tests (Frank, Lazar, & Seiden, 1992; Klorman, Salzman, & Borgstedt, 1988). ADHD children have been found to have smaller amplitudes in the late positive components of their responses. These late components are believed to be a function of the prefrontal regions of the brain, are related to poorer performances on vigilance tests, and are corrected by stimulant medication (Klorman, Brumaghim, et al., 1988; Kuperman et al., 1996). Thus, while the evidence is far from conclusive, evoked response patterns related to sustained attention and inhibition have been suggestive of an underresponsiveness of ADHD children to stimulation that is corrected by stimulant medication.

Several studies have also examined *cerebral blood flow* in ADHD and normal children. They have consistently shown decreased blood flow to the prefrontal regions and the pathways connecting these regions to the limbic system via the striatum, specifically its anterior region, known as the caudate nucleus (Lou, Henriksen, & Bruhn, 1984, 1990; Lou, Henriksen, Bruhn, Borner, & Nielsen, 1989; Sieg, Gaffney, Preston, & Hellings, 1995). More recently, studies using *positron emission tomography (PET)* to assess cerebral glucose metabolism have found diminished metabolism in 18 male and 7 female adults (Zametkin et al., 1990) and in adolescent females with ADHD (Ernst et al., 1994), but have proven negative in adolescent males with ADHD (Zametkin et al., 1993). However, significant correlations have been noted between diminished metabolic activity in the left anterior frontal region and severity of ADHD symptoms in adolescents with ADHD (Zametkin et al., 1993). This demonstration of an association between the metabolic activity of certain brain regions and symptoms of ADHD is critical in proving a connection between the findings pertaining to brain activation and the behavior comprising ADHD.

The gross structure of the brain as portrayed by *coaxial tomographic (CT) scan* has not shown differences between ADHD and normal children (Shaywitz, Shaywitz, Byrne, Cohen, & Rothman, 1983), but greater brain atrophy was found in adults with ADHD who had a history of substance abuse (Nasrallah et al., 1986). The latter, however, seems more likely to account for these results than the ADHD.

More fine-grained analysis of brain structures, using higher resolution *magnetic resonance imaging (MRI)* devices, has revealed differences in some brain regions in those with ADHD relative to control groups. Much of this work has been done by Hynd and his colleagues. Initial studies from this group examined the region of the left and right temporal lobes associated with auditory detection and analysis (planum temporale) in ADHD, LD (reading), and normal children. For some time, researchers studying reading disorders have focused on these brain regions, given their connection to the analysis of speech sounds. Both the ADHD and LD children were found to have smaller right hemisphere plana temporale than the control group, while only the LD subjects had smaller left plana temporale (Hynd, Semrud-Clikeman, Lorys, Novey, & Eliopulos, 1990). In the next study, the corpus callosum was examined in those with ADHD. This structure assists with the interhemispheric transfer of information. Those with ADHD were found to have a smaller callosum, particularly in the area of the genu and splenium and that region just anterior to the splenium (Hynd, Semrud-Clikeman et al., 1991). An attempt to replicate this finding, however, failed to show any differences between ADHD and control children in the size or shape of the entire corpus callosum, with the exception of the region of the splenium (posterior portion), which again was significantly smaller in subjects with ADHD (Semrud-Clikeman et al., 1994).

More recently, Baumgardner and colleagues (1996) studied the size of the corpus callosum in 16 children with Tourette syndrome, 27 children with Tourette syndrome and ADHD, 13 children with ADHD alone, and 27 unaffected control subjects, using MRI. Results indicated that the children with ADHD had a significantly smaller anterior region of the corpus callosum known as the rostral body. Incidentally, subjects with Tourette syndrome had significantly increased volumes of the callosum in four of the five callosal regions measured in this procedure. These results for ADHD are relatively consistent with some of the findings by Hynd and colleagues discussed above in finding the anterior (frontal) regions of the corpus callosum to be smaller in subjects with ADHD, while any findings for the posterior regions of the callosum are less consistent across these studies.

Because of the earlier research by Lou et al. (1984) demonstrating decreased blood flow in the striatal regions, a subsequent study by Hynd et al. concentrated on the morphology of this region in children with ADHD. Lesions of this region have been associated with symptoms very similar to ADHD. Results of this study indicated that children with ADHD had a significantly smaller left caudate nucleus (Hynd et al., 1993). This finding is consistent with the earlier blood flow studies of decreased activity in this brain region.

Important to understand here is the problem of very small sample sizes employed in many of these studies. Such small samples typically fall well below levels needed for adequate statistical power, and thus may obscure minor differences in brain structure and function that would be significant with larger samples. These small samples also tend to contribute to a high probability of failure, on the part of other researchers using similarly small samples, to replicate the original findings. The variability across studies using small samples has the potential to be quite large.

Fortunately, several more recent studies have used larger samples of ADHD and control subjects using quantitative MRI technology. These studies have indicated significantly smaller anterior right frontal regions, smaller caudate nucleus, and smaller right globus pallidus regions in children with ADHD compared to control subjects (Castellanos et al., 1994, 1996; Filipek et al., 1997). Interestingly, the study by Castellanos et al. (1996) also found smaller cerebellar volume in those with ADHD, possibly consistent with recent views that the cerebellum may have some role in the motor presetting aspects of sensory perception that derive from planning and other executive functions (Akshoomoff & Courchesne, 1992; Houk & Wise, 1995). Analysis of the regions of the corpus callosum found no differences between groups in either of the studies by Castellanos and colleagues (1994, 1996), as had been suggested in the small studies discussed above and found in a prior study by this same research team (Giedd et al., 1994). However, the study by Filipek and colleagues (1997) did find smaller posterior volumes of white matter in both hemispheres in the regions of the parietal and occipital lobes that might be consistent with the earlier studies, which showed smaller volumes of the corpus callosum in this same area. Castellanos et al. (1996) suggest that such differences in corpus callosal volume, particularly in the posterior regions, may be more related to learning disabilities, which are found in a large minority of ADHD children, than to ADHD itself.

The results for the smaller size of the caudate nucleus are consistent across studies but are inconsistent in indicating which side of the caudate may be smaller. The work by Hynd and colleagues (Hynd et al., 1993) discussed earlier found the left caudate to be smaller than normal in the ADHD subjects. The more recent study by Filipek and colleagues (1997) found the same result. However, Castellanos et al. (1996) also reported a smaller caudate but found it to be so on the right side of the caudate. The normal human brain demonstrates a relatively consistent asymmetry in volume, with the right frontal cortical region being larger than the left (Giedd et al., 1996). This led Castellanos et al. (1996) to conclude that a lack of frontal asymmetry (a smaller than normal right frontal region) probably mediates the expression of ADHD. However, whether this asymmetry of the caudate, with the right side greater than the left side, is true in normal subjects is debatable, as other studies found the opposite pattern in their normal subjects (Filipek et al., 1997; Hynd et al., 1993). As Filipek and colleagues have noted, many of the differences in the findings of studies regarding which side of the caudate is more affected in subjects with ADHD could readily be explained by subject and procedural differences as well as differences in defining the boundaries of the caudate. More consistent across these studies are the findings of smaller right prefrontal cortical regions and smaller caudate volume, whether on the right or left side.

Others reviewing this literature over the last 2 decades have reached similar conclusions—that abnormalities in the development of the prefrontal–striatal regions probably underlie the development of ADHD (Arnsten, Steere, & Hunt, 1996; Benson, 1991; Gualtieri & Hicks, 1985; Mattes, 1980; Mercugliano, 1995; Pontius, 1973). These regions of the brain are illustrated in Figure 2.1, where the right hemisphere of the brain is shown but the left hemisphere has been cut away to expose the location of the striatum in relation to the prefrontal regions controlling movement specifically and behavior generally.

So far, these neuroimaging studies have simply shown a difference between ADHD and control subjects in the size of particular brain regions. However, this does not prove that ADHD arises from these particular brain structures. These group differences could have other explanations, some of which may not be related to ADHD at all but to other confounding or uncontrolled variables in these experiments. To support any neurological hypothesis that ADHD arises from these brain regions, one would have to demonstrate a link between the degree of ADHD, particularly the degree of behavioral disinhibition in those with ADHD, and the size of these particular regions; in other words, demonstrate a relationship between the size of these particular regions and the extent of the deficits in behavioral inhibition in those with ADHD. A recent study appears to have done just this. Casey and colleagues (1997) used the data from the Castellanos et al. (1996) MRI study of ADHD subjects described above and correlated the size of the various brain regions of interest in that study with a laboratory measure of response inhibition from these same subjects. They found that the ADHD subjects performed significantly worse on the test of response inhibition than the

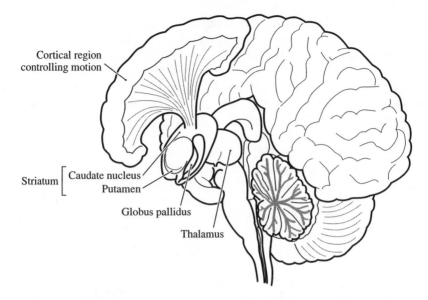

FIGURE 2.1. Diagram of the human brain showing the right hemisphere, and particularly the location of the striatum, globus pallidus, and thalamus. Most of the left hemisphere has been cut away up to the prefrontal lobes to reveal the striatum and other midbrain structures. Adapted from an illustration by Carol Donner in Youdin and Riederer (1997, p. 53). Copyright 1997 by *Scientific American*. Adapted by permission.

normal subjects; a finding consistent with many other studies reviewed in Chapter 4. More important to my purposes here, however, was their finding that performance on the test of response inhibition correlated significantly with the MRI measures of the size of the prefrontostriatal circuitry (prefrontal cortex, caudate nucleus, and globus pallidus) and that these significant correlations were more often associated with the measures of these brain structures on the right side of the brain. Such findings further support the role of the right prefrontostriatal circuitry in both response inhibition and in ADHD.

Important here is the fact that none of the neuroimaging studies found evidence of brain damage in any of these structures in those with ADHD. The regions identified as related to ADHD are simply smaller than normal, typically resulting in no asymmetry in size between the right and left frontal regions (or those of the caudate and globus pallidus) when such asymmetries are normal (right larger than left regions). This is consistent with past reviews of the literature suggesting that brain damage was probably a contributor to less than

5% of those with hyperactivity (Rutter, 1977, 1983). Where differences in brain structures are found, they are likely the result of abnormalities in brain development within these particular regions, the causes of which are unknown but are probably under genetic control. After all, genes control in large part the developmental construction of the brain.

GENETIC FACTORS

No evidence exists to show that ADHD is the result of abnormal chromosomal structures (as in Down syndrome), their fragility (as in fragile X) or transmutations, or extra chromosomal material (as in XXY syndrome). Children with such chromosomal abnormalities may show greater problems with attention, but such abnormalities are very uncommon in children with ADHD. By far, the greatest research evidence suggests that ADHD is a trait which is highly hereditary in nature, making heredity one of the most well-substantiated etiologies for ADHD.

Multiple lines of research support such a conclusion. For years, researchers have noted the higher prevalence of psychopathology in the parents and other relatives of children with ADHD. In particular, higher rates of ADHD, conduct problems, substance abuse, and depression have been repeatedly observed in these studies (Barkley, DuPaul, & McMurray, 1990; Biederman et al., 1992; Pauls, 1991). By separating the group of ADHD children into those with and without conduct disorder (CD), it has been shown that the conduct problems, substance abuse, and depression in the parents is related more to the presence of CD in the children than to ADHD (August & Stewart, 1983; Barkley, Fischer, et al., 1991; Lahey et al., 1988). Yet rates of hyperactivity or ADHD remain high even in relatives of the group of ADHD children without CD. Research shows that between 10% and 35% of the immediate family members of children with ADHD are also likely to have the disorder, with the risk to siblings of the ADHD children being approximately 32% (Biederman et al., 1990, 1992; Faraone et al., 1993; Gross-Tsur, Shalev, & Amir, 1991; Pauls, 1991; Welner, Welner, Stewart, Palkes, & Wish, 1977). Even more striking, recent research shows that if a parent has ADHD, the risk to the offspring is 57% (Biederman et al., 1995). Thus, ADHD clusters among biological relatives of children or adults with the disorder, strongly implying a hereditary basis to this condition.

Another line of evidence for genetic involvement in ADHD has emerged from studies of adopted children. Cantwell (1975) and Morrison and Stewart (1973) reported higher rates of hyperactivity in the biological parents of hyperactive children than in adoptive parents of such children. Both studies suggest that hyperactive children are more likely to resemble their biological parents than their adoptive parents in their levels of hyperactivity. However, both studies were retrospective and both failed to study the biological parents of the adopted hyperactive children as a comparison group (Pauls, 1991). Cadoret and Stewart (1991) studied 283 male adoptees and found that if one of the biological parents had been judged delinquent or had an adult criminal conviction, the adopted-away sons had a higher likelihood of having ADHD. A later study (van den Oord, Boomsma, & Verhulst, 1994) using biologically related and unrelated pairs of international adoptees identified a strong genetic component (47% of the variance) for the Attention Problems dimension of the Child Behavior Checklist (Achenbach, 1991), a rating scale commonly used in research in child psychopathology. This particular scale has a strong association with a diagnosis of ADHD (Biederman, Milberger, Faraone, Guite, & Warburton, 1994) and is often used in research in selecting subjects with the disorder. Thus, like the family association studies discussed earlier, results of adoption studies point to a strong possibility of a significant hereditary contribution to hyperactivity.

Studies of twins provide a third avenue of evidence for a genetic contribution to ADHD. Early studies demonstrated a greater agreement (concordance) for symptoms of hyperactivity and inattention between monozygotic (MZ) compared to dizygotic (DZ) twins (O'Connor, Foch, Sherry, & Plomin, 1980; Willerman, 1973). Studies of very small samples of twins (Heffron, Martin, & Welsh, 1984; Lopez, 1965) found complete (100%) concordance for MZ twins for hyperactivity and far less agreement for DZ twins. A later study of a much larger sample of twins (570) found that approximately 50% of the variance in hyperactivity and inattention in this sample was due to heredity, while 0–30% may have been environmental (Goodman & Stevenson, 1989). Examining only those twins with clinically significant degrees of ADHD within this sample revealed a heritability of .64 for hyperactivity and inattention. This implies that the more deviant or clinically serious the degree of symptoms of ADHD, the more genetic factors may be contributing to it. Other large-scale twin studies are also quite consistent with these findings (Edelbrock, Rende, Plomin, & Thompson, 1995; Gillis, Gilger, Penningotn, & DeFries, 1992; Levy & Hay, 1992; Light, Pennington, Gilger, & DeFries, 1995). For instance, Gilger, Pennington, and DeFries (1992) found that if one twin was diagnosed as ADHD, the concordance for the disorder was 81% in MZ twins and 29% in DZ twins. A more recent study of 194 MZ and 94 DZ male twins (Sherman, McGue, &

Iacono, 1997) found that concordance for ADHD ranged from 53% to 67% (teacher and mother identified, respectively) in MZ pairs and 0% to 37% (mother and teacher identified, respectively) in DZ pairs, clearly substantiating a genetic contribution to the disorder. The heritability ranged from .73 to .88 (teacher and parent identified, respectively), in keeping with other twin studies.

Stevenson (1994) summarized the status of twin studies on symptoms of ADHD by stating that the average heritability is .80 for symptoms of this disorder (range = .50–.98). More recent large-scale twin studies have been remarkably consistent with this conclusion, demonstrating that the majority of variance (70–90%) in the trait of hyperactivity–impulsivity is due to genetic factors (averaging approximately 80%) and that such a genetic contribution may increase as the scores along this trait become more extreme, although this latter point is debatable (Faraone, 1996; Gjone, Stevenson, & Sundet, 1996; Gjone, Stevenson, Sundet, & Eilertsen, 1996; Levy, Hay, McStephen, Wood, & Waldman, 1997; Rhee, Waldman, Hay, & Levy, 1995; Sherman, Iacono, & McGue, 1997; Sherman et al., 1997; Silberg et al., 1996; Thapar, Hervas, & McGuffin, 1995; van den Oord, Verhulst, & Boomsma, 1996). Thus, twin studies add substantially more evidence to that already found in family and adoption studies to support a strong genetic basis to ADHD and its behavioral symptoms.

But twin studies can also tell us as much about environmental contributions as they do about genetic factors affecting the expression of a trait (Faraone, 1996; Pike & Plomin, 1996; Plomin, 1995). Across the twin studies conducted to date, the results have been reasonably consistent in demonstrating that the shared environment contributes little, if any, explanation to individual differences in the trait underlying ADHD (hyperactive–impulsive–inattentive), typically accounting for less than 5% of the variance among individuals (Levy et al., 1997; Sherman et al., 1997; Silberg et al., 1996). Similar findings have been noted for other forms of child psychopathology (Pike & Plomin, 1996). Such shared environmental factors include social class and family educational/occupational status, the general home environment, family nutrition, toxins that may be present in the home environment (i.e., lead), parental and child-rearing characteristics that are common or shared across children in the family, and other such nongenetic factors that are common to the twins under investigation in these studies. In their totality, such shared environmental factors seem to account for 0–6% of individual differences in the behavioral trait(s) related to ADHD. It is for this reason that I stated at the opening of this chapter that little attention would be given here to discussing the role of purely environmental or social factors in the causation of ADHD.

Yet, recent research does suggest that such shared environmental factors may contribute to the persistence or continuity of behavior problems across development (van den Oord & Rowe, 1997). While this might suggest that the family social environment may have some role to play in the maintenance of behavior problems across development, it must be borne in mind that parental genetic factors contribute to family environment and child rearing (Frick & Jackson, 1993; Plomin, 1995; van den Ooord & Rowe, 1997) and so some genetic effects common to both parent and child may appear within the shared environmental effects in such studies. This issue has not been considered by earlier investigators when positing from their results that deficient parental management methods with children may be a major cause of or contributor to symptoms of ADHD and their stability over development (Jacobvits & Sroufe, 1987; Silverman & Ragusa, 1991).

The twin studies cited earlier have also been able to indicate the extent to which individual differences in ADHD symptoms are the result of nonshared environmental factors. Such factors include not only those typically thought of as involving the social environment, but also all biological factors that are nongenetic in origin. Factors in the nonshared environment are those events or conditions that will have affected only one twin and not the other. Besides biological hazards or neurologically injurious events that may have befallen only one member of a twin pair, the nonshared environment also includes those differences in the manner in which parents may have treated each child. Parents do not interact with all of their children in an identical fashion, and such unique parent–child interactions are believed to make more of a contribution to individual differences among siblings than do those factors about the home and child rearing that are common to all children in the family. Twin studies to date have suggested that approximately 15–20% of the variance in hyperactive–impulsive–inattentive behavior or ADHD symptoms can be attributed to such nonshared environmental (nongenetic) factors (Silberg et al., 1996). Research suggests that the nonshared environmental factors also contribute disproportionately more to individual differences in other forms of child psychopathology than do factors in the shared environment (Pike & Plomin, 1996). Thus, if researchers were interested in identifying environmental contributors to ADHD, these twin studies suggest that such research should focus on those biological, interactional, and social experiences that are specific and unique to the individual and are not part of the common environment to which other siblings have been exposed.

Some recent research suggests that while the nonshared environment plays a more significant role than the shared environment in the expression of behavioral problems, the shared environment, as noted above, may make a greater contribution to the continuity of behavior problems like ADHD over time (van den Oord & Rowe, 1997). And, as also noted earlier, this shared environment may well contain some genetic effects from conditions shared by both parent and child. Moreover, genetic effects on the environment by the individuals in that environment (see Scarr & McCartney, 1983) may increase rather than decrease across development (Elkins, McGue, & Iacono, 1997).

Quantitative genetic analyses of the large sample of families studied in Boston by Biederman and his colleagues suggest that a single gene may account for the expression of the disorder (Faraone et al., 1992). The focus of research initially had been on the dopamine type 2 (D2) gene, given findings of its increased association with alcoholism, Tourette syndrome, and ADHD (Blum, Cull, Braverman, & Comings, 1996; Comings et al., 1991), but others have failed to replicate this finding (Gelernter et al., 1991; Kelsoe et al., 1989). More recently, the dopamine transporter gene has been implicated in ADHD (Cook et al., 1995; Cook, Stein, & Leventhal, 1997). Another gene related to dopamine, the D4RD (repeater gene) was recently found to be over-represented in the 7-repetition form of the gene in children with ADHD (Lahoste et al., 1996). Both of these more recent findings are being replicated in an ongoing study by Swanson and colleagues (Swanson, personal communication, November 1996). Clearly, research into the genetic mechanisms involved in the transmission of ADHD across generations promises to be an exciting and fruitful area of research endeavor over the next decade, as the human genome is mapped and better understood.

ENVIRONMENTAL TOXINS

As the twin and quantitative genetic studies have suggested, the environment may play some role in individual differences in symptoms of ADHD. "Environment" should not be taken to mean, however, only those influences within the realm of psychosocial or family influences, but all nongenetic sources more generally, as noted earlier. These include pre-, peri-, and postnatal complications, and malnutrition, diseases, trauma, and other neurologically compromising events that may occur during the development of the nervous system before and after birth. Among these various biologically compromising events, several have been repeatedly linked to risks for inattention and hyper-active behavior.

One such event is exposure to environmental toxins, specifically lead. *Elevated body lead* burden has been shown to have a small but consistent and statistically significant relationship to the symptoms comprising ADHD (Baloh, Sturm, Green, & Gleser, 1975; David, 1974; de la Burde & Choate, 1972, 1974; Needleman et al., 1979). However, even at relatively high levels of lead, less than 38% of children are rated by teachers as having the behavior of hyperactivity (Needleman et al., 1979), implying that most lead-poisoned children do not develop symptoms of ADHD. Likewise, most ADHD children do not have significantly elevated lead burdens, although one study indicates their lead levels may be higher than those of control subjects (Eskinazi & Gittelman, 1983). Studies that have controlled for the presence of potentially confounding factors in this relationship have found the correlation between body lead (in blood or dentition) and symptoms of ADHD to be .10–.19; the more factors controlled, the more likely the relationship is to fall below .10 (Fergusson, Fergusson, Horwood, & Kinzett, 1988; Silva, Hughes, Williams, & Faed, 1988; Thomson et al., 1989). This suggests that lead levels explain no more than 4% (at best) of the variance in the expression of ADHD symptoms in children with elevated lead. Moreover, two serious methodological issues plague even the better conducted studies in this area: (1) None of the studies have used clinical criteria for a diagnosis of ADHD to determine precisely what percentage of lead-burdened children actually have the disorder; all have simply used behavior ratings comprising only a small number of items of inattention or hyperactivity; and (2) none of the studies assessed for the presence of ADHD in the parents and controlled its contribution to the relationship. Given the high heritability of ADHD, this factor alone could attenuate the already small correlation between lead and symptoms of ADHD by as much as a third to a half.

Other types of environmental toxins found to have some relationship to inattention and hyperactivity are prenatal exposure to alcohol and tobacco smoke (Bennett, Wolin, & Reiss, 1988; Denson, Nanson, & McWatters, 1975; Milberger, Biederman, Faraone, Chen, & Jones, 1996b; Nichols & Chen, 1981; Shaywitz, Cohen, & Shaywitz, 1980; Streissguth et al., 1984; Streissguth, Bookstein, Sampson, & Barr, 1995). Studies examining time periods other than pregnancy have shown that both parents of children with ADHD consume more alcohol and smoke more tobacco than control groups in general (Cunningham, Benness, & Siegel, 1988; Denson et al., 1975). Thus, it is reasonable for research to continue to pursue the possibility that these environmental toxins may be causally related to ADHD. However, like the lead studies discussed earlier, most research in this area suffers from two serious methodological limitations—the failure to utilize clinical diagnostic criteria to determine rates of ADHD in exposed children and the failure to evaluate and control for the presence of ADHD in the parents. Until these steps are taken in future research, the relationships demonstrated so far between these toxins and ADHD must be viewed with some caution. In the area of maternal smoking during pregnancy, at least, a recent study incorporating methodological improvements found the relationship between maternal smoking during pregnancy and ADHD to remain significant after controlling for symptoms of ADHD in the parent (Milberger et al., 1996b).

IMPLICATIONS FOR THEORY CONSTRUCTION

The research on biological and genetic factors that may be causal of ADHD, particularly the large number of twin studies and the marked consistency of their findings, has some implications for efforts to construct a theory of ADHD. First, it is clear that such a theory cannot be built purely or solely upon factors in the family environment or larger social ecology of the child, especially where such factors are likely to be shared across siblings. Family diet, common environmental toxins, family dysfunction, flawed child-rearing characteristics of the parents, social class and disadvantage, marital discord, separation, and divorce, and any of a whole host of other common environmental factors must now be ruled out as providing any credible explanation for the development of ADHD, either alone or as a major contributor in concert with other possible causes.

The studies of twins further suggest that greater hope of a causal link can be held out for those familial and social factors that may be experienced specifically and uniquely by a particular child within that family environment. Some researchers may choose to focus on the unique interaction of parent and child that is not shared by the parent's interactions with other children in the family, or even on the child's unique experiences outside of the family. That is all well and good. However, in looking for such nonshared contributory factors, one should not forget that they also include pre-, peri-, and postnatal biological hazards that may have affected this child alone in addition to the nonshared familial and social factors. Extant research suggests that maternal smoking, maternal alcohol consumption, and other risk factors during pregnancy, as well as significant prematurity of birth and smallness for gestational age, may play some contributory role, beyond that of genetic factors alone. But even then, such nongenetic, nonshared factors would appear to play only a small though significant role in the expression of ADHD in a child, perhaps accounting for 15–20% of the differences among individuals on the trait(s) comprising ADHD.

The third implication of the studies of twins is that any theory of ADHD is going to have to link up in some way with genetic factors that clearly and reliably account for the large majority of differences among children in their levels of hyperactive–impulsive–inattentive behavior. This means that psychological constructs used to build a theory of ADHD or those most proximal to its expression must have a large hereditary contribution to them as well. But genes do not directly create or alter behavior. They do so via the protein chains and other chemical processes they influence in the construction and functioning of the human body, and, in this case, the organ responsible for controlling human behavior—the brain. Mediating the expression of these genetic influences on ADHD must be neurological processes. Certain neuroanatomical structures, then, and the effectiveness of their functioning will likely be found to make a large contribution to the eventual expression of ADHD symptoms in an individual. As described earlier, research to date has repeatedly implicated the frontal lobes, and particularly the prefrontal cortex and its reciprocal interconnections with the striatum, as likely to be involved in the expression of ADHD. These neuroanatomical structures are the most likely candidates for mediating the genetic influences on inhibition and self-control that underlie ADHD. More inconsistent in the past research, however, have been findings as to whether the left or right side of these brain structures is more contributory to the disorder. Research to date favors the right prefrontal–striatal network as probably more contributory than the left side of this network in the display of ADHD characteristics. Nevertheless, neuroimaging research is rapidly homing in on the regions of the prefrontal area of the brain likely to be involved in creating symptoms of ADHD. Such findings would be consistent as well with genetic studies, particularly recent ones pursuing molecular genetic mechanisms, that focus upon the genes that build and regulate the functioning of the prefrontal–striatal network. In short, a neuropsychological model of ADHD will be the only type of model that has any hope of being reconciled with the remarkable findings about ADHD that advances in behavioral and molecular genetics and in functional and structural neuroimaging are likely to yield in the near future.

The neuropsychological model developed for ADHD will need to address the role of prefrontal lobe functions and of the striatum in order to incorporate extant research on neuroimaging and ADHD. Therefore, it will be imperative to investigate the functions of these regions. Much

information has already accumulated in the neuropsychological literature on the nature of these functions. That research can and must guide
any endeavor to construct a theory of ADHD. This will be the focus
of Chapter 5. Research to date suggests that most cases of ADHD
represent the extreme end of the dimension of a normal trait. It is
likely, therefore, that the functions of the prefrontal lobes are somehow
related to this trait or set of behavioral traits comprising ADHD.
Similarly, any credible theory of ADHD must represent the functions
of the prefrontal lobes (and the trait representing ADHD) as varying
within a normal population. As the findings of twin studies imply,
unique (nonshared) environmental contributions will affect the development and expression of the behavioral traits related to ADHD. Thus,
while a theoretical model must be essentially a neuropsychological one,
it will have to account for a certain amount of influence by unique
environmental experiences on the functions (and behavioral traits)
which it describes.

To meet these constraints, a model of ADHD must bridge the
research findings on ADHD, neuropsychology (as it pertains to the
functions of the prefrontal lobes and related structures—the executive
functions), and developmental psychology (as it pertains to the normal
development of the behavioral or psychological traits mediated by these
brain structures). As daunting as such a task of model building may
seem, advances in all of these fields have now put such a model within
reach.

CONCLUSION

It is the purpose of the remainder of this text to build a neuropsychological model of executive functions and self-control and to review
the evidence available supporting its extension to understanding the
developmental neuropsychology of ADHD. This model will provide a
very different paradigm for understanding ADHD than previous ones.
It will also yield a large number of implications for the nature of the
disorder and its assessment, diagnosis, and management. Moreover, it
will point to a sizable number of new hypotheses about deficiencies
associated with ADHD that have not been previously thought to be
involved in the disorder. Such hypotheses can drive future research into
the nature of ADHD and its clinical management, research that will
also provide a means of testing the model for its fit with the data
(falsifiability). The model to be developed here is undoubtedly incom-
plete and will surely require revision as new findings emerge pertaining
to its components and their configuration and interaction. But theory

building always needs to begin somewhere and it will begin here with the assertion that ADHD (specifically ADHD-HI and ADHD-C) is, at its core, a developmental disorder of behavioral inhibition. The terms inhibition, self-control, and executive functions are fraught with multiple meanings and uses in past research, so I will define these constructs more explicitly in the next chapter. Research supporting my assertion that ADHD is primarily a disorder of behavioral inhibition will be reviewed in Chapter 4. Chapter 5 will attempt to demonstrate how behavioral inhibition forms a bedrock functional system upon which those neuropsychological faculties (or executive functions) that permit human self-regulation are founded and necessarily depend for their own effective performance. As a result, such a model, imperfect as it undoubtedly must be at this stage of our knowledge, is at once both a theory of executive functions (prefrontal lobe faculties) and of those psychological faculties instrumental to the development of human self-regulation. Extended to ADHD, such a model asserts that ADHD is a developmental disorder of behavioral inhibition that impairs the development of effective self-regulation (executive functioning) and is not, as its name implies, chiefly a disorder of attention.

CHAPTER 3

---·---

Defining Behavioral Inhibition, Self-Control, and Executive Function

THE MODEL OF EXECUTIVE functions and ADHD to be developed in later chapters presumes that *the essential impairment in ADHD is a deficit involving response inhibition.* This deficit leads to *secondary* impairments in four neuropsychological abilities partially dependent upon inhibition for their own effective execution. Those four abilities are considered to be the executive functions, as that term is used in neuropsychology. The secondary impairments in them as well as the primary deficit in behavioral inhibition lead to decreased effectiveness in motor (behavioral) control or in guidance by internally represented information and self-directed action. Before such a model of inhibition, self-control, and the executive functions can be constructed, however, the meanings of these terms as I use them in this text need to be operationalized, that is, made more precise.

DEFINITION OF TERMS

Behavioral Inhibition

Behavioral inhibition refers to three interrelated processes: (1) inhibiting the initial prepotent response to an event; (2) stopping an ongoing response or response pattern, thereby permitting a delay in the decision to respond or continue responding; and (3) protecting this period of delay and the self-directed responses that occur within it from disrup-

47

tion by competing events and responses (interference control). It is not just the delay in responding that results from response inhibition nor the self-directed actions within it that are protected, but also the eventual execution of the goal-directed responses generated from those self-directed actions (Bronowski, 1967, 1977; Fuster, 1989). The prepotent response is defined as that response for which immediate reinforcement (positive or negative) is available or with which reinforcement has been previously associated. In both of these cases the reinforcement needs to be considered as prepotent. Some prepotent responses do not function to gain an immediate positive reinforcer so much as to escape or avoid immediate aversive, punitive, or otherwise undesirable consequences (negative reinforcement). Both forms of prepotent response will be difficult for those with ADHD to inhibit.

The inhibitory process involved in the third form of behavioral inhibition defined earlier, known as interference control, may be separable from that involved in delaying a prepotent response or ceasing an ongoing response. Indeed, as others have argued (see Engle, Conway, Tuholski, & Shisler, 1995; Goldman-Rakic, 1995a, 1995b; Roberts & Pennington, 1996; also see Chapter 5), it may be an inherent part of the executive function of working or representational memory. The second form of inhibition (ceasing ongoing responses), may arise as an interaction of the working memory function (which retains information about outcomes of immediately past performance that feed forward to planning the next response) with the ability to inhibit prepotent responses (Fuster, 1989), thereby creating a sensitivity to errors. If so, then this second form of inhibition may be distinguishable from these other forms. Nevertheless, some of the previous neuropsychological models on which the present one will be developed clustered them together as forms of inhibition. That fact, along with the research reviewed later in this chapter suggesting that all three inhibitory activities are impaired in ADHD, has led to my treatment of them here as a single global construct, for the time being.

The present definition of inhibition is not the same as that popularized by Kagan and colleagues (Kagan, Reznick, & Snidman, 1988) in their studies of shy (inhibited) and sociable (uninhibited) children. In Kagan's research, uninhibited behavior is defined by reactions to social settings involving unfamiliar people in which children are consistently sociable, talkative, and affectively spontaneous. It is the polar opposite of shyness (clinging, quiet, timid, and withdrawn). Here, in contrast, inhibition is assessed by performance on cognitive and behavioral tasks requiring withholding of responding, delayed responding, cessation of ongoing responses, and resisting distraction or disruption of performance by competing events. The social characteristics of children with low social inhibition in Kagan's research may be similar to some of the behavioral effects of the model developed here (i.e., greater initiation of social interactions). The two concepts and their correlates, however, do not appear to map precisely onto each other, nor do they seem to predict the same outcomes.

For instance, Caspi and Silva (1995) found that separate dimensions of temperament for undercontrolled behavior (impulsive, emotionally reactive, easily frustrated, and overactive) as compared to socially confident behavior (sociable, talkative, eager to explore unfamiliar contexts) could be extracted from ratings of 3-year-olds. These two dimensions (Undercontrolled vs. Confident/Resilient) predicted very different personality characteristics in adolescence (Caspi, Henry, McGee, Moffitt, & Silva, 1995; Robins, John, Caspi, Moffitt, & Stouthamer-Loeber, 1996) and adulthood, with the former associated with more maladaptive behavior than the latter (Caspi, Moffitt, Newman, & Silva, 1996). Likewise, Dickman (1994) has distinguished between functional and dysfunctional impulsiveness, with the former resembling Caspi and Silva's (1995) socially confident and gregarious type and the latter akin to their undercontrolled type. The undercontrolled behavior pattern, or dysfunctional impulsiveness, seems more closely related to the poor behavioral inhibition as described in the model to be developed in this text than is the socially confident pattern that resembles Kagan's sociable (uninhibited) children.

The distinction among three forms of behavioral inhibition (preventing prepotent responses, ceasing ongoing responses, and interference control) has been made previously in both developmental psychology (Masters & Binger, 1978) and neuropsychology (Fuster, 1989). Indeed, there may even be a fourth form of response inhibition, which Masters and Binger (1978) described as "continued inhibition" to distinguish it from "interruptive inhibition" (p. 233). The latter refers to the ability of a child to cease a behavior (playing) within 5 seconds of a command to do so, while the former represents the child's ability to sustain such inhibition over a period of 60 seconds, as indicated by the avoidance of engaging in the forbidden behavior during this period. The authors presented evidence to show that these forms of inhibition are not the same and differ in their developmental course. Continued or persistent inhibition is more difficult for 2- to 4-year-olds than interruptive inhibition, although both showed substantial improvements over this age range (see Figure 3.1).

It is not clear if this continued inhibition represents a fourth form of behavioral inhibition or if it is the same as interference control. The latter, again, refers to the ability to protect inhibitory delays in responding and the self-control occurring within those

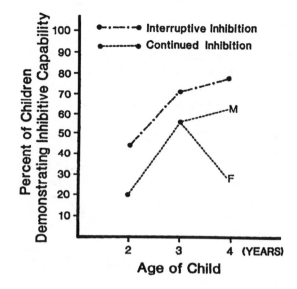

FIGURE 3.1. Percentage of children at each age demonstrating interruptive and continued inhibition. The M and F refer to the percentage of children showing continued inhibition in compliance to a male (M) or female (F) experimenter. From Masters and Binger (1978, p. 234). Copyright 1978 by *Merrill-Palmer Quarterly.* Reprinted by permission.

delays from disruption by ongoing external and internal events (Fuster, 1989). Masters and Binger (1978) likened continued inhibition to the form of inhibition displayed in delay of gratification tasks, such as those used by Mischel, Shoda, and Rodriguez (1989), which appear to involve not only response inhibition but also some form of self-directed activity during the delay (e.g., self-speech, self-distraction, visual imagery, etc.), in order to enhance success at such tasks. If so, then continued inhibition is probably the same form of behavioral inhibition as interference control, and in this text it will be treated as such.

I am hardly the first person to argue that inhibition is a central impairment in ADHD (see Douglas, 1972; Quay, 1988a, 1988b; Schachar, Tannock, & Logan, 1993; Still, 1902). Distinctive of the model to be offered later in this text, however, is its linkage of this deficiency in inhibition to the disruption of five other neuropsychological abilities that depend upon inhibition for their own efficient execution. Four of these abilities are critical for self-regulation and goal-directed persistence, and so are called executive functions here. The fifth ability is that of the motor control system. ADHD is believed to disrupt the four executive functions because the primary executive, self-regulatory act must be inhibition of responding. Such inhibition permits a delay in the decision to respond that is utilized for further self-directed, executive, or evaluative actions. Those actions and the information they yield affect the decision to respond and serve to guide, regulate, or otherwise control the eventual motor responses these executive functions generate.

This is *not* to say that behavioral inhibition directly causes these executive or self-directed actions to occur in any primary or immediately proximal sense of causation. But it does set the occasion for their performance by providing the delay necessary for them to occur. In that sense, inhibition permits, supports, and protects the executive functions. Therefore, the four executive functions I will describe later should be viewed as neuropsychological systems separable from that of behavioral inhibition yet hierarchically (or pyramidally) perched upon it and interactive with it so as to create self-regulation.

Self-Control

Self-control is any response or chain of responses by the individual which serve to alter the probability of their subsequent response to an event and, in so doing, function to alter the probability of a later consequence related to that event. There are six key ingredients implicit in this definition that deserve notice and comment.

1. As the term implies, self-regulation means responses by the individual that are directed at him- or herself, rather than at the environmental event that may have initiated them. Such self-directed action may take as its direct object of modification the individual's behavior, as when I repeat aloud to myself a telephone number I need to use in a few minutes, to increase the likelihood that I will recall it. Alternatively, they may be directly aimed at altering the environment around the individual so as to achieve a change in responding, as when I remove chocolate treats from the top of my office desk and place them down the hall with our receptionist so as to reduce my probability of consuming them excessively. In either case, the actions taken are self-directed.

2. Such actions are designed to alter the probability of a subsequent response by the individual. I rehearse a telephone number subvocally, so as to increase my chances of correctly recalling it later. Likewise, I remove the treats from my office desk to decrease the probability of my eating them. In either case, the immediate function

of the self-directed action (whether public or covert/internal) is to change the individual's behavior in some way.

3. Behaviors that are classified as self-regulatory function to change a later rather than an immediate outcome. We may think of the elements of a behavioral contingency in simple terms, such as an event, the response to it, and the outcomes of that response. Responses may have both proximal (immediate) and distal (delayed or future) consequences for the individual. Self-regulation occurs so as to achieve a net maximization of beneficial consequences across these short- and long-term outcomes of a response for the individual, particularly where there is a discrepancy between the valences of the short- and long-term outcomes. So long as there are only immediate outcomes for responding with negligible or no effects of that response over the longer term, or so long as the valence of both short-term and long-term consequences are consistent (i.e., both positive or both negative), self-regulation is unlikely to be required. Self-regulatory behaviors, therefore, can be thought of as functioning to achieve a change in the long-term best interests of that person—a net maximization of both short and long-term outcomes for behavior.

4. For self-control to occur, the individual must have developed a preference for the long-term over the short-term outcomes of behavior. Long-term outcomes may have greater reward value than short-term ones, but their value is steeply discounted by the length of time involved in the delay to that outcome (Mazur, 1993). Individuals demonstrating a preference for larger delayed rewards over more immediate ones must be discounting the value of the delayed reward less because of its delay than are people who prefer smaller, more immediate rewards. Research has documented a shift in preference for longer-term over short-term outcomes (a decrease in the discounting of the value of delayed rewards) across child development and into adulthood (Green, Fry, & Meyerson, 1994). The investigators tested samples of children, adolescents, young adults, and older adults concerning their choices between having varying amounts of money right now ($100 to $1,000) or having $1,000 later. The amount of money they would be given now varied across choice trials as did the delay (in months) to the later $1000. Individuals were found to increase their preference for the delayed reward with increasing age at each duration of delay. But individuals also showed a preference for increasingly delayed rewards with age. In a subsequent study, these authors found that, contrary to their earlier results, the preference for delayed rewards did not continue to increase across the life span. This finding had resulted from failing to take the income or economic levels of the subjects into account. When that was done in a subsequent study

(Green, Myerson, Lichtman, Rosen, & Fry, 1996), the increasing preference for the delayed reward continued only until approximately the early 30s in age. There, it leveled off and remained steady throughout the remaining age span of adults. These results are shown in Figure 3.2, where *k* represents the degree to which the delayed reward is being discounted in comparison to the immediate reward. A decrease in *k* reflects a decrease in the extent to which the individual is discounting the amount of the delayed reward compared to the immediate one (or, conversely, is expressing a preference for the delayed reward).

The authors concluded that there is an increasing preference for larger delayed rewards over smaller immediate ones across development up until approximately the early 30s. Thereafter, this preference remains at that level for the remainder of life. In other words, as individuals develop, they decrease the extent to which they discount a later reward on the basis of its delay interval, at least up to age 30 years. Moreover, individuals of higher income level demonstrate a greater preference for larger delayed over smaller immediate rewards

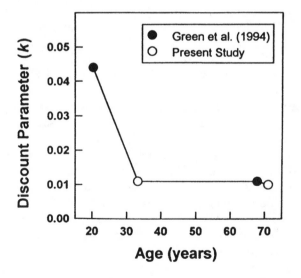

FIGURE 3.2. Estimates of the *k* parameter in the hyperbolic discounting function as a function of age. Results for the $1,000 delayed reward from both the present study and a previous study by Green, Fry, and Meyerson (1994) are shown. From Green, Myerson, Lichtman, Rosen, and Fry (1996, p. 83). Copyright 1996 by the American Psychological Association. Reprinted by permission.

relative to those of middle or lower income. The investigators interpret their findings as demonstrating an increase in impulse control (delay of gratification) across development until the early 30s. It also seems that individuals having greater preference for larger delayed over shorter immediate rewards appear to have higher income levels than those showing less of such a preference. While it is possible that people who preferred delayed rewards are thereby more likely to persist toward longer term and larger rewards and thus end up with a higher income level, it is also possible that those with higher income levels can thereby afford to defer gratification. The findings of this study are certainly consistent with Walter Mischel's (Mischel et al., 1989; Shoda, Mischel, & Peake, 1990) longitudinal research over two decades showing that children's ability to delay gratification is a significant predictor of adolescent and adult outcomes with regard to educational performance, social competence, and coping with stress and frustration.

Relying on such an interpretation of these results, I would predict that if ADHD individuals were tested using this same task, their preference for delayed rewards would be closer to that of younger individuals than to their age-matched normal peers, and would level off at the early 30s with a degree of preference below that of their peers. What is further intriguing about these findings is that they seem to parallel the developmental course of the prefrontal lobes in humans, the brain regions repeatedly described as mediating the capacity to inhibit and delay responding, thereby permitting the individual to organize behavior across temporal contingencies, as will be discussed in Chapter 5.

5. Self-regulatory actions by an individual have as an inherent property the bridging of time delays across the elements comprising behavioral contingencies. So long as there is little or no time between these events, responses, and outcomes, there is less or even no need for self-regulation. This will also be true where there is no discrepancy between the immediate and long-term outcomes for that response. Automatic responses will often suffice under such contingencies. But where time delays are introduced among these elements, self-directed actions must be undertaken to bridge them successfully and maximize the longer-term outcomes. Thus, a capacity for the cross-temporal organization of behavioral contingencies is implicit in the definition of self-regulation. It appears that this capacity is one of the most impor- tant, if not *the* most important, functions of the prefrontal lobes (Fuster, 1989, 1995), as will be discussed in the Chapter 5.

6. Some neuropsychological or mental faculty must exist that permits the capacity to sense time and the future and to put them to use in the organization and execution of behavior. To organize behavior

across time delays, to demonstrate an increasing preference for future over immediate rewards, and to direct behavior toward that future requires a sense of time and the capacity to conjecture the future. To conjecture the future, the past must be capable of recall and analysis for patterns among sequential chains of events and their behavioral contingencies, because it is from the recall of the past that such hypothetical futures can be constructed. Such capacities will demand a special kind of memory in which information about past, time, plans, and the future can be held "on-line," or in mind, while carrying out the responses needed to accomplish the goal. Discussions of self-regulation often overlook this implicit requirement for a special retrospective and prospective form of memory and the capacity to keep information about temporal sequences in mind so as to anticipate, prepare for, and respond to future events. Chapter 5 will discuss the nature of this special form of memory, but suffice it to say here that behavioral inhibition, delayed responding, delay of gratification, goal-directed persistence, and self-regulation more generally are critically dependent on the development of such a special form of memory.

The definition of self-control provided earlier is similar in many respects to that employed by others (Kanfer & Karoly, 1972; Mischel et al., 1989; Skinner, 1953). This definition also resembles Berkowitz's (1982), wherein self-control is defined as "the ability to intentionally manipulate covert mental events, most notably inner speech and images, in order to regulate one's own behavior" (p. 225). Lacking in Berkowitz's definition, however, is the key feature that such mental events are forms of self-directed behavior (self-speech, self-imaging, etc.), that they need not necessarily be covert, as is likely to be the case in young children, and that the function of such self-regulation is to alter the probability of a future as opposed to immediate outcome. We do not regulate our own behavior just for the sake of altering it, but because doing so is in our long-term best interests (maximizing net future outcomes). Nevertheless, as the model to be developed in this volume will illustrate, Berkowitz is close to the mark in specifying covert speech and imagery as two important components in human self-regulation and in recognizing that there are probably other components, as indeed I will eventually show there to be.

The terms self-control and self-regulation have often been used interchangeably, and I continue that practice in this volume. However, Diaz, Neal, and Amaya-Williams (1990) attempted to distinguish self-control from self-regulation. The former is viewed by these authors as a developmentally earlier form of self-regulation in which a child simply repeats and then obeys an adult command in the absence of the caregiver. Self-regulation, in contrast, involves more complex behavior involving self-generated plans and flexible adaptation to the changing demands of a task. Despite this difference in complexity of the self-directed activities used by the individual for self-regulation, both levels of self-regulation involve self-directed actions that serve to modify one's subsequent behavior so as to change the probability of future outcomes. Hence, they both fulfill the definition given earlier. I use the term self-control here, then, to mean both of these levels of self-regulation, admitting that there exists a developmental maturation of complexity in this process (see Kopp, 1982).

Executive Function

The self-directed behaviors occurring during the delay in the response that follows response inhibition need not be publicly observable, although it is likely that in early development many of them are so. Over development, they may become progressively more private or covert in form. The development of internalized, self-directed speech, discussed in Chapter 7, may serve to exemplify this process. Such speech remains essentially a self-directed form of behavior even when internalized, that is, disengaged from public, motor manifestation (musculoskeletal movements). *The term "executive function" refers here to those self-directed actions of the individual that are being used to self-regulate.* Most are private or covert (unobservable or cognitive) in form. The executive functions to be discussed in later chapters likely arise from: (1) the development of neural networks within the prefrontal lobes, which underlie these neuropsychological abilities and permit the acquisition of more specific skills used for self-control (Bronowski, 1977; Fuster, 1989, 1995; Goldman-Rakic, 1995a, 1995b); (2) the success these actions have had in the past for maximizing the net consequences of behavior, both immediate and delayed, when considered across long time periods (Kanfer & Karoly, 1972); (3) the socialization of the child (Berk, 1992; Kopp, 1982; Silverman & Ragusa, 1992), and (4) the ongoing reinforcement of the individual for using self-regulatory actions (Hayes, 1989; Kopp, 1982; Skinner, 1953).

In Chapters 5 and 6, I will discuss four executive functions that are fundamental to self-regulation. Suffice it to say here that this term, as used in neuropsychology, refers to the self-directed mental activities that occur during the delay in responding, that serve to modify the eventual response to an event, and that function to improve the long-term future consequences related to that event. So defined, the term executive function incorporates most of the attributes often ascribed to it by others (Denckla, 1994; Torgesen, 1994; Stuss &

Benson, 1986; Welsh & Pennington, 1988), including: (1) self-directed actions; (2) the organization of behavior across time; (3) the use of self-directed speech, rules, or plans; (4) deferred gratification; and (5) goal-directed, future-oriented, purposive, effortful, or intentional actions. In short, executive functions are those types of actions we perform to ourselves and direct at ourselves so as to accomplish self-control, goal-directed behavior, and the maximization of future outcomes.

Clearly, I make no distinction between overt (public) or covert (private, typically unobservable) actions by the individual within this definition of executive function and self-control. It has become customary in psychology to refer to overt actions as "behavior" while their covert counterparts are considered "cognitions," thoughts, or other forms of mental activity. The custom is unfortunate, in my opinion, at least for studying self-control, because it obfuscates their similarities and origins and misleads people into believing that they are qualitatively distinct forms of action by the individual that have little or nothing in common.

If my view is correct, then covert or private forms of behavior ("thinking") utilize the same or highly similar (neighboring) neurological substrates for their organization and execution as are required for their public counterparts. Admittedly, these public counterparts are also likely to activate additional brain regions related to their actual motor performance and the sensory feedback it requires, but the centers involved in organizing and preparing those behaviors are believed to be the same for both public and private forms. This appears to be the case for covert speech (Ryding, Bradvik, & Ingvar, 1996) and may well be the case for other forms of covert behavior. This would lead to the prediction that one cannot do both the identical covert and overt behavior at once, such as speaking to others while simultaneously speaking covertly to oneself. We should find a significant reduction in efficiently performing such identical types of public and covert behavior because they would demand time sharing of the same cortical and subcortical regions. Rapidly alternating between the two might occur, thereby giving the rough appearance of simultaneity, but this would result from the individual rapidly alternating between the public and covert forms of behavior. The point here is that distinguishing overt from covert forms of self-control may be more artificial than real, is probably unnecessary, and is surely confusing, causing us to overlook their strong similarities and shared origins.

If, for example, I covertly verbally rehearse a set of instructions I wish to follow some time later or choose instead to say them out loud repeatedly or even write them down and carry them with me, what practical benefit derives from referring only to the former as an executive function because it was covert? And if in following directions to a specific location while driving in a familiar city I choose to covertly visually image a map of the town with which I am familiar rather than keep the map before me on my lap, are both not acts of self-control? I would submit that they are and that both are "executive" in nature as defined here. The use of covert visual imagery to create an internally guided form of behavior is certainly impressive to the passengers riding with me. It may represent a more developmentally mature form of self-regulation if witnessed in children because of its "internalized" nature. But both external and internal forms of self-directed behavior achieve the same end result. Further, as has become evident in studying self-speech in adults, even those utilizing the more mature, covert form of self-directed behavior, such as covert self-speech, may have to fall back on its somewhat less mature public counterpart (i.e., audible self-speech) when problems of sufficient difficulty for the individual must be solved, and especially if those problems are verbal or semantic in nature (see Diaz & Berk, 1992). Both the public and covert forms of behavior are self-regulation as defined here and so are "executive" in nature.

EVENTS THAT INITIATE
INHIBITION AND SELF-CONTROL

It is possible that human adults engage nearly continuously in acts of inhibition and self-control of varying degrees. The magnitude or complexity of such actions, however, may increase or decrease depending upon the events that are occurring around and within the individual. In other words, inhibition and self-control are more likely to be a matter of more or less at any given time rather than a matter of all or none. It is worth considering what events or types of information received by the individual seem to initiate or increase behavioral inhibition, self-regulation, and the executive functions permitting self-control. Six such initiating events have been repeatedly mentioned in the literature of developmental psychology dealing with self-regulation and in that of neuropsychology dealing with the executive functions.

One such initiating event seems to occur when *the verbal instructions given in a situation or task compete with other prevailing sources of behavioral control* (Hayes, Gifford, & Ruckstuhl, 1996). The individual must now inhibit responding to the prepotent stimuli existing in that situation while adhering to the rule governing that situation. Such competing sources of behavioral control frequently arise when the situation involves *a conflict between the immediate and distal conse-quences* of a response (Kanfer & Karoly, 1972), suggesting that this may be a second type of initiating event. However, rules are often invented and stipulated so as to make the later consequences of one's actions more obvious and to help mediate the delay to those later consequences. Thus, oftentimes the apparent conflict between imme-diate and delayed consequences in a task or situation is just another way of saying that the task or situation involves a conflict between rules and competing sources of behavioral control in the immediate context. For instance, consider a situation where dull, boring, or even unpleasant work must be completed (a verbal rule) so as to have access to a later reward. The prepotent response of escape behaviors under such circumstances must be inhibited or resisted and perseverance toward the work sustained. This will require acts of self-regulation (in this case internal speech and the rule-governed behavior it permits).

A third type of event that may increase inhibition and its related executive functions may occur when *time delays are inserted into the elements of a behavioral contingency.* Delay-of-gratification tasks are of this sort. Such tasks are particularly taxing of self-control when the reward or other consequence may be visible to the individual during the delay period and hence difficult to resist. In such cases, behavior must be organized and sustained across time not only without benefit of immediate rewards for doing so, but even requiring in some cases the self-imposition of a state of deprivation—the individual must actually resist the temptation to avail him- or herself of rewards, often by doing something else so as to sustain the goal-directed activity. Thus, events, tasks, or situations that demand the cross-temporal organization of behavior require acts of self-regulation. Again, this may simply reflect a competition between rules specified in a given situation and other sources of behavioral control in that setting, for much the same reasons as noted earlier. Rules are often specified to assist individuals in bridging the temporal delays between elements of behavioral contin-gencies. The triggering event for inhibition is, once more, a reflection of competing sources of behavioral control (rules versus other control-ling events in the environment).

This implies a fourth event that may instigate self-regulation, *the specification of a future goal to be attained,* which may actually be related to the second and third factors just noted, for one could easily conceptualize a distant consequence as a goal and so formulate rules (plans) to attain that distant consequence. The insertion of a time delay among the elements of a contingency automatically results in a delay to the consequence, making the successful achievement of the delayed outcome a goal of sorts. Regardless of whether the requirement for goal-directed behavior is the same as or separate from the insertion of rules and time into a behavioral contingency, these requirements should be recognized as likely instigating events for inhibition and self-regulation.

A fifth factor to consider as a potential initiating event for inhibition and self-control is *the requirement of complexity of responding, particularly if such complex responding must be organized across time.* As Fuster (1989) has noted, complexity alone may not require the assistance of the prefrontal cortex for self-regulation, but the addition of time to complexity will most certainly do so. In fact, the addition of time to a task or behavioral contingency automatically adds complexity to the task, so it may be the element of time and not just complexity of responding that generates the need for self-regulation.

A sixth factor that may initiate or increase efforts at self-control seems to occur when *a problem arises that requires the generation of a novel response to resolve it.* Automatic responses will not suffice under such problem-solving circumstances to correctly or successfully respond to the events or tasks. Instead, the individual must engage in effortful analysis of the situation and in experimentation with various plans and simulations of solutions, and then select, execute, and monitor that solution as it is set in motion. The capacity to formulate new rules from old ones or to generalize rules from one type of problem to another may well be involved in this process of problem solving (Cerutti, 1989; Hayes et al., 1996). Once again, the first factor—a competition between rules and other sources of behavioral control in the immediate environment—comes into play here as well.

In summary, the following may serve as initiating events for the inhibition, self-control, and executive functions subserving self-regulation: (1) conflict between competing sources of behavioral control (i.e., rules vs. other sources of control), (2) conflicts in temporally separated outcomes (immediate vs. delayed), (3) time delays among the elements of a behavioral contingency, (4) a requirement for future- or goal-directed action, (5) the complexity of responding demanded by a task or situation, or (6) problem-solving situations (the demand for novelty of a behavioral structure). Other events may serve this role, particularly those that are emotionally charged (Scherer, 1994), but these may actually represent situations akin to the first and second items in the preceding list. This is so because the consequences for immediately displaying the highly charged affect will be in conflict with a rule against doing so and with the longer-term outcomes for doing so.

These, then, are at least six factors that seem to have the greatest research support at the moment for being associated with instigating acts of behavioral inhibition and self-regulation along with the executive functions the latter requires. All, as Hayes et al. (1996) noted, may reflect situations in which a competition exists between various sources of behavioral control, particularly rules that should be governing behavior versus nonverbal sources of behavioral control in the immediate situation. Also, all of them require that the individual resort to forms of self-directed behavior, often private or covert (internal) in form, in order to successfully negotiate the situation. As Hayes et al. (1996) suggest, self-directed verbal rules may be an especially important class of such private behavior that will be needed to resist the competing sources of behavior control, bridge the time delays in the elements of a behavioral contingency, and direct behavior toward a future goal. But this analysis overlooks an equally compelling class of private self-directed action—visual imagery (Berkowitz, 1982; Forisha, 1975). Covert seeing to oneself (visual imagery) as well as covert self-directed speech may be the most common means by which individuals successfully respond under circumstances where there are sources of competing behavioral control.

The future consequence that is in question in such circumstances involving self-regulation is not actively influencing this process because it has not yet occurred. Instead, conditioned signals of punishment from prior experiences, information derived from ongoing monitoring and appraisal of changing patterns of response feedback, and prior socialization may be the determinants of when inhibition and self-regulation are engaged in or increased (Newman & Wallace, 1993; Quay, 1997). A large class of such information about behavior for humans is language and the rules governing behavior that it can be used to formulate. Private, self-directed rules or private visual imagery, therefore, may function as proxies for the future events that have not yet come to pass but are anticipated.

When these initiating events arise, self-regulation can result in a reduction in immediately available rewards (self-imposed deprivation) or an increase in the aversive consequences in the immediate context (self-imposed pain or hardship) to which an individual subjects him- or herself for the sake of a better future outcome. Such self-directed acts often increase the probability of later, considerably larger rewards or the avoidance of later, greater aversive consequences, the achievement of these goals may then serve to encourage future such acts of deferred gratification or self-imposed hardship. It is the individual's evaluation of the net gain anticipated from both the immediate and delayed consequences of a response, not the gain from the immediate consequences alone, that must be appreciated as motivating such self-regulatory behavior (Kanfer & Karoly, 1972; Thoresen & Mahoney, 1974).

Circumstances or tasks that involve temporal delays, conflicts in competing sources of behavioral control (and their temporally associated consequences), or the generation of novel responses most heavily tax the type of behavioral inhibition and self-regulation described here. Resistance to temptation or deferred-gratification tasks are of this sort. Among the several dimensions of impulsivity (behavioral and cognitive, typically) discovered in past research (Milich & Kramer, 1985; Olson, 1989), the dimension reflected in deferred-gratification/resistance-to-temptation tasks, or what others have called behavioral inhibition (White et al., 1994), that is associated with the inhibitory processes described here (see also Mischel et al., 1989). Problem-solving tasks are also likely to tax behavioral inhibition and its related executive functions, such as self-speech or visual imagery (Berk, 1992; Berkowitz, 1982), so long as the level of difficulty of the problem lies within the individual's zone of proximal discovery or mastery (Diaz, 1992). By definition, problems are situations for which the individual has no readily available response and which requires the generation of a novel response as a solution. Therefore, problem-solving tasks as well as those involving temporal delays and temporal conflicts in outcomes would all prove useful in research studying not only the linkages between behavioral inhibition and the executive functions subserving self-regulation in normal development, but also their impairment in those with ADHD.

It is the "behavioral" type of impulse control that seems to be more stable over development, to correspond more closely to parent or teacher ratings of hyperactive–impulsive behavior, and to correlate more highly with later cognitive and social competence (Mischel et al., 1989; Olson, 1989; Shoda et al., 1990; Silverman & Ragusa, 1992) than does the cognitive dimension of reflectiveness (as in the Matching Familiar Figures Test, Draw-a-Line-Slowly Test; see Milich & Kramer, 1985). This may explain why methods of assessing the behavioral type of inhibition (parent/teacher ratings, delay-of-gratification tasks, and reinforcer conflict tasks, as in resistance-to-temptation paradigms) have been more useful than those assessing cognitive reflectivity in distinguishing those with ADHD from those without it, in predicting which infants and preschool children are at risk for ultimately developing ADHD, and in predicting the extent of later cognitive and social problems associated with ADHD, as will be shown later.

The immediate purpose of the executive functions that are supported by behavioral inhibition seems to be the achievement of greater prediction and control over one's behavior and environment. Ultimately, however, their overarching function seems to be the alteration of the future consequences that a response is likely to produce so as to maximize the individual's own best interests (net positive outcomes) (see Bronowski, 1977; Fuster, 1989; Skinner, 1953).

CONCLUSION

The present chapter defined behavioral inhibition as comprising three capacities: (1) to inhibit prepotent responses before they are performed, (2) to inhibit or interrupt ongoing response patterns, and (3) to protect the delay in responding so created, and the self-directed and often covert executive functions occurring within the delay, from disruption by other external and internal events (interference control). The latter form of inhibition could also be described as resistance to distraction. Self-regulation was shown to be dependent on inhibition because the first self-regulatory action must be the prevention of prepotent responses or the interruption of ongoing behavior that is proving ineffective. Self-control, or self-regulation, was then defined as any response by an individual that serves to modify his or her subsequent response to an event, thereby producing a net change or gain in the long-term outcomes for the individual. The executive functions were defined as those forms of self-directed action used in the performance of self-regulation. Although often covert or private in form, particularly in adolescents and adults, these self-directed actions need not be covert to be considered as "executive" in nature or as instances of self-regulation. Self-control and its associated executive functions appear to be most often initiated or increased by events or tasks that involve (1) temporal delays between the elements of the behavioral contingency (events, responses, and outcomes), (2) a conflict or discrepancy between the valences of immediate and delayed outcomes for a response, or (3) the requirement that the individual generate novel responses in problem-solving situations. Such situations often present the individual with competing sources of behavioral control, and that competition is often between rules and other forms of privately represented information (i.e., visual imagery) and the physical sources of behavioral control in the external setting. Acts of behavioral inhibition, self-regulation, and the latter's associated executive functions are believed to be mediated by the brain's prefrontal cortex and its interconnections with the striatum.

In the next chapter, I will argue that ADHD is a developmental disorder of behavioral inhibition in which the inhibitory deficiency creates a rippling of secondary impairments into the executive functions that depend on inhibition for their effective performance. Such impairments would then give rise to a deficiency in the individual's capacity for self-regulation, the control or guidance of behavior by internally represented information, and the direction of that behavior toward the future and away from the moment. I will examine these latter assertions more carefully in later chapters.

CHAPTER 4

────•────

Behavioral Inhibition and ADHD

THE EVIDENCE SUPPORTING a deficiency in behavioral inhibition in ADHD comes from a number of sources that will be reviewed in this chapter. I wish to emphasize again, however, that the model of ADHD that I develop in this volume does *not* refer to that subgroup whose chief problem is inattention alone (ADHD-I), as described in Chapter 1. The conclusion that inhibitory problems in ADHD are a "fact in the bag" is warranted by substantial evidence. The model to be developed in the next three chapters takes this conclusion as its starting point, assuming that *the essential impairment in ADHD is a deficit involving response inhibition.*

One consequence is that improvement or amelioration of the inhibitory deficit in ADHD should result in improvement or normalization in the four executive functions that depend upon the inhibitory capacity and also in the motor control that those executive functions afford. Another consequence is that this successive chain of impairments creates the appearance of poor sustained attention in those with ADHD, a form of sustained attention that is actually self-regulated and goal-directed persistence, as will be shown later.

EVIDENCE FOR DEFICITS IN
BEHAVIORAL INHIBITION IN ADHD
Parent and Teacher Ratings of Behavior

Many studies using parent and teacher ratings of hyperactive and impulsive behaviors in children find these behaviors to cluster into a single dimension, often called hyperactive–impulsive or undercontrolled (Achenbach & Edelbrock, 1983, 1986; DuPaul et al., 1996, in press; Goyette et al., 1978; Hinshaw, 1987; Lahey et al., 1988, 1994). It is this dimension of behavior that, virtually by definition, distinguishes those with ADHD from others without it (Barkley, 1990; Hinshaw, 1987, 1994). This argument, however, is circular; ratings of hyperactive–impulsive behavior are used to create a diagnostic category of ADHD and then those with ADHD are found to differ on such ratings. The circularity is effectively dispensed with by referring to evidence of external validation using measures other than those of parent and teacher ratings.

Behavioral Observations of ADHD Children

Many studies using objective measures have shown that children rated as being more hyperactive–impulsive or who were clinically diagnosed as having ADHD, in fact display a higher activity level than other children not so rated or diagnosed (see Luk, 1985, for a review; also Barkley & Cunningham, 1979a; Gomez & Sanson, 1994b; Porrino et al., 1983; Teicher, Ito, Glod, & Barber, 1996). ADHD children also talk more than other children, whether to others (Barkley, Cunningham, & Karlsson, 1983; Cunningham & Siegel, 1987) or out loud to themselves (Berk & Potts, 1991; Copeland, 1979), and make more vocal noises than do other children (Barkley, DuPaul, & McMurray, 1990; Copeland & Weissbrod, 1978). All of this may be taken as evidence of poor behavioral inhibition.

ADHD children also have more difficulties restricting their behavior in conformance with instructions to do so (Barkley & Ullman, 1975; Milich & Loney, 1979; Routh & Schroeder, 1976; Ullman, Barkley & Brown, 1978), deferring gratification (Campbell, Pierce, March, Ewing, & Szumowski, 1994; Rapport et al., 1986; Schweitzer & Sulzer-Azaroff, 1995), and resisting temptation (Campbell et al., 1982, 1994; Hinshaw, Heller, & McHale, 1992; Hinshaw, Simmel, & Heller, 1995). For instance, Campbell et al. (1994) evaluated 69 boys identified as ADHD in comparison to 43 non-ADHD control children, using both resistance-to-temptation and delay-of-gratification tasks. In the former, the boys were required to sit in front of a highly appealing battery-operated train that visited four rides in a pretend amusement park (Disneyland). The children were permitted to play with the toy for awhile, but when the experimenter left the room she instructed the children not to touch the toy in her absence (a period of 3 minutes). Behavioral coders observing the children from behind a one-way mirror recorded whether and how often the children touched the toy and the latency to the first touch. The strategies the children used to mediate the delay were also coded. Results indicated that the ADHD boys had a shorter latency to the first touch of the toy, touching it approximately 35% sooner than the control boys on average. The ADHD boys also touched the toy approximately twice as often as the control boys, and were less likely to use the delay strategy of attending to and talking about the toy than did control boys. In the delay-of-gratification task, the boys were instructed to wait in a room in which a cookie had been hidden under one of three cups. The boys were instructed to wait and not search for the cookie until signaled by the experimenter to do so. Then when they found the cookie, they were allowed to consume it. Impulsive responses included touching or picking up the cup and/or eating the cookie during the waiting period. The ADHD boys were found to emit such impulsive responses nearly 70% more often than the control boys. Such findings once again indicate a significant deficit in inhibition in ADHD children, especially in situations where rewards are immediately available for emitting impulsive responses. Studies also suggest that this difficulty with deferring gratification and waiting for delayed rewards worsens over time in the task and is associated with an increase in hyperactivity as time at the task increases (Schweitzer & Sulzer-Azaroff, 1995).

Laboratory Tests of Inhibition of Prepotent Responses

I indicated in Chapter 3 that behavioral inhibition largely comprises difficulty in inhibiting prepotent responses. This means that a laboratory task to detect this deficit must involve conditions in which conflicts exist between responses that have a history of being reinforced in the past or during the task itself and those responses specified in the experimental instructions. To the extent that no reinforcement is available within the task for the impulsive response one is attempting to measure, that the rewards provided are relatively weak, that no history of such reinforcement exists in the individual's experience, or that history is itself rather weak, then it will prove very difficult to document the inhibitory deficit within that experimental setting. This set of circumstances may help to explain why some studies have not been able to directly establish an inhibitory deficit in those with ADHD or found only weak evidence of such a deficit (e.g., Sonuga-Barke, Taylor, & Heppinstall, 1992; Sonuga-Barke, Taylor, Sembi, & Smith, 1992; van der Meere, Gunning, & Stemerdink, 1996). Such studies have typically fallen short of establishing a sufficient conflict between sources of behavioral control (prepotent responses vs. rules to inhibit such responses or to do something instead of those responses).

Some studies may also have failed to test the effects of signals of inhibition during the critical period when motor responses to the event are being prepared, as van der Meere et al. (1996) have noted. Laboratory paradigms that use signals to inhibit responding that occur outside of this critical period may not be able to identify differences between ADHD and normal children in inhibition. Merely setting up conditions for the subject to respond to events or to briefly delay a response will prove insufficient unless (1) the responses to be suppressed are "prepotent" as defined in Chapter 3, (2) a sufficient conflict has been created between emitting those responses and correctly following the instructions to the task that compete with them, and (3) the signal for inhibition occurs relatively close in time to the preparation of the motor response to the event. Where studies have been able to establish such task parameters, evidence for impulsive responding has been repeatedly observed.

The go/no-go task is just such a task, providing further evidence of poor inhibition in ADHD. This motor inhibition task requires subjects to emit a motor response, such as a finger tap, as fast as possible when cued to do so and then to inhibit such a movement when another cue is provided. The cues to inhibit are interspersed throughout the task in a random fashion. Subjects with ADHD are routinely found to have difficulties inhibiting responses to the no-go signal (Iaboni, Douglas, & Baker, 1995; Milich, Hartung, Martin, & Haigler, 1994; Shue & Douglas, 1989; Trommer, Hoeppner, Lorber, & Armstrong, 1988; Voeller & Heilman, 1988).

Equally convincing evidence of a response inhibition deficit in ADHD comes from studies using the stop-signal paradigm (Oosterlaan & Sergeant, 1995, 1996a, 1996b; Schachar et al., 1993; Schachar & Logan, 1990; Schachar, Tannock, Marriott, & Logan, 1995). Subjects are presented with a primary task in which they must respond to a forced-choice letter discrimination task. Periodically, they are given a signal (typically a tone) to inhibit responding in the primary task. The paradigm is based on Logan's (Logan & Cowan, 1984) race model of response inhibition. Studies have repeatedly found that children with ADHD are slower to initiate the inhibitory response when signaled to do so (show longer reaction times to the signal), are less likely to inhibit when signaled to do so, and are more variable in their inhibitory responses. The change paradigm (related to the stop-signal paradigm) has also been used to study inhibition in ADHD and other psychiatrically disordered groups of children. In this task, the subjects are required not only to inhibit their responding on the primary task when signaled to do so, but also to shift to performing another task, which consists of pressing another button when they hear the stop-signal tone.

Such research has found ADHD children to have not only the same inhibitory problems discussed with regard to the stop-signal task, but also to be slower to reengage the primary task after performance was interrupted by the stop-signal (Schachar et al., 1995).

Other tasks on which impulsive responding has been observed significantly more often in subjects with ADHD than in control subjects include delayed response tasks and those assessing reflectivity, such as Kagan's Matching Familiar Figures Test (Kagan, 1966). In the latter task, subjects must match a sample picture to one among an array of highly similar pictures. The task would seem to require some delay in responding and deliberation of the stimulus array during the delay so as to correctly perform the task in the least number of trials. Nevertheless, this task may create only a weak conflict between sources of behavioral control because the incorrect, "impulsive" response (pointing to an incorrect picture) does not seem to me to be especially prepotent. Some studies have found ADHD children to perform this task more poorly than control children (Gordon, 1979; Schliefer et al., 1975; Sonuga-Barke, Houlberg, & Hall, 1994; Sonuga-Barke, Taylor, & Hepinstall, 1992; Sonuga-Barke, Taylor, Sembi, & Smith, 1992; Weyandt & Willis, 1994), but others have not (Campbell, Breaux, Ewing, & Szumowski, 1984; Campbell, Endman, & Bernfeld, 1977; Campbell et al., 1982; Mariani & Barkley, 1997). The studies finding no differences tended to use preschool-age children, which suggests that age may be a factor in determining the sensitivity of this task to inhibitory deficits in children with ADHD. Even when ADHD subjects are forced to wait during these delay periods, they make more errors than control children and do not employ the extra time during the delay as effectively as the control group to improve their task performance (Sonuga-Barke, Williams, Hall, & Saxton, 1996; Sonuga-Barke, Lamparelli, Stevenson, Thompson, & Henry, 1994).

Blurting out incorrect verbal responses and disrupting the conversations of others with such intrusive responses are considered primary symptoms of impulsiveness in those with ADHD (American Psychiatric Association, 1994). Objective documentation of just such problems was obtained in a study by Malone and Swanson (1993) involving observations of the conversations of ADHD children compared to control children.

Numerous studies also demonstrate that hyperactive or ADHD children produce greater errors of commission on continuous performance tasks (CPT), particularly when computerized versions are employed (Barkley, DuPaul, et al., 1990; Barkley, Grodzinsky, & DuPaul, 1992; Grodzinsky & Diamond, 1992; Krener, Carter, Chaderjian, Wolfe, & Northcutt, 1993; Reader, Harris, Schuerholz, & Denckla,

1994; Robins, 1992; see also Corkum & Siegel, 1993, and Losier, McGrath, & Klein, 1996, for reviews of this extensive literature). Such errors involve pressing the response key on the computer even when no target has appeared or a false target similar but not identical to the correct one appears. Not only are such errors more common in children with ADHD, but several recent studies have found that adults diagnosed with ADHD or having a childhood diagnosis of ADHD also demonstrate more impulsive (commission) errors on CPTs (Barkley, Murphy, & Kwasnik, 1996b; Shaw & Giambra, 1993). Studies also show similar inhibitory problems on computer-simulated driving programs: An increased frequency of braking to false alarms was found in young adults with ADHD (Barkley, Murphy, & Kwasnik, 1996a).

CPT tasks can also be given using paper and pencil, such as in cancellation tasks. In these tasks, participants must scan rows of either letters, numbers, or geometric shapes as quickly as possible, placing a cancellation mark on a target stimulus. The results of studies using this task with hyperactive or ADHD children are often similar to those for the computerized CPTs (Aman & Turbott, 1986; Brown & Wynne, 1982; Carte, Nigg, & Hinshaw, 1996; Keogh & Margolis, 1976). However, some results for these paper-and-pencil tasks, particularly when self-paced, have proven contradictory (Gomez & Sanson, 1994a, 1994b; van der Meere, Wekking, & Sergeant, 1991).

Problems with response inhibition in ADHD have even been noted on tasks assessing more molecular motor movements, such as ocular gaze shifts on delayed response tasks (Pearson, Yaffee, Loveland, & Norton, 1995; Ross, Hommer, Brieger, Varley, & Radant, 1994). For instance, Pearson et al. (1995) had their subjects focus on a central fixation point (a "+") on a screen at the beginning of each trial. The children were then told that a cue (an "!" mark) would appear momentarily at either the right or left side of the fixation point and would indicate where in the periphery the target cue was likely to appear next. If the target signal was a "W," the subjects were to press a key with their left hand, and if it was an "O" they were to press a key with their right hand. They were to do so as quickly as possible. The warning cue correctly indicated the target's side of appearance on two-thirds of the trials. Results indicated that the performance of children with ADHD was much more disrupted by the appearance of the invalid cues. They made twice as many careless errors in the task than did control children. The longer the delay between the warning cue and the appearance of the target, the poorer the performance of those with ADHD. Others have found similar results on such visual attention tasks as the time delays in the task increased (Swanson et al., 1991). These results demonstrate that temporal delays pose an increased demand for the use of inhibition and executive control and that ADHD children have difficulties in performing under such task demands.

Poor behavioral inhibition likewise has been evident in deficient performances by ADHD children using passive rather than active avoidance paradigms. In these studies, passivity, or withholding a response, is required to terminate, escape, or avoid punishment. In such a task, those with ADHD have been found to show more such punished trials than normal (Freeman & Kinsbourne, 1990; Milich et al., 1994).

As discussed in Chapter 2, the study of ADHD children using MRI conducted by Casey and colleagues (1997) also found that ADHD children had significantly more problems with response inhibition than did control children. Even more important, however, is that this is the first study to show that such deficits are significantly related to the size of those structures in the prefrontostriatal circuitry that have been found to be smaller in these same ADHD children. This helps to further establish a link not only between ADHD and deficits in response inhibition, but between the latter deficits and the underdevelopment of brain regions that have been previously believed to be important in response inhibition.

Evidence for Deficits in Interrupting Ongoing Responding in ADHD

As defined in the previous chapter, behavioral inhibition also involves difficulties with interrupting or ceasing ongoing response patterns when signaled to do so. Studies using the stop-signal paradigm described earlier have found that ADHD children are less likely to interrupt their ongoing predominant response patterns, are slower in doing so, and are more variable in their inhibitory responses than are control subjects (Oosterlaan & Sergeant, 1996, in press; Schachar & Logan, 1990; Schachar et al., 1993, 1995). However, a more recent study by Jennings and colleagues (Jennings, van der Molen, Pelham, Debski, & Hoza, 1997) was not able to replicate all of these results. While these investigators did find that subjects with ADHD, particularly those with comorbid oppositional defiant disorder, had slower latencies to inhibiting their responses and were more variable in their reaction time to inhibiting responses, they did not demonstrate fewer inhibitory responses as Schachar and others have found. While Jennings et al. (1997) interpret their results as not necessarily supporting a problem with inhibition in ADHD, that interpretation must be qualified by a major methodological difference between their study and those of Schachar and others. Jennings et al. used a stop-signal procedure in which they rewarded and fined their subjects monetarily for correct inhibition of responses or failures to inhibit, respectively. Prior studies have shown that the introduction of such incentives and response consequences, particularly on a consistent and continuous basis, can significantly improve the performance of ADHD children, in some cases even ameliorating group differences on the particular cognitive task under study (Parry & Douglas, 1983; Solanto, 1990; van der Meere, Hughes, et al., 1995).

Another method for examining the capacity to inhibit or interrupt ongoing response patterns involves using a task wherein subjects must stop an ongoing response pattern and shift to a more effective one based on feedback in the task regarding correctness of the response pattern. Such a requirement is incorporated in the Wisconsin Card Sort Test (WCST; Heaton, 1981), a neuropsychological test commonly used to assess, at least in part, prefrontal lobe functioning. Patients with frontal lobe damage, particularly in the dorsolateral cortical regions, often have difficulties on this test. A recent study using neuroimaging techniques during performance of the task provides evidence that activation of the dorsolateral prefrontal cortex occurred during task performance (Berman et al., 1995).

ADHD children seem to have difficulties performing the WCST as well, often perseverating in the incorrect response pattern despite feedback about their errors. Such perseveration continues beyond the point where controls have typically shifted to a new, more effective response pattern. My colleagues and I (Barkley, Grodzinsky, & DuPaul, 1992) reviewed 13 studies that used the WCST, 8 of which found significant differences between ADHD and control groups. Perseverative errors were the most common mistakes made by the ADHD subjects. Methodological problems, such as low statistical power due to small samples and diverse age groups, may well have limited some of the studies that yielded nonsignificant findings. Performance on this test has been shown to improve with age in both ADHD and control children (Seidman et al., 1996), but even at older ages ADHD subjects have been found to make more errors on the task than control subjects. Interestingly, having a family history of ADHD may contribute to the degree to which subjects perform poorly on this task, in that individuals having more biological relatives with ADHD displayed significantly more errors on the task than those without such family histories (Seidman et al., 1996). I have been able to locate eight additional studies of ADHD using the WCST that were not included in my earlier review. Five of these (Krener et al., 1993; McBurnett et al., 1993; Reader et al., 1994; Seidman, Biederman, et al., 1995; Seidman et al., 1996) found ADHD subjects to perform the task more poorly than control groups, while the remaining three did not (Narhi & Ahonen, 1995; Pennington, Grossier, & Welsh, 1993; Weyandt & Willis, 1994). Though not entirely consistent, the weight of the evidence from this task supports the idea that individuals with ADHD have a problem with response perseveration despite feedback about errors.

In keeping with this interpretation, Sergeant and van der Meere (1988) found that ADHD children performing an information-processing task were less likely to alter their subsequent responding when they made an error than were children in the control group. Response perseveration in ADHD also has been shown in research using the Card Playing Task (Milich et al., 1994). In this task, subjects are required to bet a small amount of money on whether the next card shown on a computer display will be a face card or not. Initially, the ratio of face cards is quite high, such that subjects are more likely to be correct than incorrect if they bet on a face card appearing next. However, over the course of this task, the ratio of face cards declines such that betting on a face card becomes increasingly likely to be incorrect. Subjects with ADHD often bet on more trials than do control subjects, even though the likelihood of being incorrect is escalating across trials. Similarly, patients with prefrontal lobe injuries have also been noted to show persistence in a previously reinforced response pattern even though the contingencies may have changed and it is becoming increasingly punitive to do so. A fascinating finding in such studies is that these subjects can verbally report these changes toward increasing likelihood of being incorrect across the task, yet they still are not able to resist betting on the next trial, despite having verbalized this rule (Damasio, 1994; Rolls, Hornak, Wade, & McGrath, 1994).

According to Fuster (1989), the failure to adjust motor performance given feedback concerning its ineffectiveness may actually reflect an interaction between behavioral inhibition and working memory. The individual fails to hold in mind information on the success or failure of responding on preceding trials (retrospection), which would then be analyzed for a pattern or rule, with the information fed forward to influence or even stop future responses (prospection leading to inhibition). If correct, this view suggests that the cessation, shifting, and reengagement of ongoing responses according to task feedback is not entirely a function of behavioral inhibition, where it was placed in the definition of inhibition in the last chapter. Instead, this sensitivity to errors may result from an interaction of behavioral inhibition with one of the four executive functions, in particular, working memory. Newman and Wallace (1993) have proposed that just such an interaction, which they define as response modulation, explains much of the findings in the literature on deficits in the response patterns of psychopaths using similar tasks. They also speculated that a similar deficiency might account for the inhibitory difficulties of individuals with ADHD. I shall return to this model in Chapter 7 to discuss its similarities to and differences from the model of self-regulation (executive functions) I propose.

Schachar et al. (1995) were able to demonstrate that the capacity to interrupt an ongoing response pattern is separate from that of reengagement of the original task, and that both capacities are deficient in ADHD children compared to controls. Similarly, Lapierre, Braun, and Hodgins (1995) found that it is the power to inhibit prepotent responses (using the go/no-go test) that was more characteristic of psychopathic criminals than was the ability to shift response patterns following feedback about errors (using the WCST), although the difference between groups on perseverative responding on the WCST was marginally significant ($p < .07$). Distinguishing these two processes also suggests that the perseverative responding seen on the WCST by those with ADHD may not be an indication solely of poor inhibition but also of deficient working memory, an interpretation that is consistent with neuroimaging research involving this test (Berman et al., 1995).

More will be said about the nature of working memory and its relationship to behavioral inhibition in the next chapter. Suffice it to say here that the evidence from these studies supports the notion that those with ADHD are deficient in behavioral inhibition, even if some of the deficient performances in these tasks may also be the result of an additional difficulty with working memory. Such an additional difficulty indeed would be predicted from the model of ADHD proposed in this volume.

Evidence of Poor Interference Control

A third form of behavioral inhibition, defined in the last chapter, is the ability to inhibit responding to sources of interference while engaged in another task requiring self-control or while delaying a response. This was labeled as interference control or resistance to distraction. Evidence for poor interference control in ADHD comes from several sources. Studies using the Stroop Word–Color Association Test (Stroop, 1935) with ADHD children nearly always find them to perform poorly on this test. This test has three parts: First, the child identifies the colors of small rectangles displayed in rows across a page, then reads color names printed in black ink, and, finally, must say the name of the color of ink in which color words are printed, even though a word is the name of a color different from the color of that ink (the interference part). Subjects must inhibit the ongoing prepotent response to read the name of the word and instead emit the response of naming the color of the ink. In a previous review (Barkley, Grodzinsky, & DuPaul, 1992), six studies were located that used the Stroop test with hyperactive or ADHD subjects. Five of these six found ADHD children to take more time and make more errors during the interference portion of the task. Four more studies have since been located, and they also found similar results (Krener et al., 1993; Leung & Connolly, 1996; Pennington et al., 1993; Seidman, Biederman, et al., 1995; Seidman et al., 1996). What is striking is the consistency of such findings across studies despite differences in a number of methodological parameters, including cultures, group selection procedures, and sample sizes. Such consistency is a powerful demonstration that a deficiency in the control of interference from prepotent responses (resistance to distraction) is reliably associated with ADHD.

Important to note is that group differences between ADHD and control groups could not be attributed to comorbid learning or conduct disorders (Leung & Connolly, 1996; Pennington et al., 1993; Seidman et al., 1996), which argues for the specificity of these findings to ADHD itself. Recent neuroimaging research using the Stroop Test has identified the orbital–prefrontal regions, particularly the right prefrontal region, as involved in its performance (Bench et al., 1993; Vendrell et al., 1995). As noted in Chapter 2, other neuroimaging studies have found these same regions to be significantly smaller and less active in children with ADHD (Castellanos et al., 1994, 1996; Lou et al., 1984, 1989).

The capacity to maintain the performance of a task despite distraction might also serve as an indicator of interference control. Whether or not distracters disrupted task performance, however, would depend on at least two factors: (1) the prepotency of the response likely to be elicited by the distracting event, and (2) the extent to which any self-regulation (executive functions) was required during the task performance that required protection from such interference. Those tasks calling for such executive control, as noted in the previous chapter, might be ones involving temporal delays, temporally related conflicts in consequences, and problem-solving tasks requiring the formulation of novel, complex responses. Research on ADHD suggests that distractions outside of the immediate task materials are unlikely to detrimentally affect the performance of these children relative to normal children. Those distractions embedded within the task seem more likely to do so (Leung & Connolly, 1996). The more salient the type of distraction, the more it occurs within the task, or the more that time and delays occur within the task parameters, the greater the likelihood distracters will interfere with the task performance by ADHD children (Barkley, Koplowicz, Anderson, & McMurray, in press; Bremer & Stern, 1976; Cohen et al., 1972; Landau, Lorch, & Milich, 1992; Rosenthal & Allen, 1980; Steinkamp, 1980). These findings are in keeping with the prediction made earlier that distracters will not be found to disrupt the performance of those with ADHD on all tasks, but are more likely to do so when task performance requires self-regulation (executive control).

Other evidence of poor interference control in ADHD seems to be evident in a study of college students with ADHD (Shaw & Giambra, 1993). In this study, subjects were interrupted periodically while they performed a CPT and were asked about the nature of their thoughts at that point (on or off task). Students with a history of ADHD had more task-irrelevant thoughts during performance of a CPT than did the control group. Consistent with prior studies of ADHD children, these same students also made more commission errors on the CPT. This might imply poor interference control over internal sources of distraction.

Evidence of ADHD Symptoms in Impulsive Children

The studies reviewed to this point indicate that children and adults with ADHD have difficulties with behavioral inhibition on various tasks (see also Pennington & Ozonoff, 1996). But is the inverse relationship also true as well? That is, do children who display poor behavioral inhibition have a higher likelihood of having symptoms of ADHD? Some studies suggest that this may be the case. Young children identified as more impulsive and less able to delay responses, particularly in resistance-to-temptation and delay-of-gratification tasks, have been rated by others as displaying higher levels of ADHD symptoms both concurrently and later in development (Funder, Block, & Block, 1983; Krueger, Caspi, Moffitt, White, & Stouthamer-Loeber, in press; Mischel, Shoda, & Peake, 1988; Mischel et al., 1989; Shoda, Mischel, & Peake, 1990; Silverman & Ragusa, 1992). Likewise, children with higher levels of activity at 2 years old displayed symptoms of less self-control at 7 years old (Halverson & Waldrop, 1976). Such studies suggest that not only do ADHD children have problems with behavioral inhibition, but children identified as having poor inhibition are more likely to demonstrate symptoms of ADHD as well.

Before proceeding to a review of executive functions from which a theory of self-control and ADHD is to be built, it is first necessary to explain why a new theory of ADHD needs to be built at all.

WHY IS A NEW THEORY OF ADHD NEEDED?

A new theory of ADHD is needed for a number of reasons. *First, current research on ADHD is nearly atheoretical, at least as regards its basic nature.* Much of the research into the basic nature of ADHD has been mainly exploratory and descriptive, with two exceptions. One is Herbert Quay's (1988a, 1988b, 1996) use of Jeffrey Gray's neuropsychological model of anxiety to explain the origin of the poor inhibition seen in ADHD. This Quay/Gray model states that the impulsiveness characterizing ADHD arises from diminished activity in the brain's behavioral inhibition system (BIS). That system is said to be sensitive to signals of conditioned punishment that, when detected, result in increased activity in the BIS and a resulting inhibitory effect on behavior. This model predicts that those with ADHD should prove less sensitive to such signals, particularly in passive avoidance paradigms (Milich et al., 1994; Quay, 1988b).

The second exception to the rule of mainly descriptive research into the nature of ADHD is the work of Sergeant, van der Meere, and colleagues (1988; Sergeant, 1995a, 1995b, 1996; van der Meere, in press; van der Meere, van Baal, & Sergeant, 1989). These researchers have been successfully employing information-processing theory and its associated energetic model (arousal, activation, and effort) to the isolate the central deficit(s) in ADHD as they might be delineated within that paradigm (Sergeant, 1995b). However, this approach does not set forth a theory of ADHD. Like the Quay/Gray hypothesis of ADHD, it makes no effort at large-scale theory construction so as to provide a unifying account of the various cognitive deficits associated with ADHD. Both are attempts to document the nature of the central deficit in ADHD, and both have reached the conclusion that this deficit, at least in part, reflects a problem with the development of behavioral inhibition. I have also reached the same conclusion, based on the substantial body of research supporting it, which has been reviewed in this volume. Both of these research programs are concerned with the origin of this inhibitory deficit within their respective paradigms. They are to some extent complementary rather than contradictory approaches to understanding ADHD. Sergeant and van der Meere go further than Quay in concluding that the inhibitory deficit in ADHD is associated with additional deficiencies in motor presetting (response selection) and in effort or arousal in addition to problems in motor inhibition. I will show how such deficiencies may arise in those with ADHD in Chapter 9.

More recently, van der Meere (in press) has attempted to reduce all of these difficulties to a central deficiency in arousal. While I accept that those with ADHD may have difficulties with the regulation of arousal and alertness, as Douglas (1983) has previously noted, I would not go so far as to stipulate that this is the origin of the inhibitory deficits in ADHD, as van der Meere seems to do. As I will show in the next two chapters, deficits in the regulation of arousal and alertness in the service of goal-directed actions can arise as a secondary consequence of difficulties in behavioral inhibition and the impairments this creates within the executive functions that depend upon behavioral inhibition.

One of the foremost senior investigators in the field of ADHD over the past 25 years has been Virginia Douglas of McGill University. Douglas's (1980a) model of ADHD is not actually a theory, but is mainly descriptive. It was arrived at inductively from a review of the extant research findings on ADHD in which Douglas (Douglas, 1980a, 1980b, 1983; Douglas & Peters, 1978) discerned a consistent pattern. That pattern comprised deficiencies in four fundamental processes: (1) the investment, organization, and maintenance of attention and effort; (2) the ability to inhibit impulsive behavior; (3) the ability to modulate arousal levels to meet situational demands; and (4) an unusually strong inclination to seek immediate reinforcement. Although tremendously helpful at the time, such pattern discernment remains at a descriptive level, albeit a more synthetic level than prior efforts at conceptualizing ADHD. But it is neither explanatory nor, more importantly, predictive of new hypotheses that are testable. It still begs the question of just how the pattern itself is to be explained. Appealing to the construct of self-regulation, as Douglas (1988; Douglas, Barr, Desilets, & Sherman, 1995) has more recently done is a step in the right direction. But that step is of only modest help unless self-regulation itself is defined specifically and the manner in which it leads to the four impairments is explained. Both the pattern of deficiencies and the later use of self-regulation as an explanatory construct by Douglas fit well within the model that I develop in this volume.

The theory I propose, however, goes much further. It provides the needed definition of self-regulation (Chapter 3), articulates the cognitive components (executive functions) that contribute to it (Chapters 5–7), specifies the primacy of behavioral inhibition within the theory and the evidence for such a conclusion, and sets forth a motor control component to ADHD (Chapter 7). Most importantly, the model reveals a diversity of new, untested, yet testable predictions about additional cognitive and behavioral deficits in ADHD deserving of further study (Chapter 9).

A second reason why a theory of ADHD is sorely needed is that the current clinical view of ADHD (i.e., DSM-IV) is purely descriptive, describing as it does the two behavioral deficits (inattention and hyperactivity–impulsivity) that are believed to comprise the disorder. This descriptive approach to ADHD, helpful as it has been for the purpose of clinical diagnosis, cannot readily account for the many cognitive and behavioral deficits that have emerged in studies of ADHD. These findings were briefly noted in Chapter 1 and will be discussed in more detail in later chapters. To account for such findings, any theoretical model of ADHD must fulfill at least five key requirements:

1. It must explain why an actual deficit in attention in children with ADHD has not been found (Schachar et al., 1993, 1995; Sergeant, 1995a, 1995b; van der Meere, in press; van der Meere & Sergeant, 1988b, 1988c) even though research on parent and teacher ratings of ADHD repeatedly identifies a factor of "inattention." If attention is thought of as involving the perception, filtering, selecting, and processing of information—in other words, as involving "input" into the brain—then research on ADHD has not reliably documented such deficits. The work of Sergeant, van der Meere, and others has nicely documented that the cognitive problems associated with ADHD are within the motor control or "output" side of the brain's information processing system. While such a deficit may feed back to produce secondary impairments in the executive management of the sensory information-processing system for the purposes of goal-directed behavior (self-regulation), the origin of ADHD is not felt to reside within the sensory information processing functions of the brain. The current clinical description of ADHD (DSM-IV) makes no attempt at such delineations, important as they are for understanding the basic nature of the disorder.

2. A theory must explain the possible link between poor behavioral inhibition (hyperactivity–impulsivity) and the sister impairment of "inattention," or whatever this latter symptom turns out to be. What does this dimension labeled "inattention" represent if not a deficit in attention? Why is it associated with problems of behavioral inhibition in this disorder? Why do the apparent problems with "inattention" seem to arise later in the development of this disorder than do the problems with hyperactive–impulsive behavior (see Chapter 1)? Again, the current clinical consensus view of ADHD makes no attempt to address such questions.

3. Any credible theory of ADHD also must link the two dimensions of hyperactive–impulsive behavior and "inattention" that currently describe this disorder with the concept of executive or metacognitive functions. This is because most, if not all, of the additional cognitive deficits associated with ADHD (briefly noted in Chapter 1)

seem to fall within the realm of self-regulation or executive functions (Barkley, 1995, 1996; Denckla, 1994, 1995; Douglas, 1988, Douglas et al., 1995; Grodzinsky & Diamond, 1992; Pennington & Ozonoff, 1996; Pennington et al., 1993; Seidman, Biederman, et al., 1995; Torgesen, 1994; Welsh, Pennington, & Grossier, 1991; Weyandt & Willis, 1994). Why and how are the hyperactive–impulsive and "inattention" symptoms of ADHD linked to problems with executive functions and self-control? What are those executive functions exactly? Once more, the present clinical view of ADHD as mainly an attention deficit fails miserably in answering such important questions in psychological research on the disorder.

4. For a theory of ADHD to be persuasive, it must ultimately bridge the literature on ADHD with the larger literatures of developmental psychology and developmental neuropsychology as they pertain to self-regulation and executive functions. In most instances, past studies of ADHD have not been based upon studies of normal developmental processes, nor have efforts been made to interpret their findings in the light of extant findings in the developmental psychological literature. Likewise, researchers in developmental psychology and developmental neuropsychology have typically failed to draw upon the findings accruing in their respective literatures on self-regulation and executive functions, respectively, to enlighten each other's understanding of these processes, as Welsh and Pennington (1988) have previously noted. And rarely have researchers in these two disciplines drawn upon the substantial scientific knowledge accumulated on ADHD to illuminate the study of these normal processes. But if it is to be argued that ADHD arises from a deviation from or a disruption in normal developmental processes, then those normal developmental processes must be specified in explaining ADHD. Bridges must be built from the findings on ADHD to the findings on normal developmental processes. The current view of ADHD does not make such an attempt to link the understanding of the disorder with an understanding of normal child development in the areas of behavioral inhibition, self-control, and executive functions. This volume will do so.

5. Any theory of ADHD must prove to be useful as a scientific tool. It must not only better explain what is already known about ADHD, but must make explicit predictions about new phenomena that have previously not been considered in the literature on ADHD, or which may have received only cursory research attention. New theories often predict new relationships among constructs or elements that existing theories or descriptions did not predict. Those new predictions can serve as hypotheses that can drive research initiatives. Such hypothesis testing can also serve as attempts at falsifying the theory. The

present conceptualization of ADHD in DSM-IV provides no such utility as a scientific tool. This does not detract from the utility of the DSM-IV view of ADHD as a clinical diagnostic tool, as noted in Chapter 1, for that is a different enterprise than the one being discussed here. But as an instrument to advance the scientific understanding of ADHD, the current consensus view of the disorder is sorely wanting.

A third reason for a new model of ADHD is that the current view treats the subtypes of ADHD as sharing qualitatively identical deficits in attention while differing only in the presence of hyperactive–impulsive symptoms. As noted in Chapter 1, it is doubtful that the problems with "inattention" associated with hyperactive–impulsive behavior lie in the realm of attention. However, those problems seen in ADHD-I, the predominantly inattentive type, appear to do so, if initial research findings on this subtype are confirmed by future research.

It appears from the research discussed in Chapter 1 that ADHD-I may not, in fact, have its impairment in the same form of attention as in the other two types. Research on ADHD-I suggests that symptoms of daydreaming, "spacing out," being "in a fog," being easily confused, staring frequently, and being lethargic, hypoactive, and passive are more common in this subtype (Barkley, DuPaul, & McMurray, 1990; Lahey & Carlson, 1992), which seems to have a deficit in speed of information processing, generally, and focused or selective attention, specifically (Barkley, DuPaul, & McMurray, 1990; Goodyear & Hynd, 1992; Lahey & Carlson, 1992). The deficit in the ADHD-C, the combined type, has been characterized as being in the realm of sustained attention (persistence) and resistance to distractibility. If so, the present clinical view of ADHD may be clustering into a single set of disorders what are, in reality, two qualitatively different disorders. This distinction would also argue that children with ADHD-C who may move into the ADHD-I subtype as they get older (due to reductions in hyperactive behavior) are not actually changing types of ADHD at all. The type of inattention that they continue to manifest (lack of persistence, distractibility) would still be qualitatively different from the inattention manifested by children who were diagnosed as ADHD-I.

CONCLUSION

To summarize, the evidence that ADHD involves impaired behavioral inhibition is more than compelling, arising as it does from multiple studies, methods, and sources. Such evidence indicates that children with ADHD are more likely to have problems inhibiting prepotent responses, interrupting ongoing response patterns when signaled to do so, shifting response patterns when feedback indicates responding is becoming less effective (a sensitivity to errors), and protecting delays in responding and the periods of self-regulation (executive control) those delays permit from being disrupted by sources of interference (termed here as interference control or resistance to distraction). Thus, there is evidence that those with ADHD have deficiencies in all three elements of behavioral inhibition as defined in the preceding chapter. Evidence was also presented here that the capacity to shift or alter responding given feedback on errors, as in tasks like the WCST, may not solely reflect an inhibitory deficit but arise instead from an interaction of inhibitory ability with that of working memory (holding past information in mind that feeds forward to alter subsequent responding). ADHD subjects were found to have difficulties with such tasks in addition to those reflecting more purely a deficit in behavioral inhibition.

Emerging evidence from recent neuroimaging studies and studies of brain-injured samples suggests that the substrate mediating behavioral inhibition lies within the brain's prefrontal regions, particularly the orbital–prefrontal region and its interaction with the striatum. Such inhibitory abilities may be asymmetrically represented in the human brain, perhaps being mediated more by the right than left prefrontal regions. Such findings are consistent with neuroimaging studies suggesting that these same regions are smaller and less active in those with ADHD.

Not only is there overwhelming evidence that ADHD involves a deficit in behavioral inhibition, but there is also suggestive evidence from developmental psychology of the inverse relationship. Early deficits in behavioral inhibition appear to be associated with increased risks for later symptoms of ADHD (hyperactivity, poor persistence, reduced resistance to distraction). Taken together, the evidence presented in this chapter shows a convergence of findings across the literatures on ADHD, the neuropsychology and neuroanatomy of behavioral inhibition, and the developmental psychology of inhibition and delay of gratification. Given this foundation, the feasibility of developing a neuropsychological model of self-control and executive functions founded on behavioral inhibition will be explored in the next two chapters, and the model then constructed in Chapter 7.

CHAPTER 5

—•—

Neuropsychological Views of the Executive Functions: The Origins of a Hybrid Model

THIS CHAPTER FOCUSES on the nature of the executive functions in self-regulation as they have been conceptualized in the neuropsychological literature. In particular, four models of executive functions will be reviewed here. These were chosen because of the substantial empirical support that most of them have already amassed, the current popularity of some of them in neuropsychology, and the considerable overlap among the constructs of all four theories. Each model, however, overlooks some of the important elements of the others, so a blending of them into a hybrid theory of executive functions (the goal of Chapter 7) offers a more unifying account of those functions than does any single model alone. The hybrid model will be constructed in Chapter 7 and will then be extended to account for the nature of ADHD (Chapter 9).

THE NATURE OF EXECUTIVE FUNCTIONS

Much of the model to be developed in Chapter 7 linking inhibition to four executive functions was set forth by Jacob Bronowski (1967/1977) 30 years ago. After first reading Bronowski's paper, I was immediately struck by the usefulness of his ideas for providing a conceptual understanding of ADHD. I prepared an initial paper on the implications of his model of the unique properties of human language for understanding some of the cognitive deficits seen in ADHD (Barkley, 1994a). I then proceeded to develop Bronowski's ideas further as a model of ADHD in a second paper (Barkley, 1997), by combining them with more current theories and research on the functions of the prefrontal cortex (the executive functions). That explication differed substantially from the initial application of Bronowski's ideas to ADHD in the following respects: (1) the incorporation of portions of Fuster's (1989, 1995) theory and the views of others (Goldman-Rakic, 1995a, 1995b; Knight, Grabowecky, & Scabini, 1995; Milner, 1995) on the neuropsychological functions subserved by the prefrontal cortex; (2) the inclusion of more precise definitions of behavioral inhibition and self-regulation; (3) the addition of a motor control component to the model; (4) the inclusion of the self-regulation of drive and motivation with that of emotion in the model; (5) the reconfiguration of the components of the model to be more logical than when first presented (Barkley, 1994a); (6) the addition of numerous recent findings bearing on the linkages among these components and their applicability to ADHD; and (7) additional predictions about ADHD.

The present work represents a further effort at refinement, clarification, and even elaboration of the ideas set forth in that second paper (Barkley, 1997). Moreover, this work provides further supportive evidence from developmental psychology and neuropsychology for the hybrid model. Also discussed in this book are the larger implications of this model for the understanding, diagnosis, assessment, and treatment of ADHD, issues which were not dealt with in my earlier paper.

In some sense, the evidence reviewed later in this volume supporting the hypothesized link between inhibition and executive functions and even my extension of Bronowski's theory to ADHD would have been anticipated by his theory and could be viewed as subsequent validation of it. The model I propose in this volume also includes elements from the later theory of Joaquin Fuster (1980, 1989, 1995) on the neuropsychological functions of the prefrontal cortex, which is based on his extensive review of the animal and human neuropsychological literature. Though developed independently, and for somewhat different purposes, these two prior models have a substantial number of similarities. Fuster's ideas also overlap with the research findings and ideas of Patricia Goldman-Rakic (1995a) on the concept of working or representational memory in neuropsychology. The combination of her ideas on this concept with those of Bronowski and Fuster in the hybrid model of behavioral inhibition, executive functions, and self-control makes a great deal of sense. Finally, I will consider the somatic marker theory of Antonio Damasio (1994, 1995) as it pertains to the capacity to initiate or motivate drive states in the service of goal-directed or purposive action. My purpose in this chapter is to acquaint the reader with these other models of executive functions and to show their points of overlap and distinction.

Bronowski's Theory of the Uniqueness of Human Language

Bronowski (1967/1977) described what he believed to be the four unique properties of human language as distinguished from the languages of other animals. He argued that human language is distinctive because it is not simply a means of communication but of reflection, during which plans of action are proposed, played out, and tested. Reflection can only happen if there is a delay between the arrival of a stimulus or event and the response to that event. Therefore, Bronowski treated this capacity to inhibit and delay responses as the central and formative feature in the evolution of the four unique features of human language. These four characteristics of human language suggest the existence of four separate mental abilities that give rise to them. These mental abilities as described by Bronowski share a striking similarity to the types of executive functions that would be described 13 years later by Fuster (1980, 1989) in identifying the functions of the prefrontal lobes.

In Bronowski's thinking, it is not just the response that is being delayed by the act of behavioral inhibition, but the decision to respond (Bronowski, 1967/1977). That decision is deferred so that the four unique mental capacities (executive functions) can give rise to information that can inform that decision and also affect the execution of responses stemming from that decision. Bronowski termed the four executive functions *prolongation, separation of affect, internalization, and reconstitution.* The capacity to delay responses as well as the four consequent mental functions flowing from the evolution of that inhibitory power were attributed by Bronowski to the brain's prefrontal cortex.

Prolongation

The first of these unique properties of human language is prolongation. This refers to "the ability to refer backward and forward in time and to exchange messages which propose action in the future" (Bronowski, 1967/1977, p. 116). Such messages can only be interpreted by an animal that has a sense of the future, a sense that arises from the capacity to recall the past and manipulate the imagery of that recall so as to create hypothetical situations. This prolongation of one's reference in language, or the reliance upon past events to construct hypothetical futures and actions to be directed at them, requires a special form of memory. During the delay in responding, the features of the signal, situation, or event must be briefly prolonged, fixed, and held in some form so as to retain them for later recall when that information will serve to revive the responses associated with them in the future. From such conjecturing, plans can be formulated and anticipatory behaviors formed and initiated. This form of memory is, in a sense, remembering so as to do. It is similar to the contemporary concept of working memory in neuropsychology (see *Neuropsychology*, Vol. 8, No. 4, 1994, special issue on Working Memory, for reviews), as I will show. For now, consider the definition of working memory given by Goldman-Rakic (1995): "the ability to keep an item of information in mind in the absence of an external cue and utilize that information to direct an impending response" (p. 57).

Bronowski stated that this form of memory and the prolongation of reference it affords permitted both the gift of human imagination and the concept of time. The recall of past images surely is of self-past, giving one a sense of the past that can be used to inform ongoing behavior. The holding in mind of images of that past along with those from present events gives rise to a sense of self-present. This, I would argue, should also give humans the gift of self-awareness—a point not made by Bronowski but which I believe is evident in these concepts.

Behavioral inhibition permits a delay in the decision to respond during which images and other information from the past that are pertinent to that decision can be recalled (resensed), manipulated, and used to conjecture the future. That conjecture forms the sense of the future that will serve to initiate preparatory behavior and an anticipatory response set as the individual awaits the arrival of that conjectured event. In short, past memories are recalled so as to revive the responses associated with them in the future. Thus are the contemporary notions of working memory, hindsight, forethought, anticipatory set, sense of time, and self-awareness apparently dependent on behavioral inhibition within Bronowski's theory.

Separation of Affect

Another unique feature of human language that is a consequence of the evolution of delayed responding in Bronowski's model is the separation of affect. This refers to the separation of the emotional charge that may be triggered by a message from the content of that message. Without such separation, there is a unity of both the affective tone and the content in the response to an event; the affect and content are one and total, as they are in most other animals. Such responses tend to be automatic and carry an emotional valence that is an inherent part of the content of the motor or vocal response. Humans, by delaying their responses, can separate the information within an event or message from its affects. Such a delay in responding and the separation of the affective tone of a message from its content may be most evident and most necessary in situations that are highly emotionally charged for the individual. This separation of affect, I believe, represents the more contemporary concept in developmental psychology of the self-regulation of emotion. It affords the generation of neutral responses despite emotionally provocative events that may elicit highly charged feelings within the individual—for instance, to remain silent or speak calmly when angered. To achieve this separation and regulation of affect, Bronowski reasoned that the delay in responding must be used to refer the signal or event to more than one reference center within the brain. This serves to make an internal loop with that center's information encoding mechanism before a message or response is finally emitted. He viewed the brain's ability to process such signals through multiple reference centers (or internal loops) simultaneously as the most important property of a large brain. This ability to separate the affect associated with an event from the informational content of that event permits humans a greater degree of objectivity and even makes possible science itself.

Internalization

The delay between event and response also permits the event to be referred to more than one center in the brain, giving rise to an inner discussion of alternatives before a response is formed. This is the internalization of language, which gives a unique form to human thought and speech. During the delay in responding, language comes to be turned on the self, providing an instrument of reflection and exploration and thereby permitting the individual to construct various hypothetical messages or responses before choosing one to emit. Thus, language moves from being primarily a means for communication with others to one of communication with the self: a means of simulating hypothetical messages and responses and testing them out before one is selected to be performed. Humans, according to Bronowski (1967/1977), live with two languages—an inner and an outer one.

> They constantly experiment with the inner language, and find arrangements which are more effective than those which have come to be standard in the outer language. In the inner language, these arrangements are information, that is, cognitive assertions; and they are then

transferred to the outer language in the form of practical instructions. (p. 118)

Such instructions can be directed not only at others, but also at the self, thereby becoming a fundamental tool for self-control (Kopp, 1982). As Bronowski referenced the views of Vygotsky (1962) in supporting his assertions, I will briefly discuss them here.

Vygotsky's theory on the development of private speech remains the most accepted view on the topic at this time (Berk, 1992, 1994; Diaz & Berk, 1992; Vygotsky 1978, 1987). Such speech is defined as "speech uttered aloud by children that is addressed either to the self or to no one in particular" (Berk & Potts, 1991). In its earliest stages, it is thought spoken out loud that accompanies ongoing action. As it matures, it functions as a form of self-guidance and direction by assisting with the formulation of a plan that will eventually assist the child in controlling his or her own actions (Berk & Potts, 1991). Gradually, as speech becomes progressively more private or internalized and behavior comes increasingly under its control, such speech is now internal, verbal thought that can exert a substantial controlling influence over behavior. This internalization of speech proceeds in an orderly fashion. It seems to evolve from more conversational, task-irrelevant and possibly self-stimulating forms of speech to more descriptive, task-relevant forms, and then on to more prescriptive and self-guiding speech. It then progresses to more private, inaudible speech, and finally to fully private, subvocal speech (Berk, 1992, 1994; Berk & Garvin, 1984; Berk & Potts, 1991; Bivens & Berk, 1990; Frauenglas & Diaz, 1985; Kohlberg, Yaeger, & Hjertholm, 1968). Such subvocal or covert speech has been shown to involve multiple regions of the prefrontal cortex, particularly the left supplementary motor area adjacent to the speech planning centers and the right frontal area, which has been shown to be involved in response inhibition (Ingvar, 1993; Ryding, Bradvik, & Ingvar, 1996).

As Berk (1992) has noted, Vygotsky's theory would predict an inverted U-shaped function for the development of private speech, such that it increases in frequency (public but self-directed) across early to mid-childhood, then declines in its public form as speech becomes fully internalized. Given that research to date has not demonstrated such an inverted U-shaped function, at least across the ages studied to date, Berk (1992) has suggested that such a function is not universal. Instead, it would be seen to some extent whenever new problems are being tackled by the individual such that public self-speech is needed to facilitate problem solving and self-regulation in that particular context. Ample research exists to show that overt private speech increases with the difficulty of the task being done. This is further evidence that such private speech is serving a self-regulatory function, helping to facilitate problem solving. Its greater impact, however, may be more on the later performance of similar tasks than on the task with which the self-speech is concurrent (Berk, 1992).

Reconstitution

Bronowski believed that the internalization of language had a special structure impressed on it that was the result of two mental processes. This special structure represents the fourth consequence of the evolution of delayed responding, called reconstitution. The first of the two processes of which it is comprised is *analysis*. This is the decomposition of sequences of events or messages into their parts. Events and messages are not treated as inviolate wholes, as they are by other species, but are broken into parts. This allows the progressive redistribution of the parts of the event or message to parallel information-processing systems within the brain "so that its cognitive content becomes more particularized, and its hortative content more generalized. . . . The physical world is pictured as made up of units that can be matched in language, and human language itself thereby shifts its vocabulary from command to description or predication" (p. 121).

The second process involved in reconstitution is *synthesis,* wherein these parts can be manipulated and used to construct or reconstitute entirely new messages or responses to others. We readily recognize that phonemes can be built into morphemes that are used to create words, which are then used to build sentences. Bronowski accused linguists of concentrating more on this process and ignoring the latter process that goes with it—that of analysis. Other animals communicate in whole messages, so human communication must thus have begun as well. Such messages have the character of an entire sentence and take the form of instructions. At some later time in human evolution we developed the capacity to break down these utterances into their elements such that objects, actions, and properties could be named separately. The result of this development is that humans come to see their world as made up of separable parts. The world, along with our language, can then be taken apart through analysis but also recombined through synthesis to give humans a generative power for original productivity, both in language and the behavior it commands, that far exceeds our nearest living primate relatives.

> It is not implicit in nature that it is made up of objects, properties, and actions, and that it must be perceived in that way. We have come to perceive it so in the process of trying to command our actions on it by

the use of speech. . . . We separate reality into parts, and describe the parts by their functions, as a grammatical device which reflects its response to human actions. (p. 121)

Though this point is not heavily emphasized by Bronowski, it must be recognized that the units in such messages can represent and initiate units of corresponding behavior. As a consequence, those behavioral units, like the language that represents them, can be analyzed and synthesized (reconstituted) into entirely novel behavioral structures. The processes of taking apart and recombining gives a synthetic and increasingly hierarchical structure to both human language and behavior. Increasingly complex, novel units come to be formed out of more elemental ones, thus creating a layered structure not only to language but to behavior as well. The rules or syntax for the combining of these units of speech (and by inference their behavioral productions) follow from a conceptual description of the world as we act on it and picture it. These rules are viewed by Bronowski as an inherent part of the process of reconstitution. Thus, while this conceptual description creates an obvious grammar for speech, so must it create a less obvious grammar or syntax for behavior as well.

Reconstitution is quite evident in verbal fluency and discourse, as they represent the capacity to rapidly reconstitute parts of speech into complete messages for others. The speed, accuracy, syntax, productivity, originality, and general efficiency with which cognitive content is translated into units of speech and then into whole messages to others reflects the synthetic function of reconstitution. I would argue from Bronowski's view that verbal reconstitution should be most evident in confrontational language tasks or in goal-directed speech or writing where ideas must be rapidly conveyed to achieve the goal of the task. Such tasks require problem solving of a verbal or semantic sort, and so may provide a means of evaluating the executive function of reconstitution. But reconstitution should also be evident in nonverbal forms of goal-directed behavioral creativity more generally, as this reflects the capacity to generate a variety of novel, complex sequences of behavior directed toward goals. Combined with working memory (prolongation), reconstitution functions as the generator of diversity and flexibility in responding, permitting a variety of hypothetical futures and the potential responses to them to be internally simulated (conjectured) and tested out before one is chosen to be executed in the outer world.

Bronowski attributed these four functions to the prefrontal lobes. I have taken the liberty of calling them "executive" functions because of the common practice of describing the functions of the prefrontal lobes as being executive in nature (Stuss & Benson, 1986). It should be clear from the preceding description that such mental abilities are essential to human self-regulation, given the point made in Chapter 3 that self-regulation requires not only the ability to delay a response but also a sense of time and the future. That sense arises out of the capacity to recall the images of the past and their semantic and affective content, experiment with those images and words internally, and then employ them to construct hypothetical futures. Those hypothetical futures then can be tested out before one is selected to become the plan that will be used to organize, execute, and regulate that future-directed (goal-oriented) behavior. By this means, behavior shifts from being primarily externally guided to being planned, organized, and regulated by internally represented information—a shift from reactive to purposive or intentional actions, and from context-dependent to self-determined (internally guided) behavior.

The four executive functions identified by Bronowski are interactive and interdependent. For instance, Bronowski stipulated that the special form of memory permitting retrospective recall so as to construct hypothetical futures (working memory) and the foresight it gave rise to was dependent in an important way on visual imagery. That imagery helps not only to call up the past but to hold plans for the future in a form that readily prepares them for communication to others (permitting the prolongation of reference in human language). "This development of imagery is, in effect, the progressive internalization of speech" (p. 127). As already noted, the internalization of speech brings, as part of it, the processes of analysis and synthesis, or reconstitution.

Fuster's Theory of Prefrontal Lobe Functions: The Cross-Temporal Organization of Behavior

Fuster (1980, 1989, 1995) has proposed a theory of prefrontal lobe functions apparently independent of Bronowski's (1967/1977) model, yet having much in common with it. Fuster concludes that the overarching function of the prefrontal cortex is the formation of cross-temporal structures of behavior having a unifying purpose or goal. The prefrontal cortex is believed to encode the temporal aspects of behavior, which involves the coding of place within a sequence of actions or perceptions. It is the novelty of these behavioral structures, and especially the temporal discontiguities among their elements, that makes the prefrontal cortex essential in their formation. To a lesser extent, their complexity may additionally necessitate the involvement of the prefrontal cortex. But complexity alone is not sufficient to place such acts within the purview of the prefrontal cortex. Time, on the other hand, being inserted between the elements of the contingency (i.e., event, responses, and consequences) would be sufficient to do so. Similarly, novelty of the response demanded by the context (problem solving) would also lead to involvement of the prefrontal lobes.

It is this synthesis of novel, often complex cross-temporal behavioral structures having a purpose or goal that requires the involvement of prefrontal functions. We can recognize here some of the same elements that were described in Chapter 3 as likely to initiate inhibition, self-regulation, and the executive functions supporting self-control (i.e., time, novelty, complexity, etc.). Fuster believes that it is the goal which these cross-temporal behavioral structures subserve that defines them and gives them cohesion and direction. Smaller sequences of behavior linked over shorter time periods can be used to create longer, more complex units of behavior of increasing durations and complexities, having longer-term objectives. This pyramiding of simpler units of behavior into more complex ones produces a hierarchical structure to goal-directed behavior and bridges the temporal delays. This building up of complex behavior out of simpler behavioral elements and of reorganizing the elements in complex behavioral chains to form new ones bears some similarity to Bronowski's concept of reconstitution.

Retrospective and Prospective Functions

According to Fuster, several functions must occur to link behavioral structures across time. Two of these are temporally symmetrical and are called retrospective and prospective functions. The retrospective function entails the retention of information about past events that are held in their temporal sequence as they pertain to a goal. The memory used for this function is called provisional by Fuster because its contents have a timeliness and term about them that makes them coherent; that is, they have a purpose or goal that defines them and provides their context (timeliness), and they are discharged from that memory once the goal has been attained (term). Provisional memory permits the referring of current events to previous events in a sequence, as well as the retention of action-related information derived from that analysis. This retrospective function and the provisional memory that subserves it gives rise to a formulation and retention of a goal-directed behavioral structure—a plan of action. This, in turn, forms the prospective function as it leads to a preparation to act in anticipation of events, called *anticipatory set* or preparation by Fuster. The behavioral scheme and its relevant events are temporarily represented, deployed in the preparation to act and in the execution of those actions, and retained until the goal has been accomplished.

Delayed-response tasks, Fuster believes, are some of the best procedures for assessing the ability of animals to form cross-temporal behavioral structures and therefore for assessing the role of the prefrontal cortex in their formulation and influence over behavior. However, humans may not show as great a deficiency on such tasks after prefrontal injuries, possibly because of the availability of language to assist with mediating the delay. Even so, Fuster believes that the difficulties such patients would have with the cross-temporal organizing of behavior would be evident in their inability to execute complex plans, their temporal concreteness, and their scarcity of new and elaborate goal-directed behaviors. It would also be evident in deficits in the syntax of their speech and behavior, reflecting the impact of the deficiency in temporal organization even on thought and perception.

Important to recognize in this theory is the power of the internally represented information in provisional memory to generate preparatory motor responses as well as the execution of the goal-directed behavioral sequences once the time for their performance arrives. In Fuster's view, there is a welding of thought with action, of past experience with future behavior, of knowledge with performance, and of the "how" of behavior with the "when" of its timely performance that is provided by the prefrontal lobes. Lesions of these regions are thought by Fuster to cleave thought from action, thus resulting in a disconnection of knowledge from performance, of the "how" of behavior from the "'when" of its execution, and of past experience from present and future-directed behavior. Behavior in such brain-injured individuals is no longer under as complete or any control and guidance by the internally represented information generated by the retrospective and prospective functions. The behavior of prefrontally injured patients tends to lose its intentional, purposive, and goal-directed nature, becoming less complex or hierarchically organized and more temporally concrete, automatic, and routine as a consequence.

The executive functions as defined by Fuster are quite similar to Bronowski's concept of the special memory permitting prolongation (retrospective and prospective imagery), thereby giving rise to hindsight and forethought. They are also similar to the neuropsychological concept of working memory (Goldman-Rakic, 1995a, 1995b), which will be discussed later.

Response Inhibition/Interference Control

Fuster argued that provisional memory (the retrospective function) and anticipatory set (the prospective function) are dependent upon response inhibition and interference control. This is quite similar to Bronowski's argument that the four unique properties of human language (prolongation, separation of affect, internalization, and reconstitution) depend upon the capacity to delay a response. It is in provisional memory that goals and intentions to act are formulated and retained, according to Fuster, and their period of formulation is a critical time that is subject to sources of external interference that can pervert, distort, or completely disrupt the planning taking place. Internal sources may also interfere, such as traces of information still held in provisional memory from the formation of immediately previous behavioral structures that are now useless, their term having expired upon the completion of a previous goal. This retention of previous motor plans past their timeliness and term can lead to perseveration of responding. Old habits more familiar to the individual or having similarity to ongoing behavior may likewise disrupt this synthetic, goal-directed function, as might impulses to immediate gratification (Fuster, 1980, 1989). Studies of patients with frontal lobe injuries support Fuster's contention of the critical need for interference control during delayed response tasks (Fuster, 1980, 1989; Partiot et al., 1996; Stuss & Benson, 1986; Verin et al., 1993).

The Harnessing of Motivation and Arousal

Fuster's theory further postulates that the prefrontal cortex must make use of basic drive or arousal states so as to harness them in support of the lengthy, novel, and complex cross-temporal behavioral structures required to accomplish a goal. As Fuster (1989) states, "This attribute of prefrontal function, however difficult to define, determines the initiative, intent, motivation, and vigor with which the organism forms the behavioral structure. Without the basic drive or its cortical agent, new behavior is hardly ever initiated and, when it is, it is not driven to its intended goal" (p. 160).

Damage to the prefrontal lobes would create difficulties with drive, motivation, and arousal as they may be needed to support goal-directed behavior. The individual so injured appears to lack willpower, determination, or ambition to engage in future-oriented behavior, instead becoming more reactive to the immediate context, more controlled by immediate gratification, and more distractible and impersistent. As will be discussed in the next chapter, drive and motivation appear to be part of the same functional brain system as that governing emotion (Lang, 1995). Thus, the capacity to regulate drive and motivation in the service of goals also may entail the capacity to regulate emotional states in that service as well.

Neuroanatomical Localization of Prefrontal Functions

In Fuster's model, the dissociation of an inhibitory function from a provisional memory function is not only conceptual but neuroanatomical as well. The inhibitory functions are ascribed to the orbital–prefrontal regions of the prefrontal cortex and its reciprocal interconnections with the ventromedial region of the striatum (Fuster, 1989; Iversen & Dunnett, 1990). Other research supports the involvement of these two regions in response inhibition and interference control (Partiot et al., 1996; Verin et al., 1993), with possibly greater involvement of the right prefrontal region (rather than the left) in interference control (Bench et al., 1993; Vendrell et al., 1995). The functions of provisional or working memory are subserved by the dorsolateral region of the prefrontal cortex and its reciprocal connections to the more central region of the striatum (Fuster, 1989, 1995; Goldman-Rakic, 1995a, 1995b; Iversen & Dunnett, 1990). The harnessing of drive and arousal states in the service of goal-directed behavior is mediated by the ventromedial aspects of the prefrontal lobes (Cummings, 1995; Damasio, 1994, 1995). Substantial evidence from neuropsychological and recent neuroimaging studies (to be discussed in Chapter 6) supports this dissociation of functions (Cummings, 1995; D'Esposito et al., 1995; Fuster, 1989, 1995; Goldman-Rakic, 1995a, 1995b; Iversen & Dunnett, 1990; Knight et al., 1995; Milner, 1995; Vendrell et al., 1995; Williams & Goldman-Rakic, 1995). Even the retrospective (provisional memory) and prospective (anticipatory set) functions are likewise dissociable though interactive functions (Fuster, 1995; Goldman-Rakic, 1995a, 1995b). Each may be subserved by separate, neighboring, and interacting cortical regions in the dorsolateral prefrontal lobes. However, while these functions may be partially dissociable, they are viewed by Fuster as tightly interactive in carrying out the cross-temporal organization of behavior.

Provisional Memory: Sensing to the Self?

How might the prefrontal cortex represent the sensory information it is holding on-line, particularly after the sensory event has disappeared in the external world, so as to transfer that information across time and to prepare for an upcoming event? One possibility noted by Fuster is that this sensory information is somehow encoded in the neurons of the prefrontal cortex, but he found this to be an unlikely possibility. The more plausible alternative, more consistent with research findings in neuropsychology, is that the prefrontal cortex stimulates the posterior sensory regions associated with the type of information to be represented during the delay in responding, in a way producing a form of vague resensing of the stimulus that will eventually serve as a cue to guide the future behavior. In other words, the prefrontal lobes permit a form of sensing to oneself during delay periods that permit past events to be prolonged and transferred across time to serve as the requisite cues for preparing the motor behaviors that will eventually occur when they are timely.

This private form of sensing to oneself can be thought of as a form of internalization of sensory behavior and its associated motor responses that bears some similarity to Bronowski's concepts of the internalization of imagery and of speech. If so, then the retrospective and prospective functions of Fuster's model are actually founded on the capacity for self-directed, private behavior, especially self-directed sensing or resensing to oneself. Such a delineation and redefinition of the processes underlying provisional or working memory and the other executive functions is important as it may permit the bridging of this literature and the literature in developmental psychology on the development of visual imagery (private seeing or seeing to oneself) and private, internal speech. But it would also suggest that it is not just covert visual activity that is available to the individual during the delay period for the holding and resensing of events across time, but the entire array of human sensory behavior (olfaction, audition, touch, etc.). This would imply that individuals have the ability not only to see to themselves but to hear, smell, taste, touch, and even motorically behave or manipulate to themselves as forms of provisional or working memory. I shall return to this idea in the next chapter, that what the executive functions represent are forms of private or covert behavior that were once entirely external in early development but have now become a form of private behaving to oneself. Such behavior-to-the-self could incorporate the entire range of potential public human behaviors (sensory and motor) in a private, covert form.

Provisional Memory and Sense of Time

The capacity for holding events in mind in a correct temporal sequence in the manner that Fuster has explained could give rise to the psychological sense of time, although Fuster (1989) does not explicitly make this point. Michon (1985) and others (e.g., J. W. Brown, 1990) argue that psychological awareness of time derives from holding sequences of events in mind. If so, *time perception* would seem to be directly dependent, at least in part, on the integrity of working memory, as Bronowski claimed. A subjective sense of time would seem to be critical in Fuster's model as well, given his emphasis on the cross-temporal organization of behavior as the major function of the prefrontal cortex. Some capacity for marking time and sensing its duration and passage would be essential to anticipatory setting of motor responses in preparation for the arrival of impending events. That sense would also be necessary for programming the syntax or temporal structure of the complex behavioral chains generated in the service of goal attainment.

Influence of Prefrontal Lobe Functions on Motor Control

To summarize, Fuster recognizes three functions of the prefrontal cortex: (1) a retrospective function utilizing provisional memory, (2) a prospective function leading to anticipatory set and preparedness to action, (3) and inhibition and interference control. The last provides the delay needed for these other functions to formulate cross-temporal structures and to protect that formulation and the execution of the goal-directed behaviors so generated. These functions provide for the temporally synthetic activities of the prefrontal cortex and produce a clear influence on *motor control*. As Fuster noted, the prefrontal cortex is not particularly necessary for the performance of any motor act or even the performance of complex, overlearned responses. It is essential, however, for the orderly execution of novel, complex behaviors having a cross-temporal structure (directed toward the future).

The influence of executive functions over motor control would be seen in three ways, Fuster (1980, 1989) concludes. These would be in (1) the retention of information in provisional memory about immediate past events and acts already executed, which feeds forward to influence subsequent responding (i.e., a sensitivity to errors); (2) the anticipatory setting of the premotor and motor functions (i.e., a preparation to act); and (3) the inhibition of motor impulses inappropriate to the goal or task. A lack of the inhibitory control that provides for delaying responses, formulating cross-temporal behavioral structures, and the protection of the delay from interference would have many manifestations, Fuster reasoned, including distractibility, hyperreactivity, and impulsivity—the very symptoms attributed to ADHD.

Goldman-Rakic's Theory of Primate Working Memory

Patricia Goldman-Rakic and her colleagues at Yale University, through their elegant studies of the primate prefrontal cortex, have contributed enormously to the understanding of the anatomical and neurophysiological mechanisms underlying provisional memory, or what Goldman-Rakic calls working or representational memory (see

Goldman-Rakic, 1995a, 1995b; Williams & Goldman-Rakic, 1995). She argues that the cerebral cortex is concerned with the mental representation of the outside world and that the temporal, occipital, and parietal regions form and store these representations. A major function of the prefrontal cortex is the activation of these representations as needed, so as to hold them on-line and use them to guide a subsequent response. The prefrontal cortex therefore provides the means of regulating behavior by mentally represented stimuli rather than by the external stimuli themselves.

Using delayed-response tasks with primates, Goldman-Rakic (1995a) has shown that certain prefrontal neurons are activated only during the delay periods. The purpose of some of these delay-activated neurons is the representation of visual–spatial information about the stimulus and the response it will elicit, so as to keep it active during the delay. However, other neurons that are activated during the delay function to inhibit neurons that are associated with competing sensory input and motor responses to that input. This carrying of representations of past events forward in time throughout a delay period so as to execute a delayed response bears a striking similarity to the special memory function that Bronowski argued was necessary for prolongation of reference (the recall of past images that are used to conjecture and anticipate the future). It is also very similar to the concepts of provisional memory (retrospective) and anticipatory set (prospective) described in Fuster's theory of prefrontal lobe functions. Like Fuster, Goldman-Rakic (1995a) believes that the retrospective aspects of working memory are primarily sensory representations and are somewhat dissociable from the more prospective and anticipatory motor actions being held in mind to eventually initiate. Even so, these somewhat separable functions and their respective cortical regions are inherently interactive. The representation of a past event (retrospection) is automatically related to the preparation of the motor actions and motivational states with which it has been previously associated, although these motor representations will not be released until the delay period has ended and the time for the anticipated response has arrived. As Goldman-Rakic (1995a) has stated:

> The prefrontal centers, through reciprocal connections to motor structures, contribute to the creation of motor plans at a time when the most favorable stimulus conditions for a given action have arrived. . . . However, a wide spectrum of human responses are not memory guided or internally generated but sensory guided and implicitly learned. These latter represent a wide spectrum of behavioral control and motor action, and the machinery exists for their execution by multiple pathways that

bypass the prefrontal cortex. The prefrontal cortex is essential only when clues to the correct action to be taken cannot be found in the tangible present, and models of the past have to be consulted in order to respond effectively. (p. 61)

Despite having been developed from the study of primates, this model of working memory is in accord with neuroimaging studies of normal humans (D'Esposito et al., 1995) and studies of those having prefrontal lobe injuries and the deficits in working memory, planning, anticipatory set, and goal-directed behaviors that such patients frequently experience (Fuster, 1989; Stuss & Benson, 1986).

Others have reached much the same conclusions in reviewing the literature related to working memory (Dubois et al., 1995), stating that the dorsolateral region of the prefrontal cortex "provides the dynamic ability to disrupt automatic stimulus–response cycles, by creating a temporal buffer between the sensory and motor systems in which information is manipulated and confronted with past experiences for elaboration of a goal-oriented ongoing schema of response" (p. 57).

Goldman-Rakic (1995b) disputes the model of working memory developed by Baddeley (1986) that was comprised of three elements: (1) a visual–spatial sketchpad, (2) an articulatory or phonological loop, and (3) a central executive that manages the selection and control processes taking place in these other units. Her research suggests that there are additional domains of working memory besides those for visual–spatial and articulatory or auditory information being held in mind. These other domains correspond to other forms of sensory representation that can be held on-line during delay tasks and are represented in different regions of the prefrontal cortex than those subserving visual–spatial or articulatory representations. Recent studies using neuroimaging techniques with normal volunteers participating in delayed-response paradigms seem to support this view (Gold, Berman, Randolph, Goldberg, & Weinberger, 1996). Goldman-Rakic further argues that there is no need to postulate a central executive unit within working memory. Each of these sensory domains contains the capacity to hold that form of sensory representation on-line along with its associated motor actions, which will be prepared from that sensory information and released for execution at the most optimal time. In short, there is no need for a central executive when each domain appears to adequately manage the information being represented and the associated motor structures being prepared.

This view of working memory as having multiple domains distributed throughout the prefrontal cortex, each subserving different aspects and types of sensory representations and their associated motor elements is not inconsistent with the view I advanced above that the executive functions represent different domains of private, self-directed sensing. Different regions of the prefrontal cortex will be associated with different forms of private or covert sensing or resensing to oneself, and these sensory representations will be associated with a variety of motor, affective, and motivational elements that will be activated along with those sensory representations.

Damasio's Theory of Somatic Markers

In order to provide a theoretical model from which to understand the deficits often seen in patients with prefrontal injuries, particularly to the ventral and medial aspects of the prefrontal lobes, Damasio (1994, 1995) proposes that these patients often have a deficit in the activation of somatic markers that are normally associated with information that is stored in memory. The information about past events is capable of being reactivated into working memory, but the somatic or affective/motivational aspects of that information have been dissociated from it because of the nature of the injury. Consequently, the capacity for decision making in one's personal and social life is severely impaired because such decision making is predicated on these affective/motivational (somatic) markers, which provide some appraisal of the information for the individual. The somatic markers represent an emotional or motivational coloring to events and information that helps to constrain the process of reasoning over multiple options and multiple future outcomes that can often be far too numerous to contemplate within a reasonable time. Damasio (1994, 1995) argues that such somatic markers act to constrain decision-making space by making it manageable for a cost–benefit analysis of the options and outcomes under consideration. Without such somatic markers, all response options and their outcomes become equalized, and the individual must contemplate an excessive number of option–outcome pairs, slowing down or even halting decision making.

Patients with prefrontal lobe injuries, particularly in the ventromedial regions, can often recall previous information, but it fails to initiate a change in behavior or to motivate new goal-directed behaviors because of this disconnection from the information's affective/motivational aspects or markers. The factual knowledge component of memory can still be recalled and held in mind, but its associated somatic state is not reenacted along with it, thus precluding a rapid appraisal of the information as rewarding or punishing for the individual.

It is interesting to consider Damasio's model in light of the previous models. It would appear to be complementary to them rather than contradictory of them. Bronowski spoke of the power to separate affect from content in human language that was afforded by the capacity to delay a response. Such delays may permit the individual to partially separate the somatic markers of an immediate event from their informational or factual content. Fuster also spoke of the capacity of the prefrontal lobes to harness drive, motivational, and affective states in the service of goal-directed behaviors. This may be achieved by the recall of past events into provisional or working memory, which serves to activate their somatic markers and engenders the drive states associated with those events. Such reexperiencing or reenactment of the affective/motivational states associated with resensing past events may provide the drive necessary to carry out the prospective function of anticipatory set and preparation of future-directed behavior. Goldman-Rakic does not directly address these affective/motivational markers that are associated with the sensory information that is being held on-line and that is activating the preparation of associated motor responses, but she does acknowledge their existence as part of the sensory–motor representations held in working memory. Lesions to the ventromedial aspects of the prefrontal lobe may disconnect the working memory systems of the dorsolateral cortex, where sensory–motor representations are being held on-line apart from their affective/motivational qualifiers. This disconnection precludes the capacity to generate drive states associated with those sensory representations, which should motivate future-directed behavior (see also Tucker, Luu, & Pribram, 1995).

Others reviewing the literature on frontal lobe–injured patients have suggested that the emotional changes secondary to frontal lobe injury can be grouped into three types of disturbance: (1) disorders of drive or motivation, (2) subjective emotional experience (mood), and (3) emotional expression (affect) (Stuss, Gow, & Hetherington, 1992). Emotional hyperreactivity, irritability, low frustration tolerance, loss of emotional self-control, and lack of concern for others (Rolls, Hornak, Wade, & McGrath, 1994) are commonly noted in such patients. Thus, there seems good reason to believe that at least one executive function of the prefrontal lobes is the association of affective, drive, and arousal states with internally represented information and the self-regulation of these states in conformance with social rules and in the service of goal-directed behavior.

EXECUTIVE FUNCTIONS: A SYNTHESIS

There is much of value in these models of prefrontal lobe executive functions. While the concepts within each model may overlap to some extent with those of the others, each also seems to provide unique information about the nature of the executive functions and how human behavior becomes self-regulated or internally guided. Bronowski's model seems to be the most comprehensive of the group reviewed here, and so it will serve as the framework for the hybrid model of self-control and executive functions to be developed in Chapter 7. He left many important details of this model unspecified, but that is understandable given that the purpose of his original paper was not so much to propose a model of prefrontal lobe functions as to outline those properties that seem to make human language unique from other forms of animal communication. Nevertheless, his model maps nicely onto later, more empirically based models of prefrontal lobe functioning that can be used to complete many of the unspecified details in Bronowski's theory.

Behavioral Inhibition

If we inspect these models closely, it becomes evident that the prefrontal lobes provide at least three basic functions that create self-regulation. First, there must exist a system that provides for the inhibition of prepotent, that is, more automatic or dominant, responses that have as their function the maximization of immediate consequences. Such a system is critical if delayed consequences are to have any chance of affecting behavioral control. This inhibitory system also provides for the power to interrupt ongoing behavioral patterns should information from immediately past behaviors in the sequence be indicating errors or ineffectiveness of the ongoing pattern. Finally, it appears to be this inhibitory system that functions to control potential sources of interference that could disrupt, pervert, or destroy the activities taking place within working memory (retrospective/prospective functions and anticipatory setting of motor responses). These elements set the stage for the capacity to engage in self-regulation via the four other executive functions.

Working Memory

There is a second executive function consistent across most of these models of the executive functions. It can be considered a special form of memory that provides for the recall of past events and their manipulation so as to construct hypothetical futures. It is the provisional or working memory system, well named, I believe, because it represents remembering so as to do. Bronowski, Fuster, and Goldman-Rakic all identified two temporally symmetrical functions within this system, one of which permits the recall or resensing of the past (retrospective function) that gives rise to the second, which is the construction of hypothetical futures, the preparation of plans for attaining those futures, and the construction of behavioral structures (anticipatory set) associated with them (the prospective function). Although this second prefrontal executive system has been termed a form of memory, I believe that current evidence suggests it is actually the reactivation of previously encoded sensory–motor information, as Fuster and Goldman-Rakic have described, so that the individual is sensing and behaving to him- or herself during delay periods, in a very real sense remembering or reactivating past memories.

I believe that here we have the system that permits an important aspect of self-regulation to occur, as discussed in Chapter 3. That aspect is the capacity to engage in self-directed behavior (often covert) that will function to modify and regulate subsequent behavior and so achieve a change in the likelihood of future outcomes (the net maximization of delayed relative to immediate consequences) for the individual. This is the special form of memory that I specified would be needed to provide both for the cross-temporal organization of behavior, as in planning, and for the sense of future and its consequent preference for delayed over immediate rewards that are critical to self-control. The working memory system appears to shift behavior away from the moment and away from external control and toward the future by way of internally generated information that arises from private, covert behavior.

Internalization of Speech

Bronowski was the only theorist discussed in this chapter to have identified the internalization of speech as a critical element in a model of executive functions. Research in developmental psychology suggests that this process of turning speech on the self in a form of dialogic conversation with oneself that becomes progressively more private, covert, or internalized is a major contributor to the development of self-control (Berk, 1992, 1994; Berkowitz, 1982; Kopp, 1982). It will need to be included in any model of executive functions that is used to account for the development of human self-regulation.

Motivational Appraisal System

The third executive function is that which all authors discussed in this chapter have noted in varying degrees, but which Damasio has chosen to focus upon in his model. He recognized the importance of the other two functions but believes that the role of an affective/motivational appraisal system within models of the prefrontal lobes has not received the emphasis it deserves. This system provides for the affective and motivational appraisal of the past events being held in working memory and of the hypothetical futures created from them. By providing such affective and motivational color or tone to these events, it permits them to be immediately retained or discarded depending upon their affective and motivational value to the individual (Tucker et al., 1995). Such a system, as Damasio notes, provides the constraints that necessarily must be placed on decision making when a variety of past events and hypothetical option–outcome pairs are being considered. Put differently, this system provides for covert emotion and motivation. The individual is now capable of privately emoting and motivating to him- or herself unencumbered by the public manifestations of such activities. This, I believe, is the system that Bronowski described as permitting the separation of affect. In a sense, it separates affect by privatizing it, making it another form of covert, self-directed behavior and thereby capable of internal modulation and modification before it is publicly manifested.

Undoubtedly, this cannot be achieved apart from the working memory and inhibitory systems. As all of these authors commented, the reactivation of past sensory–motor information automatically brings with it the affective/motivational aspects linked to those events in the past (their somatic markers), and these markers are then inherently linked with those plans or hypothetical futures constructed from that past (see also Dehaene & Changeux, 1995). This process permits propositions or simulations of behavior that are internally generated to be evaluated and selected or rejected quickly and internally without having to wait for exposure to external consequences (Damasio, 1994, 1995; Dehaene & Changeux, 1995; Tucker et al., 1995). All of this is being restricted from public display and protected from external and internal sources of interference by the behavioral inhibition system.

Reconstitution (Behavioral Synthesis)

There is a fourth function that might be dissociable from the others, though that is unclear at the moment. This one was identified only by Bronowski, and it is his function of reconstitution. Fuster (1989) seems to have identified a similar process in his description of the synthetic nature of the prefrontal lobes relative to the ability of humans to generate novel, complex, hierarchically organized, and goal-directed behavior. But Fuster appears to have overlooked the analytical aspect of reconstitution, as Bronowski chided linguists of his era for doing as well. Bronowski asserted that the power to synthesize novel, complex behavioral (in his case, linguistic) structures arises out of the power to analyze or dismember past behavioral structures and their hierarchy. One can then reorganize them into novel structures, sequences, and hierarchies made up of those older structures and sequences, all of which is done mainly for the attainment of a goal. Such a function grants to humans a tremendous capacity for fluency (diversity), flexibility, and creativity in the formulation of behavioral structures aimed at the future.

This analytic/synthetic capacity of the prefrontal lobes could be viewed as simply another attribute of the working memory system. Bronowski seems to intimate such a connection when he describes the ability of individuals to manipulate the imagery of recall, giving humans the gift of imagination. This suggests that the manipulation of those images rests within the special form of memory he felt generated them. Yet Bronowski then distinguishes it as a separate and unique property when applied to human language, calling this reconstitution.

These two processes, manipulation of information and reconstitution, could be conceptualized as the same process whether applied to imagery, speech, or some other form of internal self-directed behavior, that process being the analysis, manipulation, and reconstitution of prior behavioral structures and their subunits and hierarchies to form new ones. If so, this may be a more developmentally advanced function of the prefrontal lobes than is the capacity to recall or resense past events and their associated responses and outcomes, as is done in working memory. The latter must precede the former in a developmental progression—the power to mentally manipulate and reconfigure informational units requires the requisite power first to hold such informational units in mind (Dubois et al., 1995). Later, when I construct a hybrid model of these executive functions (Chapter 7), I will delineate this reconstitutive function as a separate executive function from the other three, recognizing, however, that it may simply represent a more complex aspect of the working memory function, that is, the capacity to manipulate retained information.

Behaving to the Self

I believe it is important to rephrase these executive functions into their behavioral equivalents for several reasons. It has become commonplace in cognitive psychology and neuropsychology to use computer metaphors for the types of functions being described here. But too heavy a reliance on computer metaphors for some neuropsychological functions may also serve to disconnect the research findings in the field from those that may be pertinent in other fields of psychology, such as sensation and perception, developmental psychology, or behavior analysis, where different terms, often more descriptive of the behavior under study, are used to represent these same brain functions. If, as I suspect, nonverbal working memory, particularly covert visual imagery and audition, represents sensing to the self, then naming these activities as such may mean that those findings and limitations already documented in the psychological literature on vision and hearing are likely to apply to the study of these covert sensory activities as well (see Kosslyn, 1994, on the relation of visual imagery to visual perception).

The form of behavior directed toward the self in the case of the internalization of speech is rather obvious and requires no further comment here. But what of the motivational/appraisal function that seems to harness drive and arousal states in the service of goal-directed behavior? I believe that this represents emoting or motivating to the self. This leaves the function of reconstitution. What form of privatized behavior might this be? I have come to believe it is covert, self-directed experimentation or play—the internalized dismembering, manipulation, and reconfiguring of behavior freed of its overt, sensory and musculoskeletal manifestations. Such covert experimentation with the elements or units of behavioral structures and their sequences creates a capacity to generate a diverse range of novel behavioral sequences, or hypothetical futures as Bronowski called them. One can then test them out covertly for their likely outcomes before one is selected for controlling subsequent motor behavior. It represents a form of covert, self-directed play or simulation of behavioral sequences and their associated outcomes and provides humans with a flexibility and diversity of novel, complex response options for use in attaining goals.

CONCLUSION

In this chapter, I have reviewed four earlier models of prefrontal lobe functions, many of which have been labeled by prior researchers as the executive functions. They are so named because they appear to contribute to the capacity for human self-regulation and future-oriented, goal-directed behavior (see Chapter 3). In addition to identifying the necessity of a behavioral inhibition system in any model of executive functions, four executive functions were derived from these earlier models. Two of these are considered to be separate forms of working memory (verbal and nonverbal) by many. The third function is the motivational appraisal system that affords the harnessing of affect/motivation/arousal states in the service of future-directed behavior. Reconstitution, or the analytic and synthetic processes of the prefrontal lobes comprises the fourth executive function. In the next chapter, I will discuss further evidence that exists for the identification and independence of these four executive functions, along with behavioral inhibition.

CHAPTER 6

—◆—

Additional Evidence Supporting the Existence of the Executive Functions

THE THEORISTS DISCUSSED in the preceding chapter (Bronowski, 1967/1977; Damasio, 1994, 1995; Fuster, 1989; Goldman-Rakic, 1995a, 1995b) with the exception of Bronowski, have cited a substantial body of neuropsychological research in support of their identification of the executive functions specified within their models. It is one thing, however, to identify these functions of the prefrontal lobes and to show research that supports their existence; it is another thing entirely to show that these are separable or distinct executive functions. For instance, Fuster (1989) argues that the overarching function of the prefrontal lobes is the cross-temporal organization of behavior. However, this larger function can be subdivided into a set of subfunctions (retrospective and prospective functions, interference control, and drive/motivational control, as well as the nonexecutive function of motor control).

In Chapter 5, I identified four executive functions apart from behavioral inhibition: nonverbal working memory; the internalization of speech, or verbal working memory; the self-regulation of affect/motivation/arousal; and reconstitution. Undoubtedly, nonverbal working memory could be further subdivided on the basis of the nonverbal mnemonic content (i.e., vision, visual–spatial, audiologic, etc.) but for my purposes here these different kinds can all be subsumed under the class of nonverbal working memories. This is, admittedly, a bit of oversimplification of the executive functions, glossing over their complexities and the various subfunctions that may exist within each. But for the purpose of developing a theoretical model of the executive functions that can be extended to understanding ADHD, my painting with such broad strokes is sufficient, I believe, so long as the reader understands that my identification of these four functions does not rule out the possibility of others or the identification of separable subfunctions within each.

Accepting the existence of a behavioral inhibition system along with these four executive functions, is there evidence for independence or dissociability among them? I believe there is, to a limited extent, with the limitation being mainly the small number of studies to date that have examined this issue. Here I examine two types of evidence that may support dissociation or distinction among these functions. The first type of evidence comes from studies using factor analysis to evaluate the latent dimensions or constructs that seem to exist in batteries of tests presumed to measure prefrontal lobe or executive functions. The second type of evidence, also limited at this time, comes from neuroimaging studies that attempt to identify those brain regions that may be associated with these executive functions. If different regions participate in each of these functions, then this may be suggestive evidence that the executive functions represent relatively distinct, albeit interactive, neuropsychological processes.

STUDIES USING FACTOR ANALYSIS WITH TEST BATTERIES OF EXECUTIVE FUNCTIONS

Before proceeding to a brief review of six different factor-analytic studies of measures of executive functions, some cautionary remarks are in order pertaining to the nature of these studies and what they may be able to reveal by way of support for the distinctiveness of the executive functions.

Some Cautionary Considerations

First of all, the extant research using factor analysis to define the possible dimensions that may be present in batteries of tests of executive functions is limited in what it can tell us of these functions because of the selectivity of the dependent measures used in those studies. In other words, *these studies did not set out to directly test the question of whether there are separate dimensions that represent the different executive functions identified in Chapter 5.* Instead, this research has been mainly exploratory, merely trying to see what number and what types of dimensions emerged from the neuropsychological batteries of tests presumed to assess frontal lobe functions. For instance, none of the studies to be discussed intentionally selected measures to evaluate Damasio's (1994, 1995) somatic marker system, or the regulation of affect/motivation/arousal states. One therefore would not expect such a dimension to emerge in the analysis of these test batteries. If it did emerge, it is unlikely to have been recognized as representing drive or motivational regulation even if measures were used that unintentionally tapped this dimension to some degree, such as CPTs or sustained attention tasks might do.

Caution must also be exercised in accepting the labels assigned by researchers to the dimensions they have identified. Researchers have tended to give somewhat different interpretations to the meanings of the dimensions they exposed, based upon their understanding of what processes are assessed by the tests they found to load on a particular dimension. As an example, Mirsky (1996) has repeatedly referred to the WCST as reflecting a dimension of attention called "shift." In contrast, Levin and colleagues (1996) have recently referred to this same measure as reflecting "concept-formation, problem-solving" (p. 23), while Shute and Huertas (1990) believed that it may be reflecting the Piagetian construct of formal operational thinking in cognitive development. Thus, it is possible for investigators to identify similar dimensions yet give them quite different names and interpretations of their latent meanings. Indeed, researchers from some of the studies to be mentioned in this chapter did not intend to interpret their measures as reflecting executive functions at all; instead, they referred to these measures as assessing different aspects of attention.

This leads to a further important caution in accepting the interpretations of dimensions identified in such research at face value, and that is *the confusion evident in the literature between the constructs of attention and executive functions* (see Lyon & Krasnegor, 1996, for some excellent reviews and a discussion of this issue of overlapping meaning in constructs). To illustrate the problem, consider the long-term programmatic research of Mirsky (1996) on the components of attention. He employs a number of measures that others have frequently interpreted as assessing executive functions, including the WCST as well as a CPT. Among other things, such confusion reflects deeper problems in reaching a consensus among investigators as to the actual nature of the constructs of attention and executive functions.

I have argued elsewhere (Barkley, 1996) that executive functions constitute a special case of attention. Attention reflects a relationship between an event and the organism's direct response to it so as to achieve an immediate change in the environment (an outcome or consequence). An executive function, in contrast, is a form of behavior directed at oneself. In short, an executive function is a form of attention to the self—that is, to one's behavior, so as to modify and regulate it in order to alter a future rather than an immediate outcome.

I would assert here that the study of attention in humans, particularly those past the age of 3 years (or even earlier), is going to be hopelessly confounded with executive functions as the latter have begun to develop by that time, if not earlier (Berk, 1992; Diamond, Cruttenden, & Neiderman, 1994; Vaughn, Kopp, & Krakow, 1984). This confounding is even more evident in the fact that experiments on the construct of attention employ verbal instructions to the subjects, as of necessity they must do to complete the studies in a reasonable time. The instant that verbal instructions are used with a human subject, the specter of rule-governed behavior and the larger executive function of internalized speech is inherently embedded in such research and cannot be extricated from it in any easy way (Barkley, 1989).

It is most unfortunate that this simple fact is repeatedly overlooked not only in studies of attention, but in those of working memory and executive functions as well, illustrating, perhaps, how much we take for granted the important role of rule-governed behavior in research (Skinner, 1969, pp. 114, 120). Any study that gives an instruction to the subject, particularly an instruction that competes with other prevailing sources of behavioral control in the environment (as most studies of executive function have done; see Hayes et al., 1996) is by default studying executive functions to some extent. It is investigating the capacity of the individual to adhere to the experimental instructions in the face of competing contingencies of reinforcement for more prepotent responses. It is highly improbable that Mirsky and others (Robertson, Ward, Ridgeway, & Nimmo-Smith, 1996) studying the human attentional systems are doing so in any pure fashion, as might be done in nonverbal organisms.

At first glance, it might seem possible to circumvent the problem by performing a study of young children without using instructions and instead just using shaping and multiple reinforcement trials to teach them to do the task involved in the experiment. But even this would ignore the fact that young children, at least those of elementary age or later, are becoming adept at creating their own rules once they are exposed to intentionally ambiguous circumstances; they will try to guess the intent of the investigation, the desire of the investigator as to how they should behave, or at least the rules that may be operating in the task. Once they begin to do so, they will create and follow their own rules such that the experiment, once again, is being confounded by at least one or more of the executive functions. This illustrates not only how intertwined executive functions are with other psychological constructs being evaluated in an individual's performance of most experimental tasks, but also just how critical the executive functions are in everyday human social interactions.

For example, like most investigators in the field of ADHD as well as in the neuropsychology of attention, I have fallen prey to just such oversights in interpreting the results of CPTs, when we proclaim that omission errors reflect sustained attention and commission errors those of poor inhibition. In part what such scores reflect is the difficulty subjects are having in adhering to the investigator's verbal instructions to perform this simple, boring, unreinforcing task over a prolonged period of time (Barkley, 1989; Hayes et al., 1996). And in large part they reflect the capacity to self-regulate (sustain) motivation to the task in the absence of external sources of motivation (another executive function). Such tasks reflect the capacity for rule-governed behavior and self-motivation as much as or more than they reflect "attention."

Humans are intrinsically linguistically governed creatures from an early age. If language is becoming turned on the self and increasingly is controlling behavior in children as young as ages 3–5 years (Berk, 1992), then studying subjects of that age or later will automatically involve aspects of self-speech. We cannot as investigators continue, on the one hand, to rely so heavily on such linguistic governance of behavior, which permits us to give instructions to subjects that conveniently circumvent direct training in the contingencies of the task, and then, on the other hand, interpret the results of that study as if it were free of such executive functions. Proclaiming that one is not a behaviorist but a cognitive neuropsychologist does not discharge the obligation as a scientist to acknowledge that rules are inherent aspects of one's experiments on attention and will confound the interpretation of those experiments with this executive function. Studying nonhuman primates, as Goldman-Rakic (1995a, 1995b) and Fuster (1989) have done, may help to address this confounding to some degree. But even here the capacity of some primates to engage in visual imagery during delays in attention tasks, as Goldman-Rakic has clearly demonstrated, brings this form of executive function into play in research on attention in these species as well. For these reasons of the inherent involvement of executive functions in neuropsychological studies, I will interpret several neuropsychological studies that claim to study attention as also probably reflecting the study of executive functions.

Another methodological point that deserves consideration is that *any interpretation of prior studies using factor analysis to derive the pattern of underlying dimensions that may comprise a battery of tests must be done cautiously because of the differences in the procedures employed to carry out such statistical analyses.* This would include the types of measures used in the project and the frequent restriction of range of the executive functions they sample. It would also include the nature of the subjects and sample size, the decisions about the scores chosen for analysis from each measure (many of these tests yield several measures), the type of rotations to use in the data analyses, the thresholds chosen to permit factors to be retained or discarded in the analysis, and the very type of factor analysis employed by the investigators.

This leads to a further methodological problem that researchers rarely consider in studies of executive functions, and that is that *measures that assess executive functioning at one particular age may not do so at another.* I will make this point again in Chapter 10 in discussing research on executive functioning in ADHD. Failure to heed the issue could easily result in confusion at finding such a measure to load on a dimension reflecting a particular executive function in children of one age but not at a later stage of development. As Fuster (1980, 1989; see Chapter 5) has repeatedly noted, the executive functions provided by the prefrontal cortex are most necessary when tasks or settings demand that the individual generate novel, complex behavioral structures that organize behavior across time. What may be demands for novel, complex, or cross-temporal (time-bridging) behavioral structures at one age, and hence effortful and demanding of self-regulation, may not necessarily be so at a later age, when they have become familiar, elementary, and automatic, requiring little need for self-regulation.

To illustrate this critical issue, consider the verbal fluency test from the Controlled Oral Word Association Test (COWAT; semantic categories subtest). This test shows substantial developmental improvements in normal children from early childhood to adolescence. For young preschool-age children, the task may be quite difficult, demanding not only inhibition and due deliberation of the categories and their semantic meanings, but also posing a considerable challenge to their rudimentary reconstitutive function at this age. The time period over which the task is given (typically 1 minute for each category of animals and then of foods) might seem trivial for an older child but requires considerable effort by a young child to maintain responding of this sort across the trial period. Thus, at the preschool age, this verbal fluency test may well be reflecting executive functioning. But by, say, ages 9–12 years, or even earlier, this may not be the case any longer at all. The task now is not complex, requires little by way of novelty of responding, makes few demands on generating diversity of responses given the high familiarity of this age group with the vocabulary of each category, and will therefore demand little if any effort at self-regulation or at sustained responding across so short a temporal period. The task no longer is assessing executive functioning or is doing so very weakly. To capture fluency and reconstitution at this age, a considerably longer, more complex, and challenging task will be needed.

Therefore, I do not review the following studies to confirm a theory of executive functions, as these myriad limitations would not permit it. I discuss such studies here only to see if the information acquired through them so far might be instructive in any way about the number and types of executive functions suggested to date. Accepting the preceding procedural limitations as important, one can still search for any consistencies across studies that might be suggestive of an answer to the question posed earlier of whether there is only one executive function or many. If there are more than one, how many seem to emerge? What seems to be their nature? Do they seem to be in line with the ideas of the executive function theorists? As always, more research on the issues will be needed.

Mirsky's Model of Attention (Executive Functions)

For more than a decade, Mirsky (e.g., 1996) has been investigating a multicomponent model of attentional disorders in children and adults. Using a battery of measures presumed to assess attention, Mirsky and his colleagues have evaluated their factorial composition as well as the neuroanatomical correlates of those factors. But these same tests have been employed by others as measures of executive functions (Denckla, 1996; Levin et al., 1996; Pennington & Ozonoff, 1996), particularly in ADHD (Barkley, Grodzinsky, & DuPaul, 1992; Goodyear & Hynd, 1992; Pennington & Ozonoff, 1996). I treat them likewise here.

The factor structure for Mirsky's test battery appears in Table 6.1. As that table shows, Factor 1 consists primarily of two scores from the WCST and has been labeled Flexibility. Others consider this task to reflect concept formation and problem solving (Levin et al., 1996), in part because it loaded on a dimension assessing verbal and nonverbal fluency. Some have interpreted this test as assessing the flexibility and effectiveness of verbal regulation of behavior (Hayes et al., 1996), and still others believe it may measure the ability to inhibit prepotent responses while holding feedback in working memory from which to deduce a new rule to use in the task (Roberts & Pennington, 1996). As with many tests used to study executive functions, each likely represents several overlapping or interactive functions rather than only one. At the very least, this factor reflects more than attention. The capacity to generate a diversity of rules and to extract one quickly from feedback about performance may be involved here, giving rise to the flexibility that Mirsky identifies as involved in this dimension. But it also involves

TABLE 6.1. Rotated Factor Patterns for Child Sample from Mirsky's Research on Attention

Measures	Factors			
	1	2	3	4
CPT correct responses	−.03	−.19	.85	.01
CPT commission errors	.01	−.35	.52	−.13
CPT reaction time	−.14	.27	.65	.35
Digit Cancellation completion time	−.12	−.07	.14	.80
Digit Cancellation omission errors	−.27	−.16	.18	−.57
WISC-R Coding	.06	.38	−.11	−.58
WISC-R Arithmetic	.22	.74	−.16	.01
WISC-R Digit Span	.03	.75	−.04	−.12
WCST, % correct	.95	.10	−.03	−.01
WCST, no. of categories	.95	.11	−.06	.01
Variance explained[a]	19.7%	15.3%	15.1%	14.5%
Proposed identity of factor	Flexibility	Numerical–Mnemonic	Vigilance	PMS
Element of attention	Shift	Encode	Sustain	Focus–Execute

Note. CPT, Continuous Performance Test; WISC-R, Wechsler Intelligence Scale for Children—Revised; WCST, Wisconsin Card Sort Test; PMS, Perceptual–Motor Speed. Underlined values indicate the highest loadings within a column and were used in the interpretation of the identity of the factor. Adapted from Mirsky (1996, p. 84). Copyright 1996 by Paul H. Brookes. Adapted by permission.

[a]The total variance accounted for by the four factors was 64.6%.

a synthetic power to generate a diversity of rules for consideration, as the results of Levin et al. (1996) suggest (see discussion in the next section). Might this be the executive function of reconstitution identified by Bronowski (1967/1977) or represent the synthetic power of the prefrontal lobes, as Fuster (1989) also argued? Perhaps. However, the test–retest reliability of this task has been found to be low (see Roberts & Pennington, 1996), unacceptably so for some of its scores (perseverative errors), so the formation of a dimension comprised solely of this test should always be interpreted cautiously, if at all.

Mirsky's second factor contains two tests from the Wechsler Intelligence Scale for Children—Revised (WISC-R), Arithmetic and Digit Span. The factor was described as reflecting an encoding dimension of attention, or one of Numerical–Mnemonic Ability. Apart from involving a facility with numbers and math operations, these two tests have been interpreted by others as reflecting verbal working memory, or the capacity to hold information in mind so as to act upon it (see Becker, 1994). In either interpretation, it seems that a key element of the task is the capacity to privately represent and operate upon verbal (numerical) information, which fits Goldman-Rakic's (1995a) definition of working memory and Fuster's (1989) of provisional memory. Of course, these tests also comprise part of a larger dimension of verbal intelligence, another construct that needs to be taken into account in any interpretation of this dimension.

The third factor in Mirsky's theory of attention (executive functions) was comprised primarily of scores from the CPT. This dimension was termed the Vigilance component of attention. Such an interpretation of this test is commonplace in psychological research, although some investigators would view the errors of commission as reflecting more problems with response inhibition. Perhaps that may explain the relatively lower degree to which that score loads on this dimension in Table 6.1. But just because the test is interpreted as reflecting sustained attention does not necessarily mean that interpretation is correct. As discussed earlier, this task requires subjects to sustain their compliance to a rule (task instructions) for an extended period of time with little or no reinforcement in the task for doing so (Hayes et al., 1996). It also requires that they inhibit responding to other available and more attractive sources of behavioral control within the room or context than is being provided by the task, and so may reflect interference control to some small degree. The lack of reinforcement in the task also necessitates that subjects internally motivate themselves; that is, they must generate the drive and motivation to continue to respond to the task and adhere to the instructions on their own. Sustained effort, in short, must be derived from a process of self-regulation. Therefore, this dimension of behavior may be more reflective of the self-regulation of affect/motivation/arousal as an executive function in view of this heavy demand for sustaining behavior in the absence of reward.

The last factor in Mirsky's model of attention is represented by the Digit Cancellation scores of completion time and omission errors as well as by the Coding subtest of the WISC-R. The factor is interpreted as Perceptual–Motor Speed (PMS), and this seems to make sense, particularly given the somewhat moderate loading of reaction time on this dimension as well. Yet it has been described as reflecting the Focus–Execute element of attention in Mirsky's model, implying that selective attention may somehow also be involved in this task. It is not clear from the models of executive function discussed earlier in this book that this dimension reflects any of the executive functions described there. Therefore, it may be representing a more sluggish tempo of information processing and motor responding that has little to do with self-regulation and the executive control of behavior.

To summarize, Mirsky's model of attention may well be assessing three forms of executive functions as others have described them. Factor 1 may pertain to a capacity to generate a diversity of rules given feedback about performance and may reflect the reconstitutive or synthetic function discussed earlier. Factor 2 seems to be a verbal working memory dimension. Factor 3 may represent persistence of effort or the function related to self-regulation of motivation. Granted, there are other interpretations of these dimensions, but Mirsky's dimensions are at least not inconsistent with the major executive functions distilled from the earlier review of theories of executive functions. But it also must be recognized that Mirsky's results may simply reflect shared method variance. This is always a problem whenever a dimension is identified in a factor analysis where only the scores from a single test comprise the factor. The use of a larger test battery with multiple tests comprising each dimension would be more convincing. At the very least, however, it seems clear that Mirsky's components of attention are reflecting more than just attention. Three of them, in fact, may well represent some of the executive functions discussed earlier, masquerading here as elements of attention.

Levin et al.'s Study of Children with Closed Head Injury

Levin et al. (1996) studied 102 normal children and 81 children who had experienced closed head injury. The authors employed a large battery of measures presumed to assess executive functions, including the WCST. The results of their principal components factor analysis are shown in Table 6.2. Five factors were identified. The first factor was labeled Conceptual–Productivity and had its highest loadings from a test of design fluency, which required participants to draw as many abstract designs as possible using just four lines, within a 3-minute time period. The second highest loadings were from a verbal fluency test (COWAT). It required subjects to generate as many words as possible beginning with a specific letter and to do so within 60 seconds. Three letters were used across three trials. The other test creating this dimension was the WCST percentage of conceptual responses score. The loading of the latter test on this dimension suggests that the capacity to discover and apply rules from feedback about performance may be involved. As discussed earlier, fluency was believed by Bronowski to involve the executive function of reconstitution, or the

TABLE 6.2. Factor Loadings of Cognitive Variables Disclosed by
Principal-Components Analysis from Levin et al.'s (1996) Study of
Head-Injured Children

	Factors				
	1	2	3	4	5
Measures	Conc-Prod	Planning	Schema	Cluster	Inhibition
TOL, % solved trial 1	.05	.36	.77	.26	−.13
TOL, % solved in 3 trials	.15	.90	.11	.11	−.05
TOL, initial planning time	−.26	−.29	−.24	.31	.69
TOL, no. of rules broken	−.22	−.83	−.26	−.08	−.05
Twenty Questions Test, % of constraint seeking	.43	.09	.77	−.02	−.11
WCST, % conceptual response	.74	.22	.24	−.06	.10
Verbal fluency, no. correct	.70	.20	.29	.33	−.23
Design fluency, no. correct (fixed condition)	.85	.11	.05	.22	.00
CVLT, % of clusters	.24	.14	.13	.84	.05
Go/No-Go false alarms	−.29	−.36	−.25	.21	−.65

Note. Conc-Prod, Conceptual–Productivity; TOL, Tower of London; WCST, Wisconsin Card Sort Test; CVLT, California Verbal Learning Test. Underlined values indicate the factor loadings that define the factor. Adapted from Levin et al. (1996, p. 24). Copyright 1996 by Lawrence Erlbaum Associates, Inc. Adapted by permission.

capacity to analyze and synthesize language and to generate a diversity of novel responses quickly so as to accomplish a goal. This capacity has been interpreted as reflecting the synthetic function of the prefrontal lobes or the power to generate diverse and novel responses. Consequently, there may be more to this dimension than just conceptual reasoning, as the authors suggested.

The second factor has its primary loadings from the Tower of London (TOL) test and was interpreted as Planning ability. This task requires subjects to observe a display of three wooden pegs containing an arrangement of colored balls. They must make such an arrangement with their own set of pegs/balls within the constraints of several rules about how the balls may be moved to achieve the end result (matching the sample pattern). As in a chess game, the subject must visually represent the information in mind and then manipulate this information to evaluate possible moves or outcomes before selecting one to follow. It has been interpreted as placing heavy demands on working memory (Pennington et al., 1993; Roberts & Pennington, 1996) and probably reflects the nonverbal element of such working memory to some degree. However, this task also requires the subject to obey several rules concerning the constraints placed on possible moves. Given that the score of number of rules broken across the trials loaded heavily on this dimension, this factor may reflect the capacity of the subject to follow the rules required to solve the design problems more than it reflects working memory. The loading of another TOL score on Factor 3 suggests that this factor may represent the working memory aspect of this task more than does Factor 2.

Factor 3 in Table 6.2 has been labeled Schema and has its highest loadings from two tests: The TOL score of percentage of designs solved in the first trial and the Twenty Questions Test, which requires the subject to deduce the correct "target" picture from an array of pictures by asking as few questions as possible. The similarity of these two tasks is difficult to appreciate. The authors interpreted this factor as possibly reflecting working memory, given that problem solving on both tasks is guided by a mental representation or schema.

The fourth factor in Table 6.2 reflects only a single test, the California Verbal Learning Test (CVLT), which is a measure of verbal memory with a delayed recall element to the task. The factor, "Cluster," reflects clustering ability, but it seems to me more likely to reflect verbal working memory: the capacity to hold verbal information in mind (the internalization of speech, or Baddeley's [1986] articulatory loop).

The fifth and last factor, labeled Inhibition, receives its principal loadings from the initial planning time (time before first response) on the TOL and the number of impulsive errors (false alarms) on the go/no-go test, discussed in Chapter 4 as a measure of response inhibition. Perhaps an even more accurate label is the capacity to delay a response, given the high positive loading of the TOL score and negative loading for go/no-go impulsive errors. Either way, the dimension seems to reflect that of behavioral inhibition as discussed earlier.

To summarize to this point, this study seems to have identified a function that could be related to the concept of working memory (both verbal and nonverbal), as Mirsky's research seemed to do as well. Mirsky's research did not employ any measure of nonverbal working memory, such as the TOL, so such a factor was unlikely to emerge in that study apart from the verbal working memory (encode, or Numerical–Mnemonic) factor. Like Levin et al., Mirsky also identified a factor related to the capacity to generate a rule and follow it, using the WCST. Mirsky referred to this as a "Shift" element of attention, but the loading of verbal and nonverbal fluency measures with this test in the Levin et al. study suggests that these measures may tap a generative, synthetic process that creates and evaluates a diversity of rules before selecting one to follow, creating flexibility in responding. The placement of these fluency measures on this dimension may also indicate that it represents the function of reconstitution, as Bronowski (1967/1977) described it. Others have also argued that a rule-generative function could be used to develop a computer model of response patterns on tasks like the WCST (Dehaene & Changeux, 1995).

Levin et al. (1996) may have identified a factor that pertains to the capacity to follow rules related to constraining performance (Factor 2). Whether this is similar to Mirsky's Sustain element of attention is difficult to determine since no CPT was used by Levin et al. that might have more clearly assessed this aspect of executive functioning. Finally, Levin et al. identified a response inhibition factor that Mirsky did not, most likely because Mirsky did not employ any measures of inhibition comparable to those used by Levin et al. In short, both studies may have identified a working memory function (verbal) as well as a rule-generative function that possibly reflects the reconstitutive executive function of Bronowski. Mirsky also identified a factor related to persistence of effort (Vigilance), whereas Levin et al. appeared to employ no such measures. The latter investigators identified a response inhibition factor that Mirsky did not, most likely for the same reason. Levin et al.'s study may have also identified a nonverbal working memory function not seen in Mirsky's study, again because such measures appear not to have been used.

Taylor et al.'s Study of Children Surviving H-Flu Meningitis

In another recent study, Taylor and colleagues (Taylor et al., 1996) studied 53 children surviving H-flu meningitis along with 170 unaffected children using a large battery of measures believed to assess executive functions. The results of their principal-components factor analysis are shown in Table 6.3.

The first two factors appear to reflect the well-known dimensions of verbal and performance intelligence, given that their highest loadings come from subtests of these two forms of IQ from the WISC-R. It would have been interesting to see the factor structure had these components of IQ been removed from the factor analysis in order to see how the word fluency and verbal selective-reminding tests might have behaved without the confounding of this first factor with overall verbal ability. No other tests reflecting the generative or synthetic function reflected in the concept of reconstitution were employed, so it is not surprising that no such dimension emerged in this study.

TABLE 6.3. Factor Loadings from Principal-Components Analysis of Neuropsychological Test Battery from Taylor et al.'s (1996) Study of Children with Meningitis

Measures	Factors				
	1	2	3	4	5
WISC-R Vocabulary	.85	.06	−.06	.07	−.09
WISC-R Similarities	.78	.21	−.13	.00	.03
Word fluency	.58	−.12	.18	−.24	−.02
Verbal selective reminding	.54	−.14	.26	.03	.07
WISC-R Object Assembly	.15	.83	−.09	−.09	−.06
Grooved Pegboard Test	−.10	.64	.26	.17	.04
WISC-R Block Design	.20	.55	.10	−.29	.19
Contingency Naming, time	.00	−.04	.80	−.02	.03
WISC-R Coding	−.08	.06	.73	−.14	.05
Underlining	.17	.21	.69	.00	−.13
Contingency Naming, errors	.11	.04	.13	.66	.05
WISC-R Digit Span	.00	.05	.35	.59	.05
MTA	.26	−.05	.30	.53	.41
Nonverbal selective reminding	−.10	−.01	−.01	.11	.80
Visual–Motor Integration	−.03	.35	−.05	−.20	.51
Token Test, Part V	.27	−.11	−.01	−.35	.43

Note. WISC-R, Wechsler Intelligence Scale for Children—Revised; MTA, Microcomputer Test of Attention. Underlined factor loadings indicate those reaching statistical significance. Adapted from Taylor, Schatschneider, Petrill, Barry, and Owens (1996, p. 41). Copyright 1996 by Lawrence Erlbaum Associates, Inc. Adapted by permission.

Factor 3 is very similar to Mirsky's (1996) Focus–Execute element of attention, that is, the Perceptual–Motor Speed factor, with two of the three tests loading on this dimension being similar or identical to the two tests that Mirsky found to comprise this dimension (WISC-R Coding and Digit Cancellation; the latter is similar to the underlining test in the Taylor et al. study). As noted in the discussion of Mirsky's findings, this result probably does not reflect an executive function but one of speed of information processing and response performance, given that all of these are timed tests and that the time to perform the Contingency Naming test loaded highest on this dimension in the Taylor et al. (1996) study.

Factor 4 was believed by the authors to reflect an inhibition or interference control dimension, which may well be the case given the processes involved in two of these tests. The Contingency Naming test requires following rules and resisting prepotent sources of interference in the task, much like the Stroop test discussed in Chapter 4, while the Minnesota Test of Attention (MTA) is a CPT that assesses both response inhibition and persistence of effort. The loading of Digit Span on this dimension is puzzling, as this test has been interpreted by others as reflecting verbal working memory. Its failure to load on the verbal IQ dimension (Factor 1) and the fact that interference control is important in working memory (Fuster, 1989) make the interpretation of this dimension as one of interference control more plausible.

Finally, the fifth factor was interpreted as reflecting a planning dimension; this would be consistent with the interpretation given for planning ability in the Levin et al. (1996) study as indicative of nonverbal working memory. Supportive of this interpretation was the high loading of the Nonverbal Selective Reminding Test (a nonverbal memory task) and of the Visual–Motor Integration (VMI) design copying test on this dimension.

In summation, this study found a set of executive functions— working memory (nonverbal, in this case) and response inhibition (interference control)—similar to the studies reviewed earlier. The failure of a separate verbal working memory function to emerge may have been the result of including tests of verbal IQ that seemed to have pulled the verbal selective-reminding test (verbal memory) and word fluency test to this dimension. These latter tests otherwise might have reflected verbal working memory and reconstitution.

Shute and Huertas's Study of Normal College Students

Shute and Huertas (1990) reported a factor analysis of a smaller battery of measures presumed to assess frontal lobe functions using 58 subjects. Such small samples often do not auger well for the stability of any dimensions that might be found in the battery of tests, but, again, the purpose here is merely exploratory, to see if any of these factors are consistent with those found by other researchers. The results of this factor analysis appear in Table 6.4, which identifies four factors from this test battery. The authors did not interpret these factors, but I will hazard some guesses here as to what they may represent from the standpoint of the models of executive functions discussed earlier.

The first factor comprises four tests: the Category Test from the Halstead–Reitan neuropsychological test battery (given in booklet form here), Part B of the Trail Making Test from the same battery, the perseverative errors score from the WCST, and the cognitive development measure. The latter measure is the Shadows Task and is a

TABLE 6.4. Varimax-Rotated Factor Loadings for Measures of Frontal Lobe Function from Shute and Huertas's (1990) Study of Normal Young Adults

Measures	Factors			
	1	2	3	4
Category Test	.78	.14	.08	−.18
Trail Making Test, Part B	.64	.48	.27	.03
WCST, perseverative errors	.52	−.11	.28	.34
Cognitive development	−.74	.01	.07	.01
Trail Making Test, Part A	.12	.82	.10	.02
Digit Symbol	.00	.85	−.08	−.13
Internal Attention, error score	.11	.09	.88	−.02
Selective Attention, error score	.05	.10	.87	−.10
Average time estimation error[a]	−.10	−.01	−.02	.88
Average time estimation error in selective attention	.06	.46	−.20	.71
Percentage of variance	19%	19%	17%	15%

Note. N = 58; WCST, Wisconsin Card Sort Test. Underlined factor loadings indicate those reaching statistical significance. Adapted from Shute and Huertas (1990, p. 8). Copyright 1990 by Lawrence Erlbaum Associates, Inc. Adapted by permission.

[a]This measure is scored with either a negative sign indicating that the average time period was underestimated or a positive sign indicating that the average time period was overestimated.

Piagetian measure of formal operational thinking. It includes a group of logical reasoning abilities that allows one to construct totally hypothetical mental representations and then operate upon them and manipulate them to examine the range of possible relationships. Like the WCST and the verbal and design fluency tests that characterized their concept formation dimension in the Levin et al. (1996) study, or like Mirsky's (1996) Flexibility factor, such formal operational thinking reflects the flexibility of rule generation and rule application. It may therefore represent Bronowski's (1967/1977) concept of reconstitution or Fuster's (1980, 1989, 1995) view of a function that generates a diversity of behaviors, including rules. I interpret the first factor as reflecting the inverse of such generative flexibility—the perseveration of the individual in previous response patterns. I do so because the first three measures loading positively on this dimension reflect impaired performance (greater perseverative errors on Category and WCST and greater time on Trails B). The negative loading of the Shadows Task (cognitive development) supports this interpretation. This pattern of inflexibility in following a rule, or perseveration of previous response patterns in the face of feedback to the contrary, may result from the failure to clear working memory of past rules and other representational information that controlled previous behavior so as to allocate this memory capacity to the formulation of a new rule (Dunbar & Sussman, 1995).

Factor 2 consists mainly of two tests that could easily reflect the Perceptual–Motor Speed factor once again. It is comprised of Trails A, which requires subjects to connect a sequence of numbers in sequence as quickly as possible, and Digit Symbol, which is similar to the WISC-R Coding used by Mirsky and interpreted by him as reflecting Perceptual–Motor Speed. Both tests reflect, again, a speed/accuracy trade-off in performance of an information-processing task, both are timed, and both load positively on Factor 2. All of this suggests that this factor is the inverse of Perceptual–Motor Speed, that is, perceptual–motor sluggishness. It is, once again, a nonexecutive function.

Factor 3 includes two rather simple tests that probably comprise verbal working memory. The Internal Attention test requires subjects to count the number of times the letter E occurs in the first two lines of the chorus of "Jingle Bells." The Selective Attention test is almost the same, except that subjects now count the number of times the letter L occurs and *also,* simultaneously, must indicate each time 15 seconds has elapsed throughout the task (a time estimation task). Shute and Huertas (1990) note that both tasks require the mental representation of information, thus, my interpretion of this factor as a working memory (verbal) function seems consistent with their interpretation.

The fourth factor in Table 6.4 is an interesting one, given that it is comprised of time estimation tasks. The authors' description of these tasks is not quite correct, however, as tasks requiring subjects to produce a specified time interval are time production tasks. They are believed to place demands on short-term memory for temporal sequences of events (Zakay, 1990). Consequently, while this dimension may well reflect that of time production, such production depends on working memory (most likely nonverbal) as Bronowski (1967/1977) and Michon (1985) have both suggested. In other words, this factor may involve the executive function of nonverbal working memory.

Robertson et al.'s Study of Normal Adults

In another recent study of human attention, Robertson and colleagues (1996) conducted an exploratory factor analysis of a battery of measures thought to assess different components of attention. They employed a sample of 154 normal adult subjects and a range of tests, some of them cleverly devised to reflect more ecologically valid attention tasks, similar to those required in everyday adaptive functioning. The test battery and results of the factor analysis (principal-components analysis) are shown in Table 6.5.

Factor 1 was primarily comprised of five tests, and was labeled Visual Selective Attention/Speed. The fact that two of the tests loading negatively on this dimension represent time to complete the task (Trails B, Telephone Search) may well support this factor as being simply a Perceptual–Motor Speed factor, thus placing it outside the realm of executive functions. The identification by Taylor et al. (1996) of a Perceptual–Motor Speed factor (Factor 3) comprising several similar tests would further support the idea of such a nonexecutive nature to this factor.

TABLE 6.5. Factor Analysis of Attention Tests for Standardization Sample from Robertson et al.'s (1996) Study of Normal Adults

| Measures | Factors | | | |
	1	2	3	4
Map Search	.84	.09	.02	.00
Stroop	.72	.19	.05	.10
Telephone Search, time to target	−.80	−.25	−.09	−.21
Trails B	−.74	−.19	−.27	−.22
d2 total	.67	−.13	−.02	.43
Visual Elevator, no. correct	.22	.78	.19	.22
WCST, categories	.29	.68	.00	.21
Lottery	.25	.18	.70	.10
Elevator Counting	−.27	.28	.56	.12
Dual Task Decrement	−.21	.24	−.72	−.31
Auditory Elevator Reversal	.49	.12	−.10	.62
Auditory Elevator with Distraction	.03	.32	.28	.52
Digit Span Backward	.04	.14	.06	.77
PASAT-2s	.33	.18	.10	.58

Note. N = 154. Stroop, Stroop Word–Color Association Test; WCST, Wisconsin Card Sort Test; PASAT, Paced Serial Auditory Addition Test. Total variance explained by factors 1–4 = 62%. Underlined factor loadings indicate those reaching statistical significance. Adapted from Robertson, Ward, Ridgeway, and Nimmo-Smith (1996, p. 532). Copyright 1996 by Cambridge University Press. Adapted by permission.

Alternatively, this dimension might reflect the function of interference control (resistance to distraction) and the larger construct of behavioral inhibition. The nature of some of the tests could support this interpretation. For instance, performance on the Stroop Word–Color Association Test, Part III (interference) has been repeatedly interpreted by others as reflecting the capacity to inhibit prepotent responses (reading the word) while persisting in following a rule (describe the color of ink in which the word is printed). It is a test that pits sources of behavioral control against each other (Hayes et al., 1996), so interpreting it as a test of interference control and persistence of rule following makes some sense. But Robertson et al. do not describe which scores from the Stroop were used in this study or which parts were scored. Parts I and II are essentially timed tests involving more automatic behaviors (color naming, reading single words) that would be more consistent with the interpretation of this factor as indexing perceptual–motor speed. The d2 measure is based on a letter cancellation task, which is a form of paper-and-pencil CPT. As noted earlier (Taylor et al., 1996), such cancellation tasks may reflect perceptual–motor speed, but they may also involve persistence in rule following (the instruction to locate the target) and resistance to the distracting influence of other letters within the cancellation task. The Map Search measure requires the subject to search for the knife-and-fork symbol indicative of a restaurant on a colored map of the Philadelphia area. It is a timed test, and so not only requires perceptual-motor speed but also careful searching of the map and resistance to distraction from competing symbols of information while doing so. Like the Map Search test, the Telephone Search test involves searching a simulated telephone directory for plumbers (or restaurants or hotels) while also looking for key symbols. A similar interpretation could be given to the Trails B test of the Halstead–Reitan neuropsychological test battery as well. Thus, while there is good reason to consider this factor as reflecting the nonexecutive function of perceptual–motor speed, one could also argue that it might also reflect the executive function of resistance to distraction (interference control) and persistence in rule following. I believe that the first interpretation is more correct; these tasks involve a speed/accuracy trade-off in information processing and so probably reflect a nonexecutive function having to do with such processing, rather than reflecting interference control.

The second factor, labeled Attention Switching, is comprised of two tests, one of which is the WCST. That test has been interpreted by others studying executive functions (see the preceding discussion of studies) as reflecting the capacity for flexibility in generating rules from performance feedback. It may involve, at least in part, the generative, synthetic, or reconstitutive function, and it permits a diversity of new rules to be considered based upon the nature of the performance feedback. One rule is selected and employed until feedback suggests that a new rule is now required. Supporting this interpretation is the nature of the second test loading on this dimension, the Visual Elevator test. On this task, subjects count up and down as they follow a series of visually presented floors in the simulated elevator. The requirement of reversal of direction of counting in the task was interpreted by the authors as assessing flexibility or attention switching. Both tasks require flexibility, to be sure, but not flexibility of attention. It is a flexibility related to the verbal regulation (rule governance) of behavior during the task.

Factor 3 in this study was termed Sustained Attention, and was comprised of three tests that demand persistence of effort and rule-following behavior, although persistence seems to be key in these tasks. The Lottery task is very similar to an auditory CPT. Subjects must listen for 10 minutes to a series of letter–number combinations played on a tape player so as to detect their winning lottery number (55). They must write down the two letters that preceded each occurrence of this winning number (only 10 of which occur in the 10-minute interval). Elevator Counting is, likewise, a form of CPT in that subjects must pretend to be in an elevator and determine which floor they are on by counting tones that signal arrival at the next floor. As a measure of sustained responding, it makes sense that it would load on the same dimension as the CPT-like Lottery task. Similarly, the Dual Task Decrement score is the difference between the Telephone Search task and performance on this same task given again, but with the added requirement of counting simultaneously presented strings of tones played by a tape player. Like previous CPTs, such tasks place heavy demands on self-motivation (persistence of effort) and, to some extent, on adherence to a rule in the absence of reinforcement. They may reflect the executive function of self-regulation of affect/motivation/arousal as discussed earlier in this chapter, rather than just sustained attention.

As I mentioned briefly in Chapter 1 and will discuss at length in Chapter 7, investigators must recognize that at least two forms of sustained responding exist. One is contingency-shaped and reflects the prevailing reinforcement schedule in the task. It is externally governed sustained responding. The other arises out of self-regulation and is best termed goal-directed persistence. It reflects internal governance of behavior by the goal (the rule in this case) and the power to self-motivate or renew the drive state toward the goal. Given that CPTs typically lack external reinforcement schedules, individuals must generate motivation in support of the goal of the task. Factor 3, therefore, is more likely to reflect this form of goal-directed persistence (an executive function) than that of sustained attention (a nonexecutive function).

The fourth and last factor is labeled Auditory–Verbal Working Memory and seems appropriately named, given the nature of the tasks that comprise this dimension or component. Digit Span Backward and the Paced Auditory Serial Addition Test (PASAT-2s) both have been interpreted by others as reflecting verbal working memory (Levin et al., 1996; Mirsky, 1996). The Auditory Elevator with Distraction task is like the Elevator Counting task in that subjects must count up the tones in the imaginary elevator while ignoring a high tone that may occur throughout the task as well. While involving some resistance to distraction, the requirement of mental addition in the task would seem to be the greater demand and explain its relationship to the PASAT-2s and Digit Span Backward tests loading on this same component. The Auditory Elevator Reversal is the same as the Visual Elevator task discussed earlier except that it is presented by audiotape rather than visually. It thus requires as the major demand of the task that subjects again count to themselves. I would agree with these investigators that this most likely represents the verbal working memory function. But I would disagree with their consideration of working memory as an element of attention when most researchers view it as an executive function instead.

As with the other studies reviewed in this section, the study by Robertson and colleagues identifies a working memory function (verbal), a sustain function likely reflecting goal-directed persistence (persistence of effort/motivation), a rule-generative/flexibility function (reconstitution), and an interference control (inhibitory) function.

Mariani and Barkley's Study of Preschool ADHD Boys

Mary Ann Mariani and I (1997) have recently reported a study of preschool ADHD (*n* = 34) and control children (*n* = 30) in which we employed a battery of 25 tests of academic achievement, measures of neuropsychological functions, and some behavioral observations taken during task performances. To reduce this battery to a manageable size for interpretive purposes, we conducted a dimensional (factor) analysis of the tests and found a four-factor solution that accounted for 45% of the variance. These tests and the factors on which they loaded are shown in Table 6.6. Tests having a loading of at least .53 on a particular factor have their factor loadings underlined, while those tests having their highest loading on a factor are marked with an asterisk beside their factor loading.

The first dimension extracted from this analysis was labeled *Motor Control,* given the high loadings of the scores from the Purdue Pegboard Test on this dimension. The K-ABC Spatial Memory test, Color Form test, and the number of (colored poker) chips sorted during a work period all involve aspects of perceptual–motor speed and so would fit with such an interpretation of this factor. The second factor was clearly a dimension reflecting verbal learning and memory. It was composed entirely of the three measures from the Wisconsin Selective Reminding Test (WSRT), a verbal memory test very similar to that developed by Buschke (see Buschke & Fuld, 1974) for use with adults. Consequently, this factor was labeled *Verbal Learning–Memory.* Factor 3 had major loadings from tests that require subjects to recognize and label pictures (the K-ABC Gestalt Closure and the Faces and Places subtests) and draw upon factual knowledge (K-ABC Vocabulary subtest). This dimension was therefore called *Picture Recognition–Factual Knowledge.*

Factor 4 received major loadings from a number of tests which, at first glance, seemed quite unrelated. However, the K-ABC Hand Movements, Number Recall (digit span), Arithmetic (mental), and Spatial Memory subtests all require the fixing and holding of information in mind while acting upon it and using it to execute tasks. Therefore, these tasks could be considered ones involving working memory. This would be consistent with the other studies reviewed, in which a factor comprising digit span and mental computation was similarly interpreted. While two academic achievement tests load on this dimension (K-ABC Arithmetic and Reading/Decoding), the other K-ABC achievement tests did not, raising doubt that this dimension simply reflected one of academic achievement. It would seem that the tests from the K-ABC stressing factual knowledge load on another dimension, whereas those involving skills used to correctly obtain an answer load here. Moreover, the high loadings on this dimension of some measures (Disruptive Behavior during the CPT, Number of chips sorted, K-ABC Hand Movements) and marginally significant loadings of others (CPT Number Correct, Disruptive Behavior during Chip Sort) thought to assess sustained attention and behavioral control further question interpreting this as a purely achievement dimension. *Working Memory–Persistence* was chosen as the label for this dimension, recognizing that its validity and content are in need of more research.

It is interesting to find in this study of preschool-age children that separate dimensions for verbal and nonverbal working memory did not seem to emerge from the analysis. The fourth factor, labeled working memory, appears to contain tests thought to evaluate both nonverbal and verbal working memory. The loading of the K-ABC

Spatial Memory and Hand Movements subtests as well as Porteus Mazes on this dimension implies that nonverbal representational memory may be a part of this dimension given the reliance of these tests on more nonverbal, spatial test materials. However, the loading of K-ABC Number Recall and Arithmetic subtests implies that some element of verbal working memory is involved here as well. The finding of the high loading of the K-ABC Reading/Decoding test on this dimension would seem consistent with that view. Of course, given the small sample size and potential instability of the dimensions that might result, the relationship could simply be a method artifact. However, it may also be explained by the fact that early reading of common words at the ages studied here is based considerably less on phonetic decoding and more on sight-word or whole-word recognition.

Novice readers seem to identify common or "sight" words as whole visual patterns (Ehri & Wilce, 1985; Olson, Forsberg, Wise, & Rack, 1994), the memory of the whole word's visual pattern must be held in mind while linking it to its phonological memory. If so, then it is not surprising to find that a measure of reading taken in these preschool-age novice readers would load so heavily at this developmental stage with some measures of nonverbal working memory—a functional system in which the picture of the word must be sustained while searching for its complete sound in memory.

All of this may suggest one of two things. One is that nonverbal and verbal working memory are not yet distinct from each other at this preschool-age range. Given that speech is just beginning to be turned on the self at this age level and has not yet become fully covert or internalized in form (Berk, 1992; see also Chapters 5 and 8), this might make sense. It would imply that working memory at this stage is a general representational memory system relying more heavily on the earlier developing forms of covert seeing and hearing (nonverbal working memory) than on covert self-directed speech. As speech becomes fully internalized, it will come to form a separate working memory system from this more general, nonverbal representational one. If so, this line of reasoning suggests that when preschool children perform tasks like digit span and mental arithmetic, they are relying on visual/auditory resensing of this material to aid with task performance, rather than on a private, covert speech system.

The alternative interpretation of this dimension is that it actually represents traditional nonverbal working memory while the dimension represented in Factor 2 of Table 6.6 is the verbal working memory system. I find this a less satisfying interpretation than the first one for several reasons, not the least of which is the loading of so many tests

TABLE 6.6. Factor Structure of the Dependent Measures
from Mariani and Barkley's (1997) Study of Preschool ADHD Boys

Dependent measures	Dimensions			
	I	II	III	IV
Purdue Pegboard, dominant	.59[*]	.24	−.21	.19
Purdue Pegboard, nondominant	.80[*]	.29	.04	.39
Purdue Pegboard, both hands	.91[*]	.38	.11	.47
K-ABC Spatial Memory	.68[*]	.28	−.12	.55
Color Form	−.61[*]	−.19	.21	−.41
Number of chips sorted	.62[*]	.30	.03	.55
WSRT Recall	.43	.95[*]	.08	.35
WSRT Long-Term Storage	.34	.90[*]	−.02	.36
WSRT Long-Term Retrieval	.36	.87[*]	.06	.39
K-ABC Gestalt Closure	.21	−.09	.53[*]	.08
K-ABC Vocabulary	−.08	.28	.59[*]	.03
K-ABC Faces and Places	.19	.17	.70[*]	.30
K-ABC Riddles	.16	.23	.39[*]	.37
K-ABC Number Recall	.28	.27	.05	.59[*]
K-ABC Arithmetic	.32	.16	.17	.69[*]
K-ABC Reading/Decoding	.18	−.03	.28	.61[*]
K-ABC Hand Movements	.38	.25	.03	.67[*]
Porteus Mazes	.54	.42	−.09	.59[*]
Disruptive behavior (CPT)	−.38	−.47	.23	−.64[*]
Disruptive behavior (chip sort)	−.26	−.36	.05	−.48[*]
CPT correct responses	.44	.19	.02	.47[*]
CPT commission errors	−.13	.22	−.14	−.24[*]
MFFT latency	.28	.22	−.22	.36[*]
MFFT errors	−.33[*]	−.33[*]	−.18	−.31
Beery DTVMI	.06	−.04	−.05	.08

Note. WSRT, Wisconsin Selective Reminding Test; K-ABC, Kaufman Assessment Battery for Children; CPT, Continuous Performance Test; MFFT, Matching Familiar Figures Test; DTVMI, Developmental Test of Visual–Motor Integration. Coefficients are correlations. Measures having correlations > .53 with a dimension are underlined. Asterisks indicate dimension on which each measure had its highest loading. From Mariani and Barkley (1997, p. 121). Copyright 1997 by Lawrence Erlbaum Associates, Inc. Reprinted by permission.

having a verbal component to them on this factor rather than on the verbal memory dimension. Second, fully covert self-speech has not yet developed in such young children. Consequently, a verbal working memory system independent of that for nonverbal working memory would be inconsistent with my earlier interpretation that verbal working memory originates from the internalization of speech. A separate verbal memory storage system may well exist at this age, and that may be what is reflected in Factor 2. But it is verbal memory that is assisted by the public recitation of the word list required in the performance of the WSRT and by the examiner reminding the subject of those words that were missed. This is a public, dialogic interaction using speech, and it directly assists with long-term storage of verbal material. It is not working memory, but long-term memory. It may well be that this represents the early beginnings of what eventually will become covert self-speech and the verbal working memory system later in development. The notion that a verbal working memory system has not yet been added to the earlier existing nonverbal one at this age is intriguing and worthy of future research.

The identification in this study of a dimension that potentially couples traditional working memory tasks with measures frequently used to assess sustained attention (persistence) and behavioral control in the developmental psychopathology literature pertinent to ADHD is likewise intriguing. If it can be replicated in other studies, it suggests that general representational memory may give rise to the capacity for goal-directed behavioral persistence, as others have previously argued (Fuster, 1989). Not only must the goal of the task be retained in mind and self-motivation to persist toward the goal be activated, but interference control, also integral to an effective working memory system, bears a heavy demand from any given task. Perhaps it is this aspect of behavioral inhibition that is common to the tests loading on this dimension. If so, then working memory–interference control may be the better label applied to this dimension.

Also of interest was the fact that this study was unable to identify a separate dimension of cognitive impulse control in this sample apart from that of working memory–persistence. Perhaps this resulted from our failure to use more than a few measures of this construct or because the measures we did use assessed a heterogeneous set of mental functions. The finding that the highest loadings of these measures on the working memory–persistence dimension were still of a modest size implies such a measurement problem. Even so, the individual measures of impulsiveness taken here (Matching Familiar Figures Test [MFFT] latency, MFFT errors, and, particularly, CPT commission errors) did not distinguish these two groups of young children to a statistically significant degree. The latter finding is in agreement with the inconsistency observed in prior studies regarding whether the MFFT distinguishes ADHD from comparison children at this age. The preschool version of the CPT task used here also may simply be too easy for preschool children of this age to perform to be of much value in differentiating ADHD from non-ADHD children.

As discussed in Chapter 3, it appears to be the component of impulse control, comprising behavioral observations of disruptive, undercontrolled conduct, restlessness, and impersistence that reflects the dimension of behavioral inhibition. That is also the component of inhibition believed to be more involved in ADHD, as noted in Chapter 4, than is the cognitive form of impulsiveness versus reflectiveness, as assessed by the MFFT.

Grodzinsky and Diamond's Study of ADHD Boys

Grodzinsky and Diamond (1992) reported a study conducted in my clinic using 66 boys with ADHD and 64 control boys from the community, all between the ages of 6 and 11 years, who were administered a large battery of tests presumed to assess frontal lobe functions. With the permission of Gail Grodzinsky, I conducted a factor (dimensional) analysis of the data from this study, so as to compare the resulting factor structure with that obtained in the other studies reviewed here. The dimensional analysis was conducted using Gorsuch's UniMult program with both a varimax and then ProMax Rotation, much as was used in the study by Mariani and Barkley discussed above. The results of this analysis are shown in Table 6.7.

The first factor is composed entirely of scores from the WCST and, as in the study of Mirsky (1996) discussed above, seems to form a dimension of behavioral inflexibility, given the high positive loading of perseverative errors and responses on the dimension and the equally strong yet negative loading of categories and concept formation scores. It could also be interpreted as reflecting an insensitivity to errors as well as an inability to learn and apply a rule or strategy (concept formation), as described earlier, when given feedback about performance.

The second factor is difficult to interpret. While the high positive loadings of the verbal fluency measures here suggest that this dimension reflects the capacity to generate a diversity of responses (verbal) on demand, the equally high loadings of Porteus Mazes (age score) and the Stroop test words score cloud this interpretation. Also puzzling is the negative loading of the Trails A and B scores on this dimension, to a degree comparable to that of the verbal fluency measures. Perhaps it is best not to interpret this dimension at this time.

TABLE 6.7. Factor Structure of the Dependent Measures from Grodzinsky and Diamond's (1992) Study of ADHD Boys

Measures	Dimension					
	I	II	III	IV	V	VI
WCST, no. correct	−.76					
WCST, total errors	.94					
WCST, no. of categories	−.91					
WCST, perseverative errors	.92					
WCST, concept formation score	−.95					
Trails A, time (seconds)		−.73				
Trails B, time (seconds)		−.70				
Porteus Mazes (age score)		.70				
Rey–Osterrieth (age score)		.48				
Stroop, words		.66				.62
Verbal fluency, FAS		.70				
Verbal fluency, animals		.65				
Verbal fluency, foods		.68				
Verbal fluency, names		.71				
Pegboard, dominant			.94			
Pegboard, nondominant			.92			
WCST, nonperseverative errors				.97		
CPT, commissions					.73	
CPT, omissions					.70	
Stroop, color						.73
Stroop, interference						.76

Note. WCST, Wisconsin Card Sort Test; Trails, Trail Making Test; Verbal Fluency, Controlled Oral Word Association Test, Verbal Fluency Subtests; Pegboard, Grooved Pegboard Test (time in seconds); CPT, Continuous Performance Test; Stroop, Stroop Word–Color Association Test. Coefficients are correlations. From Grodzinsky and Diamond (1992). Reprinted by permission.

The third factor seems to be a relatively straightforward one to interpret, given that it contains the two scores from the Grooved Pegboard Test. It most likely reflects a fine motor speed/coordination dimension of performance.

The fourth dimension to emerge from this analysis was formed only by the high loading of the nonperseverative errors score from the WCST, reflecting mistakes made by the subject of a nonperseverative nature. Whether it is comprised of responses reflecting a trial-and-error or random responding strategy is not clear at this time.

The fifth factor to be found in this analysis is comprised mainly of the two scores from the CPT. It seems to reflect difficulties with both impulsive and inattentive errors on the test and is consistent with the dimension of Vigilance, or persistence, found in Mirsky's (1996) study.

The sixth and last factor discovered in this analysis is composed of the scores from the Stroop Word–Color Association Test. While it is tempting to interpret this as reflecting the function of interference control, the nearly equivalent loading of the color and word scores for this test on this same dimension would challenge such an easy interpretation. In fact, given that most of the dimensions in this analysis are comprised, like this one, primarily of scores from the same test, these dimensions could just as conceivably reflect shared method variance.

Summary of Findings

The findings of all of the studies reviewed here could be considered in some ways as being consistent with the executive functions extracted from the theories discussed in Chapter 5. Moreover, where tasks have been used that involve visual imagery or other forms of nonverbal working memory, a separate or dissociable dimension representing this form of working memory may emerge apart from those tasks comprising a verbal working memory dimension, at least in children older than the preschool-age group and in adults. Evidence for a working memory dimension has also been found in other studies using confirmatory factor analysis (Daigneault, Braun, & Whitaker, 1992), so the place of that particular function within a theory of executive functions seems secure.

The executive function of reconstitution was not always evident in these studies or was more difficult to discern from the few measures of it that may have been used and the fact that they measured more than just this function. For instance, measures such as the WCST involve aspects of response flexibility but also require working memory and behavioral inhibition, making it difficult to interpret the factors this test may load on as purely reflecting reconstitution (response flexibility). It is unclear from these studies whether a separate factor of reconstitution exists apart from that of working memory, though the research studies discussed in this chapter imply that it might. Likewise, no executive function of the self-regulation of affect, motivation, and arousal was obvious in these studies. This was chiefly the result, however, of these studies not employing measures intended to assess this domain of functioning. Even so, the emergence of a factor labeled persistence or "sustain" in Mirsky's research and in the other studies intimates that this factor may represent more of a motivational function (persistence of effort) than an attentional one.

To the extent that relatively simple tasks are employed that require automatic responses and speed of perceptual–motor responding, then a corresponding perceptual–motor speed factor emerges in these data as well. Such a factor would not qualify as executive in nature, however, as that term was defined in Chapter 3. It does not seem to involve any form of covert self-directed action, such as self-directed sensing, self-speech, self-motivation, or self-experimentation (reconstitution) that defines the other functions as being executive in form. Rule following is certainly inherent in these tasks as well because of the role of experimental instructions in their procedures, as noted earlier; this suggests that the executive function of rule governance may be involved in such tasks. But such rules are simple and, more importantly, the instructions they convey do not set up competing sources of behavioral control between the rule and more external sources that promote the occurrence of prepotent responses that conflict with it. Such competition between internal (rules) and external sources of control often characterize a task as being executive in nature (Hayes et al., 1996). Therefore, a perceptual–motor speed factor would not fall into the realm of executive functions.

NEUROIMAGING STUDIES USING MEASURES OF EXECUTIVE FUNCTIONS

As discussed in Chapter 5, substantial research studying human patients and primates with lesions to the prefrontal cortex have suggested a tripartite distinction among the executive functions and the regions that mediate them. Studies of brain injuries in humans are problematic, however, because the lesions are not likely to be as discrete as one would like in order to establish for certain what role different regions play in what functions. Moreover, as is well recognized in neuropsychology, the area that has been damaged may not necessarily account for the behavioral changes in evidence after the injury because of the distributed networks likely involved in complex human mental abilities. The behavioral changes could be the result of the release of other brain systems from the control exerted by the injured region, rather than indicating that the injured region is purely responsible for the function that has been lost or impaired. For these and other reasons, the study of normal brain function in noninjured humans using modern neuroimaging techniques may give another means by which to evaluate the involvement of different prefrontal regions in various tasks.

The images created from modern brain scanning technology can be collected while the subjects are performing the tests of executive functions so as to indicate which regions of the brain (with particular interest on the prefrontal cortex) may be mediating these functions. This approach to studying executive functions is still in its relative infancy, but some of the findings of studies already completed support the differentiation among some the executive functions.

The executive functions discussed in the previous chapter were believed to be localized to different regions of the prefrontal cortex. Figure 6.1 illustrates these regions of localized functions. I have taken the same figure used in Chapter 2 to illustrate these important brain regions. It may be helpful to refer to this figure throughout the

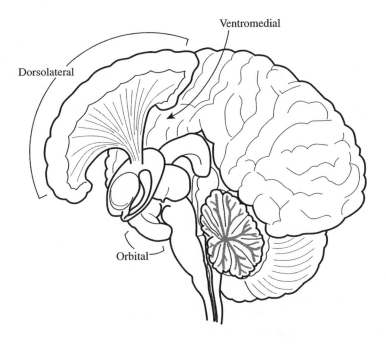

FIGURE 6.1. Diagram of the human brain with most of the left posterior hemisphere cut away to expose the right hemisphere. Illustrated here are the areas of the prefrontal lobes that correspond to the dorsolateral, ventromedial, and orbital regions. Adapted from an illustration by Carol Donner in Youdin and Riederer (1997, p. 53). Copyright 1997 by *Scientific American.* Adapted by permission.

following discussion when reference is made to these brain regions. Recall that the function of behavioral inhibition was believed to be localized to the orbital–prefrontal region, shown toward the bottom of Figure 6.1. Both nonverbal (internalized sensing) and verbal working memory (internalized speech) were believed to be localized to the dorsolateral regions of both frontal hemispheres. This region is indicated over the frontal portion that remains of the left hemisphere in Figure 6.1, the remainder of that hemisphere having been cut away. As discussed in the last chapter, it is likely that the function of reconstitution takes place within this same dorsolateral region of both hemispheres. Finally, the function of the self-regulation of affect, motivation, and arousal has been attributed to the ventromedial regions that are contained on the inner or midline surfaces of both hemispheres. We will see that neuroimaging research tends to support this same localization of functions hypothesized to exist by theorists in the previous chapter.

Behavioral Inhibition

Do neuroimaging studies support the involvement of a distinct region of the prefrontal lobes in behavioral inhibition and interference control separate from the regions supporting the other functions? As noted in Chapters 3 and 5, studies of humans with brain injuries suggest that the orbital–prefrontal region is involved in behavioral inhibition (Cummings, 1995; Truelle et al., 1995). To the extent that inhibitory behavior must be sustained over extended periods of time, the right prefrontal region may also be involved, given its role in sustained persistence of responding and interference control.

A neuroimaging study by Bench et al. (1993) using PET scan to study the brain regions related to performance of the Stroop Word–Color Association Test (Interference part) appears to be consistent with earlier studies of brain-injured patients. In one experiment, performance of this part of the Stroop test resulted in activation of the right orbital–prefrontal regions (in addition to the posterior parietal structures likely to be involved in the sensory–perceptual requirements of the task). In a second experiment in which parameters of the Stroop test were altered so as to create a faster presentation rate of stimuli and thus create a greater demand for persistence of attention and effort, findings indicated that the right frontal polar cortex and the right anterior cingulate were now more likely to be activated. Such findings are consistent with the view that prefrontal executive functions are not only interactive but involve a distributed network of brain regions, with some regions being more or less involved depending on the nature of the executive functions demanded by the task. Once again, when sustained attention, persistence of effort, and resistance to distraction must be maintained as more important aspects of the task, the right prefrontal region appears to become more involved. When the major demands of the task seem to involve response inhibition, as in the first experiment, the orbital–prefrontal cortex is more likely to be activated, particularly on the right side.

Working Memory

The inhibition of prepotent responses seems to be localized to the orbital–prefrontal regions and in particular the right prefrontal region when demands for interference control are inherent in a task. Is there evidence from neuroimaging studies that working memory is localized to a region distinct from this one, in support of factor-analytic studies buttressing such a distinction? After all, a large number of studies of frontal lobe–injured patients have suggested that the dorsolateral regions of the prefrontal cortex are instrumental to the performance of working memory tasks (see Chapter 5; also Cummings, 1995; Fuster, 1989, 1995; Goldman-Rakic, 1995a, 1995b). Such lesions also tend to produce a simplification of motor behavior to more automatic, context dependent, or field driven and generally less complex behavior than normal (Cummings, 1995; Milner, 1995; Truelle et al., 1995). I believe that the evidence available from neuroimaging studies quite strongly supports an affirmative answer to this question.

Smith, Jonides, and Koeppe (1996) recently reported three separate experiments in which subjects performed working memory tasks while brain activity was being evaluated using PET scan. In the first experiment, the subjects were required to retain either the names of four letters in mind or the positions of three dots across an interval of 3 seconds. The former assessed verbal working memory and the latter nonverbal (spatial) working memory. Results indicated a clear-cut double dissociation between the regions activated during these tasks. Regions within the left hemisphere were activated during the verbal task while areas of the right hemisphere mediated performance of the spatial position task. In the second experiment, the same four letters were employed as in the first task except subjects either had to remember the names of the letters, as in experiment 1, or they had to remember the positions of the letters in a display. In this case, the verbal task once again activated left-hemisphere regions. However, the spatial task was found to result in activation of both hemispheres, though activity was somewhat greater in the right than left hemisphere. In the final study by these authors, a continuous verbal memory task was employed, which found the same regions of the left hemisphere to be activated as in the discrete verbal memory task of letter naming. The authors concluded that verbal and spatial working memory were being mediated by different neuronal structures. Such findings are consistent with my position in this volume that verbal and nonverbal working memory are distinct executive functions.

Another study addressed the distinction between spatial and nonspatial working memory using functional magnetic resonance imaging (FMRI). In this study (McCarthy et al., 1996), subjects performed tasks that required them to remember either the location or the shape of successive visual stimuli presented to them during the imaging procedure. Results indicated that the spatial location memory task preferentially activated the middle frontal gyrus of the right hemisphere, while the shape (nonspatial) working memory task activated this same gyrus in both hemispheres. The latter finding may have resulted from the fact that geometric shapes can be considered either nonverbal, spatial forms of information or, if they have a readily recognizable shape, as involving both verbal and nonverbal information during the memory task. Consequently, it is not surprising to see that both hemispheres may have been activated by this task. In conjunction with the results of Smith et al. (1996), this study again points to the right hemisphere, in this case the right prefrontal cortex, as more activated during spatial working memory tasks than is the left prefrontal cortex. Moreover, McCarthy et al. (1996) were able to show that the mnemonic nature of the task greatly activated the prefrontal cortex in contrast to a perceptual target detection task, where activation of these regions was considerably less. This study also suggests that different regions of the prefrontal cortex will be activated as a function of the content of the information that must be retained during delay periods. Such a finding is supportive of Goldman-Rakic's (1995a) assertion, discussed in Chapter 5, that there can be many different forms of working memory and different regions of the prefrontal dorsolateral cortex subserving them as a result of the nature of the information requiring retention during delay intervals.

Further support for Goldman-Rakic's (1995a) view of working memory as being multifaceted comes from a recent study by Courtney, Ungerleider, Keil, and Haxby (1996) that used PET scan to evaluate those brain regions involved in working memory for faces in contrast to those regions involved in working memory for spatial location. These tasks were believed to distinguish two important forms of nonverbal working memory that both human and primate studies have identified, memory for objects (or the "what" pathway) and for the locations of objects (the "where" pathway). Compared to memory for faces, spatial-location memory tasks activated the superior and inferior parietal cortex as well as the superior frontal sulcus. During the working memory task for faces, the inferior frontal and anterior cingulate cortices, among other areas, were more activated than during the spatial memory task. Such findings again suggest that working memory for spatial location involves frontal regions, among other brain regions, that are distinct from those frontal regions activated by object memory tasks.

Other studies using neuroimaging during working memory tasks have continued to support the involvement of the dorsolateral prefrontal cortex in such tasks (Gold, Berman, Randolph, Goldberg, & Weinberger, 1996; Milner, 1995). The content of the information to be retained in working memory, as well as the actions to be taken with it, appear to determine which of the regions within the lateral prefrontal cortex are involved in the performance of such tasks and whether left or right prefrontal regions play a more active role. Thus, all of the studies reviewed so far support the conclusion that the dorsolateral aspects of the prefrontal cortex are involved in the executive function of representational or working memory. Different dorsolateral prefrontal regions, and even some subcortical structures, will be involved as a function of the mnemonic content of the memory task. The same is true when considering which posterior hemispheric regions will be activated during the task.

Most of the aforementioned studies on working memory dealt with various forms of nonverbal working memory. Is there evidence of different neural regions of the prefrontal cortex being involved in private speech and verbal working memory? The studies cited earlier imply that verbal working memory is more likely to be asymmetrically represented in the left than the right dorsolateral prefrontal regions, in keeping with the lateralization of the neural mechanisms underlying speech to this hemisphere in most individuals. If, as I believe, private or covert speech is involved in verbal working memory, then the study by Smith et al. (1996) suggests that the left cerebral hemisphere is more likely to participate in this type of working memory than the right hemisphere. Are the same regions involved in covert speech? Perhaps. Ryding et al. (1996) used a measure of regional cerebral blood flow to investigate those brain regions that may mediate silent or covert speech as compared to public or overt speech. In both of their studies, the silent speech task resulted in a pattern of activation that involved the left hemisphere speech perception and speech motor control areas, consistent with the well-known involvement of the left prefrontal regions in speech production. The prefrontal cortex appeared to be significantly activated in this silent speech activity (silent counting) relative to audible (overt) speech (counting). However, activation of the right dorsolateral prefrontal cortex also occurred in this task, perhaps as a result of the requirement to retain the position within the sequence in mind as well as to sustain attention toward the task. The latter interpretation is based on other studies that have shown this region to be involved in sustained attention tasks (Pardo, Fox, & Raichle, 1991) in addition to the retention of position information in mind while performing a task (Courtney et al., 1996; McCarthy et al., 1996; Smith et al., 1996). These findings for internalized or self-directed speech implicate different regions of the prefrontal cortex than would be involved in the internalized visual–spatial sensing that appears to be involved in spatial working memory tasks discussed earlier.

It would appear then that working memory is associated with a region of the prefrontal cortex that is distinct from that of behavioral inhibition. The former appears to necessitate activation of the dorso-lateral regions of the prefrontal cortex while the latter appears more likely to activate the orbital–prefrontal regions. However, persistence and interference control may be asymmetrically represented, localized more to the right anterior regions than to the left.

Reconstitution

As I discussed in Chapter 5, it is not clear whether reconstitution, or the generation of novel behavioral rules, response diversity, and behavioral flexibility, is distinct from or is simply a more complex stage of representational activities within working memory. Is there evidence to localize the executive function of reconstitution as I have extracted it from earlier theories?

Evidence from such studies suggests that if the information being retained in working memory must be manipulated during the delay period, different regions of the prefrontal cortex are activated than when working memory is involved in the organization of a sequence of responses. Petrides (1994) has argued that lateral aspects of the prefrontal cortex, well substantiated as being involved in working memory, may be subdivided into two separate systems. Recently, Owen, Evans, and Petrides (1996) found evidence for this argument when they found, using PET scan, that the ventrolateral regions were more likely to be activated when a sequence of responses had to be planned and executed using working memory than when spatial information within working memory had to be manipulated. The latter task was more likely to activate the middorsolateral frontal cortex.

Such findings could be viewed simply as being consistent with the observations of Fuster (1989, 1995) and Goldman-Rakic (1995a) that working memory is comprised of two processes, one associated with sensory representations during delay periods and the other with the motor representations that preset the motor system for responding to the anticipated event. However, these neuroimaging studies may also suggest that within the working memory system, the manipulation of sensory representations may be carried out by somewhat separate regions within the dorsolateral cortex from those that maintain the sensory representations on-line during delay periods. This would argue for a two-stage process in working memory, the first of which involves the representation of information and the organization of a sequence of responses as a function of it, while the second stage involves the manipulation of the information being represented, as Petrides (1994) has suggested.

Various forms of fluency were mentioned in Chapter 5 as reflecting the function of reconstitution as Bronowski (1967/1977) construed it. Neuroimaging studies using this type of task might shed some light on the issue of whether this executive function is the result of brain regions distinct from those involved in working or representational memory. Cardebat and colleagues (Cardebat et al., 1996) used single photon emission computed tomography (SPECT) scanning to evaluate changes in regional cerebral blood flow in normal subjects during performance of two fluency tasks. One was the more traditional or formal verbal fluency task that requires subjects to generate as many words as possible that begin with a particular letter in a short time period (2 minutes). The other was a semantic fluency task requiring subjects to generate as many words as possible belonging to a particular semantic category, such as animals and fruits, using the same 2-minute period. A baseline condition was used in which subjects had to repeat words for a 2-minute period. The activation by this task was then used as the comparison condition for the two fluency tasks.

Results indicated no significant increase in frontal lobe activity during the letter or formal fluency task over this baseline condition; however, this may be a consequence of the use of a verbal task that required repetition of words, thereby producing some activation of the left frontal region associated with speech planning and production. This might have obscured any activation of this region by the letter fluency task when compared to it, given that such a fluency task is believed to be associated with more left than right frontal lobe activity. Other neuroimaging studies using verbal fluency tasks have shown greater activation in the dorsolateral prefrontal regions, particularly on the left, underscoring this point that the baseline task used in this study may have obscured such a finding (Friston, Frith, Liddle, & Frackowiak, 1993; Frith, Friston, Liddle, & Frackowiak, 1991).

The semantic fluency task, in contrast, resulted in a significant increase in the right dorsolateral and medial frontal regions relative to the baseline task. Such findings are consistent with studies of brain-injured patients that have suggested greater involvement of right than left prefrontal regions in using semantic knowledge for categorization. The regions activated in these fluency tasks, however, are comparable to those that have been found in verbal and nonverbal working memory tasks, suggesting that the function of reconstitution (behavioral diversity and flexibility) is housed within the same regions as those subserving working memory. This evidence would argue that reconstitution may not be so much an executive function distinct from working memory as a later, more advanced developmental stage of it.

Certain WCST scores from the factor-analytic studies discussed earlier also may reflect the executive function of reconstitution. Recall that several of those studies identified a dimension that some researchers, such as Mirsky (1996), termed flexibility. Measures of the number of categories (sorting rules) correctly identified by subjects appeared to load heavily on this dimension. Such flexibility of behavior in tasks having ambiguous rules that must be both detected by the individual and then changed as feedback for behavior is changed have been attributed by both neuropsychologists (Dehaene & Changeux, 1995) and behavior analysts (Cerutti, 1989; Hayes et al., 1996) to the capacity of humans to formulate rules. The synthesis of such rules and the novel, complex behaviors they permit I have assigned to the reconstitutive function derived from Bronowski (1967/1977). By this line of reasoning, one might consider the WCST to reflect, in part, this executive function, though, as I have argued in this chapter and in Chapter 4, it also reflects working memory to some extent, given the need to hold feedback in mind so as to construct a rule that will shift behavior in a new direction (Marenco, Coppola, Daniel, Zigun, & Weinberger, 1993). Neuroimaging research using the WCST therefore may shed some light on the localization of the working memory system (particularly verbal) as well as on the reconstitutive function dependent upon it.

Nine studies were found that used neuroimaging methods to study those brain regions that seem to mediate the WCST (Berman, Zec, & Weinberger, 1986; Berman et al., 1991, 19955; Daniel et al., 1991; Marenco et al., 1993; Osmon, Zigun, Suchy, & Blint, 1996; Rezai et al., 1993; Rubin et al., 1991). All of these studies found that regions of the prefrontal cortex mediated task performance, particularly the dorsolateral regions.

Supporting the interpretation that several executive functions are involved in the WCST, several distinct regions of the prefrontal lobes were activated during task performance, in addition to posterior hemisphere regions that would be involved in the perceptual demands of the task. One study (Marenco et al., 1993) found activation of the right anterior prefrontal area, which, as noted earlier, seems to be involved in both persistence of responding and interference control. The second region activated in that study comprised the more posterior dorsolateral regions of the prefrontal lobes, which have been associated with working memory functions, as noted earlier. This region has been found to be most commonly activated during the WCST across these studies (Berman et al., 1995). The third region found to have increased activation in the Marenco et al. (1993) study was the medial regions of the frontal lobes, to which Damasio (1995) and others have ascribed affective, motivation, and arousal functions. Osmon et al. (1996) were able to demonstrate that the rule-learning function of the task was more related to dorsolateral prefrontal regions than was the attribute-identification aspect of the task. That aspect was less likely to be associated with prefrontal activation than with posterior hemisphere activation.

Across these studies, there has been a trend toward somewhat greater activation of the left dorsolateral prefrontal regions during this task (Rezai et al., 1993), although the results are quite mixed (see Berman et al., 1995, for a review of most studies). This tendency toward greater left prefrontal involvement could be the result of the subject having to construct a verbal rule from the performance feedback that will subsequently guide responding, as Dunbar and Sussman (1995) have suggested. While such asymmetrical activation may also stem from the subject's use of the right (typically dominant) hand in task performance, Berman et al. (1995) subtracted out such sensorimotor involvement in the task from their analysis of activation patterns and still found somewhat greater left prefrontal involvement in its performance. Nevertheless, both dorsolateral prefrontal regions become activated during the task, most likely reflecting the task's requirements for both verbal and nonverbal working memory and the need to extract a verbal rule to guide behavior (Berman et al., 1995; Dehaene & Changeux, 1995; Dunbar & Sussman, 1995).

Berman et al. (1995) also identified some degree of increased activation of the orbital prefrontal regions in performance of the task in their study. Perhaps this was a result of the task requirements for inhibiting prepotent responses so as to shift to following a new rule. As noted earlier, and in Chapter 5, the orbital–prefrontal region has been frequently associated with task demands for response inhibition (Cummings, 1995; Truelle et al., 1995).

Taken together, such research indicates that the WCST does not cleanly measure one type of executive function nor one specific prefrontal region. Instead, the test seems to involve several or even all of the executive functions I identified in Chapter 5 and their respective prefrontal regions. This makes sense given the complex demands of this task. Nevertheless, the study by Osmon et al. (1996) implies that the dorsolateral regions are more involved in the rule-formulation aspects of the task. Studies of brain-injured samples likewise attribute the flexibility aspects of the WCST to these same regions (Grattan, Bloomer, Archambault, & Eslinger, 1994). Given that this area has been most often associated with working memory, this finding would imply that the reconstitutive function is part of the working memory components of the model rather than dissociable from it. Thus, although the factor-analytic studies of neuropsychological test batteries indicate support for a separate factor of reconstitution and response flexibility, neuroimaging studies do not. Instead, the latter research appears to show such executive activities to be mediated by the same prefrontal regions subserving a psychological dimension of working or representational memory.

Planning

Planning is considered by many neuropsychologists to characterize the executive functions. This ability has been thought to involve the manipulation of events being held in working memory so as to guide an effective response to a task. In that sense, planning involves several executive functions—inhibition and interference control, working memory, and reconstitution. The TOL has been frequently used in neuropsychological research to study planning ability. Four neuroimaging studies using this task were located. Two of these employed SPECT scan to evaluate cerebral blood flow during the task, and one employed PET scan to evaluate brain metabolic activity. Rezai and colleagues (1993) used SPECT scan to study frontal lobe activation while subjects performed a variety of executive function tasks, including the TOL. Findings suggested that the TOL was more likely to activate mesial regions of the prefrontal cortex bilaterally than was the WCST, which was associated with dorsolateral activation, primarily on the left side. The fact that performance on a CPT in the Rezai et al. (1993) study activated the same prefrontal region as the TOL may suggest that such activation comes more from the cingulate gyrus than the mesial cortex. SPECT scans have some difficulty distinguishing activity in these regions, and the cingulate gyrus is believed to be involved more in sustained attention. Both tasks require persistence as well as interference control; the authors suggest that the former might explain this activation finding.

Morris, Ahmed, Syed, and Toone (1993) also employed SPECT scanning to evaluate neural activation patterns during performance of the TOL. These investigators employed a motor control procedure and subtracted out activation that may have been a function of the motor requirements of the TOL. In contrast to that of Rezai et al. (1993), this study found that the left prefrontal region was activated during the performance of this task. The more time the subjects took in planning their moves before responding as well as the fewer moves they employed in solving the problem, the greater was the activation in this region. Although the TOL has often been viewed as placing greater demands on visual–spatial working memory and the manipulation of sensory representations of objects within space, this finding might suggest that covert self-speech may also be involved during the planning stages of the task. As discussed Chapter 5, children and adults often employ self-speech during problem-solving tasks as a means of elaborating possible response options via verbal description of the task. But self-speech also permits self-questioning, the development of possible rules that may solve the problem, and the deployment of those rules during the motor performance of the task (Levin et al., 1994).

Perhaps helping to integrate the findings of the preceding studies is the PET scan study by Baker and colleagues (1996). These investigators found that performance on the TOL activated three separate prefrontal regions, apart from the activation of posterior parietal and occipital cortices that would be needed for the sensory perceptual (visual–spatial) demands of the task. The authors found significant activation in the dorsolateral prefrontal regions bilaterally, and interpreted this finding as reflecting both the nonverbal and verbal working memory demands involved in this task. The second region activated was the rostrolateral prefrontal cortex, a finding the authors interpreted as reflecting the generation of imagined response sequences and their evaluation and selection. The third region involved the anterior insula and inferior frontal gyrus; their activation was interpreted as reflecting automatic sequencing of moves required within the task and imagining of their movement.

Such findings illustrate that the TOL, like the WCST, involves multiple executive functions. Thus, its performance may not be localizable to a single region, but reflects the interactive nature of the executive system when performing complex problem-solving activities. Information that would involve both nonverbal and verbal working memory systems must be held in mind and manipulated; the performance of such covert, self-directed actions must be protected from interference, and prepotent responses must be inhibited, thereby involving the behavioral inhibition system (see Goel & Grafman, 1995); multiple response possibilities must be generated and evaluated, involving reconstitution, rule generation, and response flexibility; and the sequence of behaviors involved in the chosen option must then be communicated to the premotor planning and motor execution areas for performance. These neuroimaging studies clearly indicate, then, that tasks such as the TOL that are believed to assess planning ability involve multiple executive functions that must interact in concert to perform the task, rather than just reflecting spatial working memory, as some researchers have previously believed. Consistent with this view of the TOL, recall the results from the factor-analytic study by Levin et al. (1996) that different scores from the TOL loaded on different dimensions: response flexibility (reconstitution) and working memory.

Such flexibility has been shown to be hampered in practice, however, by injuries to the medial or mesial aspects of the prefrontal cortex (Grattan et al., 1994). This may be because of its contribution of the affective/motivational outcomes to these response options that permits decision making among them to occur (Damasio, 1995).

Summary of Findings

In summarizing the foregoing neuroimaging studies, it should be noted that this relatively recent approach to the study of brain functions in normal individuals has resulted in findings that are relatively consistent with earlier lesion studies of humans and animals. Though far more research using these new technologies remains to be done to pinpoint more precisely the brain regions and their networks involved in various aspects of executive functioning, more general, tentative conclusions are possible at this time. These conclusions seem reasonably consistent with the studies of brain-injured patients that suggest that orbital-prefrontal regions are more involved in behavioral inhibition (Cummings, 1995; Truelle et al., 1995; Vendrell et al., 1995), while dorsolateral prefrontal regions may be more involved in various forms of representational or working memory (Cummings, 1995; Fuster, 1989; Goldman-Rakic, 1995a, 1995b). Where behavior must be sustained along with inhibition and resistance to distraction, the right prefrontal region, particular its most anterior polar region, may be more involved in performance of such tasks (Knight et al., 1995; Pardo et al., 1991; Rueckert & Grafman, 1996). This is not to ignore some of the inconsistencies across these studies seeking to evaluate the brain regions associated with the same task or executive function under study. But these inconsistencies do not contradict the issue here, which is that different brain regions in the prefrontal lobes appear to be associated with different executive functions. More to the point of this chapter, however, such findings speak not only to the separate existence of some of the executive functions, but are in keeping with the results of the factor-analytic studies reviewed. Thus, neuroimaging studies further support distinctions among the basic executive functions, especially behavioral inhibition, verbal and nonverbal working memory, and maintenance of drive and effort in support of a goal (persistence of responding to verbal rules). Neuroimaging studies, however, are not able to show that a separate executive function of reconstitution and the response flexibility it permits are subserved by prefrontal regions distinct from those involved in working memory.

As many of the investigators conducting these neuroimaging studies noted in their articles, tasks involving working memory do not simply activate the prefrontal regions subserving this executive function. They also activate a variety of posterior hemisphere as well as subcortical regions. The latter areas of activation are often interpreted as reflecting the particular sensory–motor processing demands being made by the particular working memory task. This is certainly likely to be the case. Yet the activation of these posterior regions, particularly those involved in complex sensory phenomena, may in part be reflecting the various forms of sensing to the self I described in Chapter 5. For instance, the TOL places heavy demands on working memory, both verbal and nonverbal. We should not be surprised then to see that visual–spatial association regions of the posterior cortex are activated by this task, not just because the subject is looking at the stimulus array, but also because the subject is actively engaged in private imagery and the manipulation of that imagery in covertly testing out various simulations or rearrangements of the stimulus array. Surely the subject is also engaging in private, self-speech as part of this testing out of various response options in order to discover the rules or steps to follow in achieving the correct design arrangement. This self-speech would, likewise, activate not only anterior regions related to subvocal speech to the self but also posterior speech association regions related to the covert perception and comprehension of that speech. Therefore, I believe that the neuroimaging studies cited in this chapter give testimony not only to those regions of the prefrontal lobes subserving the executive functions, but also to the forms of private sensory–motor behaviors directed at the self of which those functions are comprised.

RELATIONSHIP OF INTELLIGENCE TO EXECUTIVE FUNCTIONS

The skeptic may suggest that many of the functions described as executive sound a lot like intelligence, particularly the major subtypes of intelligence often called verbal and performance IQ (nonverbal, visual–spatial–constructional ability). How can we be sure that the executive functions, as set forth in Chapter 5 and discerned in the factor-analytic and neuroimaging studies discussed in this chapter are distinct from IQ? After all, many studies exist in neuropsychology to show that verbal abilities are asymmetrically represented in the left hemisphere and that visual–spatial–constructional abilities are more likely to be represented in the right hemisphere. Could not these two major, well-established patterns of abilities and their asymmetrical representation in the cerebral hemispheres account for many of the findings, particularly those concerning verbal and nonverbal working memory? To address such skeptics, research must show that these executive functions are reasonably distinct from traditional measures of intelligence.

The literature that supports such a distinction is far more vast and complex than space or reason would permit reviewing here. I will simply cite a few lines of evidence to support the contention that the executive functions cited in this and the previous chapter are not just forms of verbal and performance intelligence masquerading under another name (i.e., executive functions, or EF).

One line of evidence supporting the IQ–EF distinction is represented in the large number of studies of patients suffering injuries to the prefrontal lobes. Such patients often show little or no alteration in their IQ scores as a function of such lesions (Stuss & Benson, 1986), depending in large part on how IQ is defined and measured. If measures of fluid intelligence are used, which have a closer similarity to the executive functions of planning, working memory, impulse control, flexibility, concept formation, and the like, then frontal lobe patients may well show impairments in this form of IQ (Duncan, Burgess, & Emslie, 1995; Stuss & Benson, 1986).

A second line of evidence comes from studies of the factorial structure of IQ tests themselves. For instance, research on the development of the Wechsler Intelligence Scales has repeatedly identified a third factor separate from that of verbal and performance IQ, which Kaufman once named the Freedom-from-Distractibility factor (see Kaufman, 1975, 1980, for the children's versions as well as test manuals for WISC-R, WISC-III, and WAIS-R). This factor is often comprised of tests of Arithmetic, Digit Span (forward and backward), and Coding/Digit Symbol. Tests of mental arithmetic and recall of digit span have often been used to assess verbal working memory and frequently formed such a dimension in those studies. This finding has led some theorists to suggest that these three tests are assessing more than just freedom from distractibility (see Ownby & Matthews, 1985;

Stewart & Moely, 1983). However, in keeping with both Fuster's (1980, 1989, 1995) and Goldman-Rakic's (1995a, 1995b) concepts of provisional or working memory as discussed in Chapter 5, interference control is critical in working memory. Thus, these IQ subtests may well reflect both the ability to represent information in mind so as to act upon it (working memory) as well as resistance to distraction (interference control). Related to these findings of a separate dimension of working memory from IQ are the results of the Taylor et al. study (1996; see Table 6.3) that separate dimensions of verbal working memory and nonverbal working memory (Factors 4 and 5) were distinguished from those of verbal and performance IQ (Factors 1 and 2). In any case, such studies suggest that at least the construct of working memory is dissociable from that of intelligence as traditionally assessed (i.e., crystallized), as others have concluded as well (Embretson, 1995; Miller & Vernon, 1996).

Studies using factor analysis with intelligence tests and tests involving executive functions so as to evaluate the heritability of both general intelligence and specific cognitive abilities also shed some light on this issue. Cardon, Fulker, DeFries, and Plomin (1992) studied adopted and nonadopted children in the Colorado Adoption Project. The authors not only found that a separate factor for working memory was distinguished from that for verbal and performance intellectual abilities, but that the pattern of heritabilities varied across these domains of functioning. These heritabilities were independent of those affecting general cognitive ability, or *g*. Environmental influences were found to make little contribution to explaining individual differences on these more specific cognitive abilities. Similar results were found by Pedersen, Plomin, and McClearn (1994) using samples of twins and adoptees from the Swedish Adoption/Twin Study on Aging, and by Luo, Petrill, and Thompson (1994) using twins from the Western Reserve Twin Project. These and other studies suggest that a factor of cognitive abilities is associated with representational or working memory but is distinct from general cognitive ability (*g*) as well as more specific measures of verbal and performance intelligence. Moreover, genetic influences make the largest contribution to individual differences on the working memory factor, while common environmental factors explain little of this variance among individuals (see also Wadsworth, DeFries, Fulker, Olson, & Pennington, 1995). Studies also suggest that individual differences in verbal working memory explain most of the differences among individuals in reading performance, especially in reading comprehension (Swanson & Berninger, 1995; Wadsworth et al., 1995), and that both share common genetic influences (Wadsworth et al., 1995).

These findings are important because they demonstrate not only that working memory as an executive function is dissociable from general intelligence, but also that individual differences in working memory are largely determined by genetic factors. Recall that genetic factors likewise explained the largest proportion of individual differences in the etiologies of ADHD, as discussed in Chapter 2. As a result, I conjectured that any theoretical model of ADHD using neuropsychological constructs would have to involve components that would, likewise, be shown to have a substantial hereditary contribution to them. The evidence for working memory is in keeping with this theoretical supposition.

What of the other executive functions? Are they also relatively free of contamination by IQ or general cognitive ability? Again, the factor-analytic studies reviewed earlier would suggest that this is the case, in that studies such as that by Taylor et al. (1996) and others find dimensions for executive functions such as behavioral inhibition and response flexibility or reconstitution that seem to be separable from those for verbal and performance IQ. Psychological research also shows that the correlations of measures of inhibition (such as the Stroop test), measures of persistence of effort (such as CPTs), and tests of behavioral flexibility and rule discovery (such as the WCST) with measures of IQ are statistically significant but are rather modest in size. IQ appears to account for less than 10–12% of the variance typically found in these other measures (Dempster, 1991), suggesting that individual differences in these executive functions are not primarily explained by differences in general intellectual ability. As McCall (1994) has argued, it may be from a developmental psychological perspective that the direction of contribution here is from the executive functions to that of intelligence rather than vice versa.

CONCLUSION

This chapter has reviewed additional evidence in support of both the existence of and the distinction among the constructs of behavioral inhibition and the four executive functions derived in Chapter 5 from reviews of theories of these functions. Studies using factor analysis of neuropsychological test batteries seem to identify separate dimensions of performance related to behavioral inhibition, working memory, behavioral fluency/flexibility (reconstitution), and persistence of responding and effort (the self-regulation of motivation/arousal). Some of these studies also suggest that working memory can be subdivided into two separate factors related to nonverbal and verbal working memory abilities. The results are not always consistent across studies, however, and the interpretations given to these psychological dimensions by the authors of these studies are not necessarily the same as those I have given them here. Nevertheless, it seems to me that there is sufficient consistency across studies to conclude that these executive functions exist and may be dissociable from one another. Such psychological dimensions do not appear to be explained by general cognitive ability or intelligence (*g*) and, at least for working memory, have been shown to be separable from a dimension representing such general ability. Studies using neuroimaging procedures seem to have identified distinct regions of the prefrontal cortex that mediate several of these executive functions, particularly response inhibition, nonverbal and verbal working memory, and even persistence of effort and responding. The study Mariani and I (1997) conducted using preschoolers intimates the possibility that a general working memory system exists in the preschool years, from which a separate verbal working memory system has not yet emerged. It may be that attempts by children in this age group to perform verbal working memory tasks are likely to rely more heavily on nonverbal visual and auditory resensing than on truly covert self-speech (verbal working memory), which has not yet developed in such children in its fully covert form.

Less clear from these studies is whether behavioral flexibility or reconstitution is subserved by prefrontal brain regions distinct from those for working memory. This may indicate, as I discussed in Chapter 5, that reconstitution may represent a more advanced stage in the development of working memory rather than representing an entirely distinct executive function.

I believe that the evidence reviewed in this chapter and the previous one is sufficient to accept the existence of these rather general executive functions and the likely dissociation among them. I also believe that such evidence is sufficient to permit the formulation of a general model of these executive functions that is a hybrid of models developed previously by others and reviewed in Chapter 5. The construction of that hybrid model is the goal of the next chapter.

CHAPTER 7

———•———

Constructing the Hybrid Model of Executive Functions

IN THE PREVIOUS TWO chapters, I reviewed several models of the executive or prefrontal lobe functions, noted their points of overlap and distinction, and discussed evidence for the existence of behavioral inhibition and four separable executive functions. These functions have been consistently shown in research to be mediated by the prefrontal regions of the brain and to be disrupted by damage or injury to these various regions. The hybrid model to be developed in this chapter specifies that behavioral inhibition, representing the first component in the model, is critical to the proficient performance of the executive functions. It permits them, supports their occurrence, and protects them from interference, just as it does for the generation and execution of the cross-temporal behavioral structures developed from these executive functions. I have taken Bronowski's (1967/1977) lead here in separating the internalization of speech (verbal working memory) from nonverbal working memory even though I view both as being a part of a larger system of working or provisional memory, as described in Chapter 5. This division results in four executive functions in the hybrid model dependent on behavioral inhibition, namely, (1) nonverbal working memory, (2) internalization of speech (verbal working memory), (3) the self-regulation of affect/motivation/arousal, and (4) reconstitution.

These executive functions, despite having distinct labels, are believed to share a common purpose—to permit self-control so as to anticipate change and the future, thereby maximizing the long-term outcomes or benefits for the individual. These four functions also share a common characteristic—all represent private, covert forms of behavior that at one time in development were entirely public and outer- or other-directed in form. They have become turned on the self to control behavior, and have become covert or internalized in form as maturation proceeds. As Michon and Jackson (1984) noted:

> Life distinguishes itself from inorganic nature in its potential for *self-organization,* the ability to develop an internal structure that creates a certain, growing independence from the vicissitudes of the environment. Greater independence is usually achieved by *internalizing* the environment. . . . At one stage in their evolution, it has occurred to most species that one of the most powerful aids for self-organization is the *internalization of change as such.* This allowed them to anticipate certain regular changes in the environment and to return, for instance, to their lair before it became dark in the evening. (p. 299)

I believe that the executive functions represent the internalization of behavior so as to anticipate such change in the environment. That change is essentially the concept of time. Therefore, what the internalization of behavior achieves is the internalization of a sense of time, which is then applied toward the organization of behavior in order to anticipate sequences of change in the environment, events that probably lie ahead in time. Such behavior is therefore future-oriented, and the individual who employs it can be said to be independent, goal directed, purposive, and intentional in his or her actions. This process of internalization has received almost no attention in neuropsychology, but it has been studied to some extent in developmental psychology as it may pertain to the internalization of speech (Diaz & Berk, 1992), and, to a much lesser extent, to the internalization of sight, or visual imagery (Berkowitz, 1982). Yet it is a rather miraculous process that must have some neural mechanisms and neuropsychological system responsible for it. It is a developmental neuropsychological process deserving of far greater study in its own right, apart from any specific executive function, for I believe it provides the origins of the executive functions identified in the last chapter. As I discuss in Chapter 8, I believe that, like language and its internalization during child development, this process is universal and instinctive, not merely a product of cultural training. It makes some sense, then, that inhibition should be instrumentally related to this process, for behavioral inhibition probably assists with the suppression of the observable motor accompaniments associated with each form of executive function, thus facilitating the internalization of behavior.

Behavioral inhibition and at least three of the executive functions identified in the previous chapter appear to be mediated by separate but surely interactive regions of the prefrontal lobes. Behavioral inhibition and its three-component processes seem to be localized to the orbital–prefrontal regions and associated interconnections to the striatum. There is accumulating evidence that persistent inhibition or resistance to distraction (interference control) may be somewhat more lateralized to the right anterior prefrontal region, while the capacity to inhibit prepotent responses so as to delay the decision to respond is situated in the orbital–prefrontal region. Working memory (both verbal and nonverbal) seems to be associated with the dorsolateral regions. And the regulation of affect/motivation/arousal has been attributed to the ventral–medial regions.

While I believe that each of these functions is capable of being dissociated from the others, as studies both of patients with frontal lobe injuries and of normal patients using modern neuroimaging techniques suggest, all of these functions are interactive and interreliant in their naturally occurring state. This is a critical point. *It is the action of these functions in concert that permits and produces normal human self-regulation.* Deficits in any particular executive function will produce a relatively distinct impairment in self-regulation, different from that impairment in self-control produced by deficits in the other functions. For instance, the loss of the capacity for internalized speech or for visual imagery may produce a pattern of self-regulatory deficits quite different from that created by an impairment in the ability to generate the somatic markers (affective/motivational states) typically associated with and arising from such internally generated forms of information.

Behavioral inhibition and the four other executive functions it supports influence the motor system, wresting it from complete control by the immediate environment so as to bring it under the control of time (change) and the future and to put it in to the service of goal-directed behavior. I have labeled the motor component of the model as *motor control/fluency/syntax.* The latter component emphasizes not only the features of control or management of the motor system which these executive functions afford, but also the synthetic capacity for generating a diversity of novel, complex, publicly observable motor responses and their sequences in a goal-directed manner. Such complex behavior requires the generation of an ideational syntax, an activity placed for now within the reconstitution component of the model, which must be translated into the actual execution of motor sequences, an activity placed within the motor control component.

These executive functions and the internalized forms of behavior they represent originate within the brain's motor system, broadly construed (prefrontal and frontal cortex). But they may also produce effects beyond the motor system, such as upon the sensory–perceptual, linguistic, memory, emotional, and other brain systems in an executive, managerial manner to the extent that the regulation of those other brain systems is necessary for the execution of goal-directed behavior (Fuster, 1989). Thus, while memory, linguistic, spatial, emotional, or even perceptual systems are viewed as brain systems that are relatively independent from those of the prefrontal cortex, these nonexecutive systems may be influenced or enslaved by the executive system as needed in the service of goal-directed behavior.

I will build the hybrid model one piece at a time. Although I represent the components of the model as geometric shapes (see Figures 7.1–7.8), they are not meant to be stages in an information-processing model. Such cognitive or information-processing models tend to use computers as a metaphor for brain functions, and I do not wish to employ that metaphor here. I prefer, instead, to think of the rectangular boxes as representing simply different forms of private, self-directed, and often covert behavior. Nor is the particular configuration of these boxes intended to be a critical element of the model. Other configurations would do just as well. It is the functions these boxes represent that I wish to emphasize here, as well as their hierarchical configuration. The executive functions are dependent on behavioral inhibition. The motor control component depends on both inhibition and those executive functions if behavior is to be internally guided (self-regulated) in the service of a goal. Beyond intending to convey this set of conditional relations, the exact arrangement of the boxes in the model is unimportant.

The goal here is admittedly ambitious; perhaps overly so, for the proposed model may be potentially misconstrued as a "theory of everything." Yet its boundaries are generally circumscribed to the domain of self-regulation in developmental psychology or executive functions in neuropsychology. Albeit a broad domain, it is not unlimited. It can be readily distinguished from other major domains of neuropsychological functioning, such as sensation and perception, memory, and so on. The model may overlap with these other domains, however, to the extent that self-regulation employs them in its goals. Let me reiterate that I fully recognize this model to be a relative simplification of a complex set of brain functions. The model is admittedly imperfect, but it will suffice to show (1) that a hybrid model of executive functions, broadly defined, can be discerned within current theoretical writings on these functions, and, more to the point of this book, (2) that such a model can be extended to understanding ADHD, a step of tremendous heuristic value.

BEHAVIORAL INHIBITION

The first piece of this model, and probably its most important, as Bronowski (1966/1977) had recognized, is the capacity for behavioral inhibition. The first executive function must be inhibiting the prepotent response from occurring or interrupting an ongoing response pattern that is proving ineffective. This creates a delay in responding during which the other executive functions (self-directed, covert actions) can occur, as they are dependent upon behavioral inhibition for their effective execution and their regulation over the motor programming and execution component of the model (motor control). This component of the model is shown in Figure 7.1. It exerts a direct influence over the behavioral programming and motor control system of the brain, as indicated by the downward arrow between these two systems. As previously defined, behavioral inhibition refers to three inhibitory functions: (1) the *inhibition of prepotent responses,* (2) the *interruption of ongoing responses* that are proving ineffective, and (3) the protection of the delay created by these forms of inhibition, the self-directed actions occurring within the delay (the remaining executive functions), and the goal-directed behaviors they generate from disruption by external and internal sources of interference (*interference control*).

As noted previously, behavioral inhibition does not directly cause the four intermediate executive functions to occur, but merely sets the occasion for their performance and protects that performance from interference. To visibly represent this crucial point, the lines I will use to eventually connect the component of behavioral inhibition to those other four executive functions will be blunted. But because these executive functions themselves produce direct and causal effects on the motor programming and execution system, lines with arrowheads will be placed between each of these executive functions in the figure and aimed at the motor control system to convey that direct, controlling influence.

Preventing a prepotent response from occurring is critical to self-control (see Chapter 3). The individual cannot engage in self-control so as to maximize later outcomes related to a particular event if he or she has already acted to maximize the immediate ones related to that event or context. This is particularly evident when there is a conflict between the valences of the immediate versus later outcomes (imme-

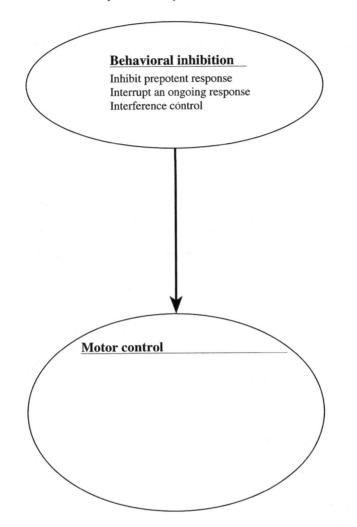

FIGURE 7.1. The influence of the behavioral inhibition system on the motor control system.

diately rewarding outcomes that lead to later and larger punitive ones or immediately aversive ones that lead to later and larger rewarding ones). As discussed in Chapter 3, such situations create a conflict for the individual between sources of behavioral control (typically external vs. internal) and so impose a demand on him or her to utilize self-directed, private forms of behavior and information to manage that situation successfully.

The capacity to interrupt an ongoing sequence of behavior is likewise critical to self-regulation. If the individual is currently engaged in a pattern or series of responses, and feedback for those responses, such as a shift in the schedule of the consequences toward apparently greater punitiveness or errors, is signaling their apparent ineffectiveness, then this sequence of behavior must be interrupted, the sooner the better. There must exist a flexibility in ongoing behavior that allows it to be altered quickly as the exigencies of the situation change and those changes are detected by the individual. This presupposes a degree of self-monitoring and awareness of immediately past responses and their outcomes, which permits the individual to read the signs in the trail of past behavior for information that may signal the need to shift response patterns. As discussed in the previous chapter, the nonverbal working memory component of the model probably contributes to this self-monitoring function, so the capacity to interrupt ongoing response patterns likely reflects an interaction of the behavioral inhibition system with working memory to achieve this end. This creates both a sensitivity to errors and the appearance of flexibility in the individual's ongoing performance in a task or situation. Once responding is interrupted, the delay is, once again, used for further self-directed action by the executive functions that will give rise to a new and, ideally, more effective pattern of responding toward the task or situation. The detection of the errors in the past and ongoing behavioral performance and the new pattern of behavior that will eventually be generated from analysis of that pattern of feedback both are believed to arise from the working memory component. However, the behavioral inhibition component must nevertheless become engaged to halt the current stream of responses in order to permit such analysis, synthesis, and midcourse correction to occur and to thereby redirect the motor programming and execution system to this new tack of responding.

The third inhibitory process in this component of the model is interference control. Interference control is as important to self-regulation as are the other inhibitory processes, especially during the delay in responding, when the other executive functions are at work. As Fuster (1980, 1989) noted, this is a time that is particularly vulnerable to both external and internal sources of interference. The world does not stop changing around the individual just because his or her responses to it have temporarily ceased and covert forms of self-directed behavior have been engaged. New events playing out around the individual may be disruptive to those executive functions taking place during the delay; the more similar those events are to the information being generated by these executive functions (private behaviors), the more difficult it is to protect those functions from disruption, distortion, or perversion. We all recognize this when we attempt to talk covertly to ourselves in a room full of loud conversation—and often state that we find it difficult to hear ourselves think in such situations. Likewise, sources of internal interference may arise, such as other ideas that occur in association with the ones that are the focus of the executive actions yet which are not relevant to the goal. In addition, the immediate past contents of working memory must be cleansed or suppressed, to prevent them from being carried forward into the formulation of the new goal-directed behavioral structure and thereby disrupting its construction and performance. All of this requires inhibition, which protects the self-regulatory actions of the individual from interference.

This aspect of the model is shown in Figure 7.2. The schematic diagram of the model now shows the behavioral inhibition system having not only a direct influence over the motor control system, but also a supportive and protective role with regard to the other four

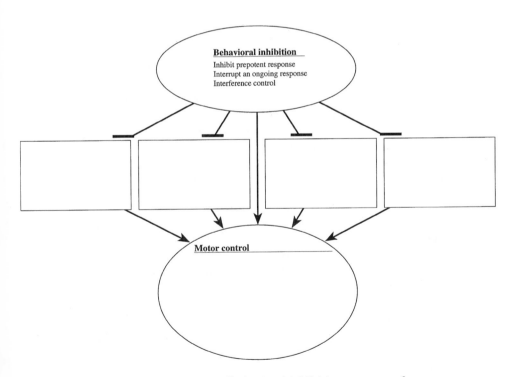

FIGURE 7.2. The relationship of behavioral inhibition system to four executive functions (boxes) and their relationship to the motor control system.

executive functions, the boxes for which have been left blank for the moment.

NONVERBAL WORKING MEMORY: COVERT SENSING TO THE SELF

Nonverbal working memory represents covert sensing to oneself. What is being resensed by this process is not just the event or its sensory representations but the entire behavioral contingency related to the event (event, response, and outcome). This component of the model is shown in Figure 7.3. It includes all forms of sensory–motor behavior of which humans are capable, two of which are particularly important to human self-regulation: covert visual imagery (seeing to oneself) and covert audition (hearing to oneself). These two internalized, covert sensory–motor behaviors or actions, along with the other types of sensory behavior, comprise a form of internal information or stimuli that is then used to guide behavior across time toward a goal. Although I use the neuropsychological term "nonverbal working memory" to represent these self-directed forms of sensory–motor behavior in this discussion, it is important to keep in mind the forms of private behavior that term represents. This will be critical to bridging the neuropsychological literature to those of developmental psychology and modern behavior analysis, where more behaviorlike descriptions of these same executive functions prevail (i.e., Berk, 1992; Hayes et al., 1996).

Given the preceding characterization of working memory as representing private, covert forms of sensing to oneself, I believe that Goldman-Rakic (1995a) is more likely to be correct than is Baddeley (1986; Baddeley & Hitch, 1994) about the nature of the working memory system.

Baddeley (1986) has described three components in the working memory system, these being (1) the visual–spatial sketch pad, (2) the phonological loop, and (3) the central executive. The visual–spatial sketch pad is a form of short-term memory that serves to hold and manipulate visual and spatial information. The phonological loop provides much the same functions for verbal or speech-based information. The central executive is an attentional control system, and it is the most complex yet least understood component. It coordinates the operations of the other two systems, in essence setting their goals or purposes. In a way, as discussed earlier, there are as many forms of working memory as there are forms of human sensory–motor behavior that can become self-directed and private or covert. There is not just a visual–spatial sketch pad and an articulatory loop, as Baddeley pro-

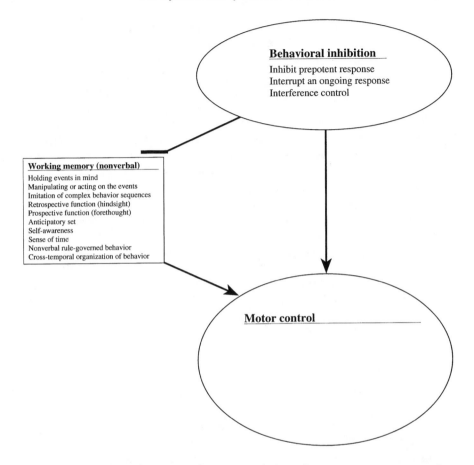

FIGURE 7.3. The functions of the nonverbal working memory system and its relationship to the behavioral inhibition and motor control systems.

posed, which corresponds in my thinking to visual imagery and self-speech. There are also likely to be found olfactory, gustatory, auditory, tactile, proprioceptive, and kinesthetic forms of working memory as well as combinations of these to the extent that sensory behavior is capable of cross-modal integration. Even so, while they may be dissociable, these various forms of private sensing to the self are likely to be occurring simultaneously in varying degrees as a function of the demands of a task or setting. Similarly, we are not likely to engage one form of working memory (sensing to the self) exclusively in any given task, though some may be emphasized to greater degrees than others as a function of those same demands of task and setting.

The retention and reactivation of prior sensory representations is the means by which events or information is "held in mind." When we "see" to ourselves, we are covertly reactivating the images of the past, just as when we hear, or taste, or smell to ourselves we are reactivating and maintaining prior sensory representations within these modalities. *Nonverbal working memory, then, is the capacity to hold events in mind so as to use them to control a response* (Goldman-Rakic, 1995a). In more common parlance, it is actually comprised of covert sensing to oneself that will serve to initiate the motor responses associated with those sensory representations when the situation calls for them. The number and types of such past events that can be reactivated and held on-line at any one time as well as the length or complexity of their temporal sequence likely increases with development. Eventually, individuals develop the capability not only to hold such events or series of events in mind (reactivate and maintain prior sensory events), but also to *manipulate or act upon the events* as task demands may necessitate. This ability to manipulate, analyze, and synthesize such sensory representations is likely to represent a later, more highly developed ability of the working memory systems, which will be discussed further in the discussion of the reconstitution component of the model.

Imitation and Vicarious Learning

Important to note but often unspecified in modern neuropsychological conceptualizations of working memory is that this ability underlies *the imitation of complex sequences of behavior* by individuals. Imitation is a powerful tool by which humans learn new behaviors. The power to imitate another person's behavior requires the capacity to retain a mental representation of the behavior to be imitated. In many cases, that representation will be made through visual imagery or covert audition.

For instance, to imitate a sequence of gestures, as in the Kaufman Hand Movements Test (Kaufman & Kaufman, 1983), the subject of that test must be able to mentally represent (privately re-image) the observed sequence of hand gestures during the delay between demonstration and the required reproduction of that sequence. Alternatively, he or she must in some way fix the sequence in mind using self-speech by labeling each gesture in the sequence and then restating the labels covertly. In either case, forms of working memory (private, self-directed imagery or speech) will be needed in order to correctly imitate the sequence of hand movements; the longer that sequence, the greater the demand for such covert representations so as to correctly perform the task. Thus, one can predict that the more lengthy and complex the sequences of new behavior that individuals are expected to imitate, the greater will be the demand of such tasks on working memory systems.

Imitation is likely but a part of the larger domain of behavior known as vicarious learning. Individuals are able not only to acquire new behaviors by imitating others, but to acquire more information in general about environmental contingencies through the observation of others. What the individual adopts for imitation through the observation of the experiences of others is not just their behavior, but the larger contingency arrangement in which that behavior takes place. The individual learns not only what to do, but when to do it and, just as important, what will happen if he or she does it. Critical to understand here is not so much the acquisition of the information through observation, which is probably related more to storage of sensory information in long-term memory, but the reactivation of that stored information into working memory in the formulation of and control over ongoing behavior. Therefore, working memory may not be critical to the acquisition of information through vicarious learning but through its application in adaptive performance. Neuropsychologists have not given much emphasis to this phenomenon of imitation and vicarious learning or noted its likely dependence on working memory when vicariously learned information is put into the service of the individual who has acquired it. Given the importance of imitation and vicarious learning to the development of the human behavioral repertoire, such emphasis is certainly warranted.

Hindsight

As both Bronowski (1967/1977) and Fuster (1989) discussed, the ability to reactivate past sensory events (such as the images and sounds of the past) and to prolong their existence during a delay in responding is the basis for *hindsight,* aptly named because of its proper association with the re-imaging of past events. But, as noted previously, we also have hind-sound, hind-taste, hind-smell, and so on, representing the reactivation of the variety of past sensory experiences the individual may have. Fuster (1989) called this the *retrospective function,* by means of which the individual's pertinent past history comes forward into the moment to inform the selection of a response to an event and to aid in guiding that eventual response at some future point. A delay in responding is critical to engaging in hindsight.

Delayed-response tasks, as Fuster (1980, 1989) noted, may be some of the best tasks designed for assessing working memory. During the delay in responding, the subject must mentally represent an immediately prior event. Current analysis indicates that this is likely being achieved through the prolongation of the sensory representation of that event within the pertinent sensory cortices and their association areas; the subject is seeing or sensing to him- or herself during the delay. Delay tasks, then, are assessing a rudimentary form of hindsight. Over development, the individual builds up a progressively larger archive of such past sensory representations that can be reactivated during delay periods as they may be pertinent to the formulation of a response in the present situation. Important in such recall is the ability to keep the temporal sequence of these past events in a correct order so as to guide the correct sequence of responses based upon them. There must exist a syntax for recall and ongoing representation of events within working memory, as many others studying working memory and the functions of the prefrontal cortex have theorized (Butters, Kaszniak, Glisky, Eslinger, & Schacter, 1994; Fuster, 1989; Godbout & Doyon, 1995; Grafman, 1995; McAndrews & Milner, 1991; Milner, 1995; Sirigu et al., 1995).

Forethought

Bronowski (1967/1977) and more modern writers on the subject of working memory have all described a parallel or temporally symmetrical function that arises out of hindsight, or the retrospective function—*forethought, or the prospective function*. The reactivation of prior sensory representations appears to simultaneously activate the motor response patterns associated with those prior events, undoubtedly learned as a result of those events. In a sense, what is being reactivated is not just the individual's sensory experience of the past event but a relational network of that sensory information with prior motor responses to it and their associated somatic markers (affective and motivational tones). Sensory events are reactivated along with the entire behavioral contingency of which they were a part. Through this mechanism, the reactivation and prolongation of past sensory events will be associated with a priming of the motor responses associated with those events, should their associated somatic markers bias toward their selection rather than their inhibition. In this way, hindsight creates forethought.

Anticipatory Set

The recall of the past permits the anticipation of a hypothetical future, which acts to prepare or prime a set of motor responses directed toward that future. Fuster (1989) referred to this as *anticipatory set*. Both Fuster and Goldman-Rakic (1995a, 1995b) noted that hindsight, or the retrospective function, represents the sensory aspects of this process (the reactivation of past sensory experiences), while the prospective function linked with it represents the motor aspects, or the presetting and priming of motor response patterns associated with those sensory events. To eventually initiate these primed or preset motor responses, there must also exist an ongoing comparison of the sequence of events playing out in the external world with the sequence of sensory events being represented in working memory. Such a comparative process will instruct the timing of the release of the primed responses (Goldberg & Podell, 1995). The mechanism for this comparison of external versus internal states of information is not well described but has been assigned to the right prefrontal regions of the brain by some researchers (see Dehaene & Changeux, 1995; Goldberg & Podell, 1995, for a discussion). Negative feedback or information about one's errors during task performance should be a particularly important source of self-regulating information as such feedback indicates a discrepancy between the actual current state (external situation) and the internally represented desired state of affairs (outcome) and the adequacy of the current plans for achieving that outcome. That feedback must be temporarily held in mind so as to assist with correcting and refining the internally represented plans, which then feed forward to result in changes in behavior that may better achieve the desired state. Thus, a sensitivity to errors and a flexibility of behavioral responding should be a consequence of effective self-regulation.

Self-Awareness

The referencing of the past so as to inform and regulate the individual's present behavior and aim it toward the future events anticipated from such a process most likely contributes to *self-awareness*. Past events and behaviors involving oneself are being reactivated and prolonged (held in mind) so as to prepare for a future for oneself, out of this process likely arises an awareness of oneself, a feeling of the sense of the self as the agency of behavior change and self-control. Kopp (1982) has made this same point in discussing the essential role of representational (working) memory in the development of self-awareness, as did Charles Darwin (1871/1992) over a century ago.

Humphrey (1984) has theorized that self-awareness may have evolved in humans as a means for predicting the intentions of others and their behavior and thus as a means of anticipating and even controlling the behavior of others. Through examining one's own behavior and motives covertly, the individual is able to conjecture the intentions, motives, and possible behavior of others, permitting the individual to anticipate and prepare for such social eventualities and even to attempt to control them in the process. If Humphrey is correct, it would mean that the evolution of covert self-directed sensory–motor behavior, as is represented in the executive functions, provides both a means of self-control and of social control over others.

It seems to me, however, that it is also likely that covert self-directed behavior as involved in working memory and in the other executive functions arose for an another reason as well. The behavior that is turned on the self in self-control was probably at some time earlier in evolution entirely public, much as it may be in its earliest forms in child development. It may have evolved to being entirely covert or private because of selection pressures that stem from intraspecies competition. That is, if others witness how an individual uses his or her behavior to achieve a change in subsequent behavior, they have obtained information about how they might more effectively control that individual. It seems to me that there would have been heavy selection pressure for moving to suppress or inhibit the public manifestations of these self-directed behaviors, so as to prevent the individual from being at a competitive disadvantage in this way. Publicly emitted self-control was undoubtedly better for the individual than no self-control, but covert self-control would have been even better, minimizing as it would any cues to others about how the individual was regulating his or her behavior and toward what goals that behavior was intended. I can see no reason why both Humphrey's explanation of self-awareness and my own explanation of the internalization of the executive functions could not be considered compatible.

Self-awareness may have arisen in evolution for its social advantages, but its movement toward covertness would have enhanced those advantages considerably. Moreover, as others have suggested (Dennett, 1995; Gregory, 1987; Popper & Eccles, 1977); the move to internal, self-directed sensing permits the simulation and testing out of imagined environments and the behavioral contingencies within them that would have provided individuals with a selective advantage over those less able or even unable to mentally simulate such information so as to preselect responses before they are emitted. I will return to this point later (in Chapter 11), but suffice it to say here that covert, self-directed sensory–motor activity as seems to comprise working memory would have a number of selective advantages in the evolution of the human mind.

Sense of Time

The retention of a sequence of events in working memory appears to provide the basis for the human *sense of time* (Bronowski, 1967/1977;

J. W. Brown, 1990; Michon, 1985). By holding such sequences in mind and making comparisons among the events in the sequence, a sense of both time and temporal duration appears to arise (Brown, 1990; Michon & Jackson, 1984). The human perception of time as having a characteristic flow or stream of directionality to it may arise out of the constraints that exist in human perception, attention, and working memory. The focus of human perception and attention is limited, and so is the storage capacity for working memory. To gain more information about the environment, attention must be shifted about, creating a sequence of events that may not necessarily exist in the larger physical universe precisely as we have perceived it or precisely as others may be experiencing it (Davies, 1995). The "flow" of the stream of time is an artifact of having to inspect events in a sequence as they recede from the temporal "now." This sense of time having a direction is further enhanced by our inability to recall our entire past at once, but rather as moments in a sequence.

Davies (1995) illustrates the point with an example. Imagine that the universe is represented by a wall in a dark room containing a matrix of single-digit numbers on it. You, the observer, enter this room; your limited attentional focus is represented by a small flashlight that you carry. As you shine your light about to inspect the wall, only one number can be illuminated at a time. The result will be the perception of a sequence of digits, creating a sense of time and a directionality to it. You will perceive the universe as represented by a sequence of digits giving rise to a sense of time's arrow or directionality, when in reality all digits exist on the wall simultaneously. All possible events in the universe may exist simultaneously in space–time, but we will perceive time as a separate dimension representing a sequence of events with a directionality to it, all of which arises out of our cognitive limitations. The perception of time, therefore, arises out of the perception of sequences and their ordering. As Davies (1995) quotes an anonymous source, "Time is just one damn thing after another" (p. 40). A memory capacity that permits the retention of such event sequences and their ordering "on-line" or "in mind" appears to give rise to the human sense of time.

The memory capacity in which event sequences in the present are stored or into which past event sequences are reactivated appears to be what neuropsychologists have called working memory and time psychologists have called sequential memory (Michon, 1985). This perception of events as a sequence requires a sense of spatial position and change in spatial position (recall the changing positions of the flashlight on the wall of the universe). It is fair to say, then, that the human sense of time is actually based on the perception of change and may derive from the need to perceive and predict the motion of objects in space. To perceive such change, a prior event must be held in mind and compared against more immediate events in this perception sequence. The perception of events in a sequence permits the analysis of those sequences for patterns of recurrence, which in turn allow for the prediction of future such patterns when events found to exist early in the pattern are detected in the environment. The processing of events in a sequence, or what is essentially temporal information, is not automatic but requires effort (Michon & Jackson, 1984; Michon, Jackson, & Vermeeren, 1984). This effort reflects attention and that attention, is likely afforded through the working memory system.

Knowledge of patterns of events can be stored and retrieved at a later time to permit prediction of and anticipation of impending events in the environment. This may be how the sense of past event sequences gives rise to a sense of future event sequences and thus the ability to preset motor responses in anticipation of those impending events. The retention and storage of increasingly longer patterns of event sequences over development creates the capacity to anticipate events further ahead in time, and may be the basis for the increasing sense of future and its time horizon across human maturation, as I will discuss later in this chapter.

This perception of time as a change in the relative position of things probably creates the need for parietal lobe involvement to some degree in the sequencing tasks designed to evaluate frontal lobe functions and in tasks assessing time perception. The parietal lobes mediate visual–spatial abilities, accounting for their involvement to some extent in studies of time perception and sequential ordering of events, as some neuropsychological researchers have recently noted (Godbout & Doyon, 1995; Sirigu et al., 1995).

The positioning of event moments in a sequence as well as the number of other event moments that may fall between these events appears to be the basis for judging temporal durations (J. W. Brown, 1990). Attention to internal and external sources of temporal information (change) must be increased while that paid to purely spatial information must be decreased in the judgment of temporal durations. Such attention to and retention of that temporal information can be readily disrupted by distracting events (S. W. Brown, 1985; Zakay, 1990, 1992). This suggests that the sense of time, as a result of its dependence on working (sequential) memory, requires the protection from interference that is provided by the behavioral inhibition system. It also may help to explain why behavioral inhibition appears to be related to the capacity to accurately estimate and reproduce temporal durations (Gerbing et al., 1987; White et al., 1994).

The retrospective and prospective functions of working memory (hindsight and forethought) and the sense of time they permit may contribute to or even underlie the development of an increasing preference for delayed over immediate rewards, as discussed in Chapter 3 (Green et al., 1994, 1996). As I noted in that chapter, such a preference would seem to be a prerequisite for the development of self-control, given that the ultimate function of self-control is the maximization of future over immediate consequences. Measures of impulsiveness therefore should not be found just to be related to measures of sense of time, but also to the temporal discounting of delayed rewards, as Green et al. (1996) have noted.

The sense of the future that working memory promotes could be conjectured to be associated with a number of aspects of daily adaptive functioning. Inhibition and the preference for delayed rewards associated with it would be expected to be correlated with level of educational attainment (deferred gratification within the educational system), persistence in goal-directed behavior, level of occupational attainment, and even monetary saving practices (see Green et al., 1996, for supportive research). It would also be predicted to be involved in preference for positive health practices, given that such practices often require restraint from immediate gratification and even exposure to effortful and aversive circumstances (i.e., exercise) so as to reduce or avoid the later harm that less healthful practices would entail. Such a relationship seems to be the case, albeit weakly, in adolescents (Mahon & Yarcheski, 1994), in whom working memory and a preference for delayed rewards are not yet fully mature.

The gradual awareness of time and the future afforded by the development of working memory probably underlies the growing awareness of one's mortality. This has been referred to in developmental psychology as the universality concept of death. It seems to emerge at 5–7 years of age (Speece & Brent, 1984), but with a considerable range around this period that seems partly to be a function of the stage of a child's cognitive development. Children apparently need to have achieved at least the stage of concrete operational thinking, in Piagetian theory, to have developed the universality concept of death (Speece & Brent, 1984). Undoubtedly, the arrival of that stage has much to do with the development of working or representational memory as well as the internalization of speech (discussed later) that seems to characterize the "5-to-7 shift" taking place at this age (Berkowitz, 1982).

Cross-Temporal Organization of Behavior

In a way, the development of hindsight and forethought creates a window on time (past, present, future) of which the individual is aware. The temporal opening of that window probably increases across development, at least up to age 30 years, if the development of a preference for delayed over immediate rewards is any indication (Green et al., 1996). This might suggest that across child and adolescent development, the individual develops the capacity to organize and direct behavior toward events that lie increasingly distant in the future. By adulthood (ages 20–81), behavior is being organized to deal with events of the near future (8–12 weeks ahead) most often but can be extended to events later in time if the consequences associated with those events are particularly salient (Fingerman & Perlmutter, 1994).

If, as Fuster (1989) has suggested, the overarching function of the prefrontal cortex is *the cross-temporal organization of behavior,* then the period over which such cross-temporal behavior can be organized could be expected to be considerably shorter in young children and increase across development as the prefrontal cortex matures. Young children will be capable only of anticipating and preparing behavior toward events in the future that are near in time, in contrast to older children, adolescents, or adults, who can prepare for events far more distant in time. This suggests that one means of judging the time horizon for individuals of differing ages is to examine the length of the average period prior to an event that typically results in the initiation of preparatory behaviors. Of course, this time horizon will vary as a function of the saliency of the consequence associated with the hypothetical event. The point here is that, given a particular event, adults will engage in preparatory behaviors toward that event at foreperiods (time horizons) typically much greater than those for adolescents, whose preparatory foreperiods in turn will be larger than those of younger children. Moreover, according to the present model, differences among individuals at the same age in terms of their preparatory foreperiod are likely to be, at least in part, a function of differences in their capacity for behavioral inhibition and working memory.

Neuroanatomical Localization

As discussed earlier and in Chapters 5 and 6, working memory or the capacity to engage in self-directed, covert behavior appears to be mediated by the dorsolateral regions of the prefrontal cortex. Some research suggests that verbal working memory and the temporal ordering of verbal material may be lateralized more to the left than the right dorsolateral prefrontal regions. The opposite may be true for nonverbal forms of working memory and the temporal ordering of visual–spatial or nonverbal material, though it seems likely that both prefrontal hemispheres contribute to some degree to both forms of working memory (Goldberg & Podell, 1995; Milner, 1995). Also of interest are research findings suggesting that the left prefrontal region may be more involved than the right in the internal generation of plans and temporal ordering of these events as well as the control of behavior by them. In contrast, the right prefrontal region may be more involved in attending to the ordering of external events, with the comparison of these events with the internally represented plans and their ordering controlled by the left prefrontal regions (Goldberg & Podell, 1995).

Lesions to the right prefrontal region produce forms of behavior in humans that are characterized as stimulus bound or excessively controlled by external events relative to internally generated information and plans (Fuster, 1989; Goldberg & Podell, 1995; Stuss & Benson, 1986). On tests such as the WCST, individuals with such lesions tend to produce more perseverative errors, persisting in an ineffective response pattern despite feedback concerning their errors. They may also be more likely to engage in utilization behavior, in which they have difficulties resisting manipulating and interacting with objects in their visual field, often demonstrating their appropriate use, but at times when such demonstrations are inappropriate to the context. Left prefrontal lesions, in contrast, result in an inability of the individual to persist in following plans and rules generated internally and greater nonperseverative errors on the WCST (Drew, 1974; Goldberg & Podell, 1995). Regardless of the side to which these functions may be localized, there is ample evidence to suggest that the prefrontal cortex is involved in the generation of internal simulations of behavior, the monitoring of events in the external world, and the cross-checking of these internal simulations with events taking place in the external world (Knight et al., 1995).

Nonverbal Rule-Governed Behavior

If the mental representation of past events in working memory serves ultimately to initiate and guide motor responses associated with those events, then such mental representations take on the power of rules in governing behavior. Rules have been defined as contingency-specifying stimuli (Skinner, 1953, 1969). Language comprises a large part of such stimuli for humans but it need not be, nor is it the only form such stimuli can take. Images, signs, symbols, and their sequences can all serve to specify behavioral contingencies. Therefore, mental representations of such stimuli also could come to serve as a rudimentary form of rules, in keeping with this definition. For instance, a line drawn on a map can come to serve as a form of rule for governing behavior within the terrain represented by that map (Skinner, 1969). If the map can serve such a behavior-controlling function, then so can the covert visual image of that map when it is privately resensed or held in mind. For convenience, I have deferred the discussion of rule-governed behavior to the next section, dealing with private speech, given the large role that language plays in rule-governed behavior. However, the features to be described as characteristics of rule-governed behavior are just as likely to be applicable to behavior under the guidance of nonverbal working memory, or covert self-directed sensing, given that such covert sensory stimuli can serve effectively as rules that govern behavior.

Summary

The executive function of working memory can be seen to provide individuals with the capacity to resense information during delays in responding, and even to manipulate that information into sequences of events. These event sequences are held in mind or on-line so as to guide the execution of a subsequent response to an event. This capacity to resense event sequences provides not only the power to imitate others' complex actions and their sequences, learning vicariously from their experiences. But it also provides the template for the human sense of time and the means by which that sense can be used to regulate subsequent behavior. A sense of time, timing, and timeliness can now be imparted to motor actions. Working memory also provides the capacity to re-experience relevant past information (retrospective function), or to have a sense of the past, out of which arises the capacity to construct hypothetical futures, or a sense of the future. The individual is now bestowed with the power to anticipate probable future events and to prepare for them, even setting in motion a series of behaviors timed to meet the arrival of the anticipated event. Human behavior is now controlled not only by a sense of time, but a sense of past and future giving rise to goal-directed, purposive, and intentional behavior driven to its destination by the information being internally represented in working memory. Human self-control can be said to originate here, through the mechanisms of covert self-directed sensory behavior that comes to regulate motor actions.

INTERNALIZATION OF SPEECH
(VERBAL WORKING MEMORY)

Fuster's (1989) model has little to say about the internalization of speech as a function of the prefrontal cortex. Bronowski (1967/1977), however, stressed the uniqueness and importance of the self-direction and internalization of speech and the profound control it may produce upon the individual's behavior. Developmental psychologists (Berk & Potts, 1991; Kopp, 1982) and developmental neuropsychologists (Vygotsky, 1978, 1987) have, likewise, emphasized the importance of this process for the development of self-control. Yet the internalization of speech seems to have gone relatively unnoticed or underemphasized, particularly its role in the governance of motor behavior, in most modern neuropsychological models of the executive functions, despite Luria's (1961) emphasis of it in earlier conceptualizations of the executive functions. Berk and Potts (1991) argued that the influence of private speech on self-control certainly may be reciprocal—inhibitory control contributes to the internalization of speech, which contributes to even greater self-restraint and self-guidance. Despite this reciprocity, initial primacy within this bidirectional process is given here to behavioral (motor) inhibition.

This component of the hybrid model is shown in Figure 7.4. Although it will be discussed as representing the internalization of speech, this component is believed to comprise what some neuropsychologists have considered verbal working memory, or the articulatory loop (Baddeley, 1986). The capacity to converse with oneself in a quasi-dialogic fashion has a number of features important for self-regulation. Self-directed speech is believed to provide a means for *description and reflection* by which the individual covertly labels, describes, and verbally contemplates the nature of an event or situation prior to responding to that event. Private speech also provides a means for *self-questioning* through language, creating an important source of *problem-solving* ability as well as a means of *generating rules* and plans (Skinner, 1953, 1969). Eventually, rules about rules (*meta-rules*) can be formulated into a hierarchically arranged system that resembles the concept of metacognition in developmental psychology (Flavell, Miller, & Miller, 1993).

The interaction of self-speech (verbal working memory) with nonverbal working memory may contribute to three other mental abilities: delayed performance of a current instruction containing a future reference for that performance (see the following discussion of rule-governed behavior), reading comprehension, and moral reasoning. Among these various functions, however, rule-governed behavior may be among the most important. *Reading comprehension* has been shown to have a significant relationship to measures of working memory (Swanson & Berninger, 1995; Wadsworth, DeFries, Fulker, Olson, & Pennington, 1995), with the prefrontal lobes playing a critical role in this process (Frisk & Milner, 1990). This relationship may exist because what is read to the self must be held in mind if maximum semantic and inferential content is to be extracted from it.

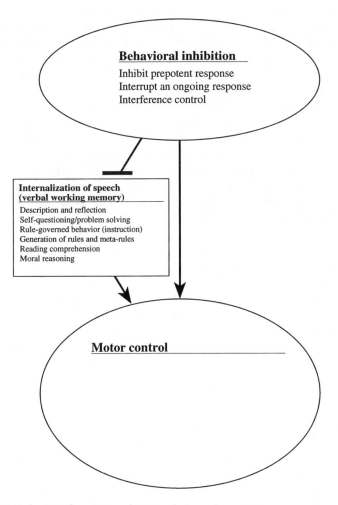

FIGURE 7.4. The functions of the verbal working memory system and its relationship to the behavioral inhibition and motor control systems.

Rule-Governed Behavior

Although the progressive shift from public to private speech is fascinating in its own right, a more important aspect of this privatization may be the increasing control language comes to have over motor behavior with development (Berk, 1992, 1994; Berk & Potts, 1991; Luria, 1961; Vygotsky, 1978). This control has been referred to within the field of modern behavioral analysis as *rule-governed behavior* (Cerutti, 1989; Hayes, 1989; Skinner, 1953). As noted earlier, rules are contingency-specifying stimuli; they specify a relationship among an event, a response, and the consequences likely to occur for that response. Language provides a substantial amount of such stimuli. Skinner (1953) hypothesized that this influence of language over behavior occurs in three stages: (1) the control of behavior by the language of others, (2) the progressive control of behavior by self-directed and eventually private speech, as discussed earlier, and (3) the creation of new rules by the individual, which came about through the use of self-directed questions (second-order rules). Both Bronowski (1967/1977) and Skinner (1953) stressed two important aspects of internalized speech. One was informational—the power of self-directed speech for description, reflection, and the creation of new rules by which to guide behavior (problem solving). The other was instructive—the power of these messages to actually control motor responses.

Rule-governed behavior appears to provide a means of sustaining behavior across large gaps in time among the units of a behavioral contingency (events, responses, outcomes). By formulating rules, the individual can construct novel, complex (hierarchically organized), and prolonged behavioral chains. These rules can then provide the template for reading off the appropriate sequences of behavioral chains, guiding behavior toward the attainment of a future goal (Cerutti, 1989; Hayes, 1989; Skinner, 1969). By this process, the individual's behavior is no longer under the total control of the immediate surrounding context. Behavior is now shifted to control by internally represented information (in this case, verbal behavior and the rules it generates).

In order for self-directed speech to make any sense to the individual in its use of prolonged references (to past and to future), the individual must also have a capacity for working memory that gives rise to the sense of past and of future, as Bronowski (1967/1977) suggested. It is by this means that a rule can be issued in the moment yet make reference to performance of behavior at a later time. Through the use of such rules employing temporally prolonged references, the individual may be able to bridge the delay between the now and the future time when that performance will be required.

Specific Characteristics of Rule-Governed Behavior

Hayes (1989) and Cerutti (1989) have stipulated a number of specific effects on behavior that rule governance produces. These will become important later in this volume as predictions from the model about ADHD. Behavior that is rule-governed rather than contingency-shaped is likely to have the following characteristics: (1) The variability of responses to a task will be greatly reduced when rule-governed behavior is in effect than when behavior is contingency-shaped (developed and maintained by the environmental contingencies alone); (2) rule-governed behavior may be less affected or entirely unaffected by the immediate contingencies operating in a situation or by momentary and potentially spurious changes in those contingencies; (3) where rules and immediate contingencies compete in a given situation, the rule is more likely to gain control over behavior, and progressively more so as the individual matures; (4) rule-governed responding under some conditions may be rigid or inflexible even if the rule being followed is eventually shown to be incorrect; and (5) self-directed rules permit individuals to persist in responding under conditions of very low levels of immediate reinforcement or even the absence of reward, as well as during extreme delays in the consequences for responding. To this list might be added some of the additional characteristics of rule-governed behavior cited by Skinner (1969): (6) Rule-governed behavior is likely to be associated with less emotion or passion, given that the individual has not been exposed to the actual contingencies in the setting, which would give rise to greater affect associated with responding; and (7) the behavior is likely to appear conscious, intentional, deliberate, and purposive rather than impulsive, reactive, and ill-considered.

In short, self-directed rules assist with bridging temporal gaps in behavioral contingencies and thus contribute to the cross-temporal organization of behavior. The motor execution of such verbal rules appears to be partially dependent on the capacity to retain them in working memory (to restate the rule) and to inhibit prepotent or irrelevant responses that compete with the rule (Zelazo, Reznick, & Pinon, 1995).

Stages of Rule-Governed Behavior

Hayes et al. (1996) have described three levels of functions within a hierarchy of the development of rule-governed behavior that they hypothesize may reflect corresponding stages of moral development. These levels are as follows.

1. *Pliance.* This represents responding to rules on the basis of being previously socially rewarded for doing so. It represents compliance to directions, instructions, commands, and other forms of rules on the basis of socially mediated reinforcement for rule following, and is believed to represent the most rudimentary form of rule-governed behavior.

2. *Tracking.* At this level, rules are followed because of a history of agreement or correspondence between those rules and the actual contingencies to which they pertain. In other words, such behavior reflects the success of the rules in predicting the actual contingencies and the individual's prior history of being rewarded by the contingencies when following such rules. If one has been told to do something so that some outcome will happen, and when one does so the predicted outcome occurs, the next time a similar rule is given it is likely to be followed. This is a form of tracking.

3. *Augmenting.* This form of rule-governed behavior is the result of rules that alter the capacity of particular events to function as consequences. Some augmentals are motivative; such rules serve to increase or decrease the degree to which previously established consequences serve as rewards and punishments. Other augmentals are formative; they establish new consequences as being rewarding or punitive. Hayes et al. (1996) give the example of "if 'being good' has developed reinforcing functions over a period of time, and 'sharing' is identified as being good, then 'sharing' may function as a formative augmental, as it has now acquired some of the functions of 'being good' " (p. 292). It is possible that the capacity to generate or create one's own rules and to adhere to them may represent a fourth level of the development of rule-governed behavior within this developmental hierarchy, as Skinner (1953) suggested.

Moral Reasoning

Moral reasoning is the internalization of community norms, mores, or morals about how one ought to behave, both now and in the future (Berk, 1992; Hayes et al., 1996; Kohlberg et al., 1968). The control of behavior by the sense of past and future that arise from working memory as well as by the more general rules or meta-rules formulated from them through internalized speech or acquired via socialization most likely makes a contribution to the development of conscience and moral reasoning (Hoffman, 1970; Kochanska, DeVet, Goldman, Murray, & Putnam, 1994; Kohlberg, 1963), as noted earlier. In this way, moral development arises as a consequence of the interactions of the executive functions, with a heavy contribution made by internalized speech. Even Darwin (1871/1992) made this observation in *The Descent of Man*:

> As soon as the mental faculties had become highly developed, images of all past actions and motives would be incessantly passing through the brain of each individual; and that feeling of dissatisfaction, or even

misery, which invariably results . . . from any unsatisfied instinct, would arise, as often as it was perceived that the enduring and always present social instinct had yielded to some other instinct, at the time stronger, but neither enduring in its nature, nor leaving behind it a very vivid impression. . . . After the power of language had been acquired, and the wishes of the community could be expressed, the common opinion how each member ought to act for the public good, would naturally become in a paramount degree the guide to action. (pp. 304–305)

A moral being is one who is capable of comparing his past and future actions or motives, and of approving or disapproving of them. (p. 311)

Summary

One can appreciate the substantial contribution that private self-directed speech comes to make to self-regulation as well as to civilized and moral conduct. Whereas language begins as a form of public behavior that comes to inform, influence, and even regulate the behavior of others, through the process of internalization it then becomes turned on the self. It is now a means of informing, influencing, and controlling one's own behavior, eventually passing on to becoming fully private, covert speech or verbal thought that is integrated with action. To follow rules is to guide behavior with a strategy.

SELF-REGULATION OF AFFECT/MOTIVATION/AROUSAL

We not only privately sense and behave to ourselves but also emote or motivate ourselves as an integral part of this process of private, self-directed actions. It is this power to emote to/motivate ourselves that provides the drive, in the absence of external rewards, that fuels the individual's persistence in cross-temporal behaviors and thereby bridges the delay to the future outcomes. This may explain why children, as they mature, become increasingly less dependent on external forms of immediate reinforcement in order to persist at tasks and activities and to defer gratification—they are developing the capacity to motivate themselves.

This component of the hybrid model is shown in Figure 7.5. It combines Bronowski's (1967/1977) concept of the separation and self-regulation of affect along with Damasio's (1994, 1995) theory of somatic markers. Everyone recognizes that external events elicit emotional reactions of varying degrees along with the motor responses to those events. But, as Damasio and others (Fuster, 1989) have noted, the internally generated events arising from nonverbal working memory and self-speech are also paired with affective and motivational tones, or somatic markers. Covert visual imagery and covert self-speech, among other forms of covert self-directed behavior, produce not only

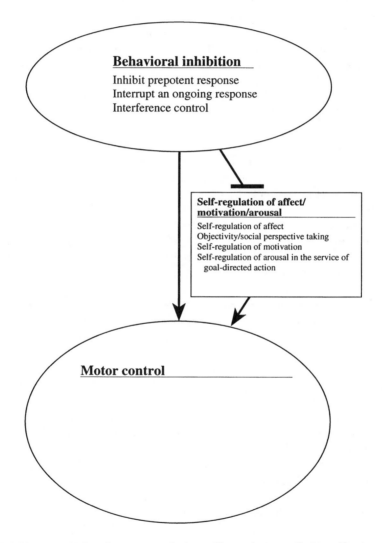

FIGURE 7.5. The functions of the self-regulation of the affect/motivation/arousal system and its relationship to the behavioral inhibition and motor control systems.

private images and verbalizations but also the emotional charges associated with them. For instance, try imaging your fingertip being sliced open by a razor and you will notice how it elicits a degree of emotional reaction to that privately visualized event.

Emotional Self-Control

The power to inhibit and delay prepotent responses to events brings with it this power to delay the expression of those emotional reactions that would have been elicited by the event and whose expression would have been a part of the expression of those prepotent responses. Just as the delaying of the prepotent response permits a period for self-regulation through the use of internally generated and self-directed behavior (e.g., imagery, private speech, etc.), so the delaying of the affective response to the emotional charge of that event permits it to likewise undergo a change as a function of self-directed, private action. The covert deliberations concerning the decision to respond will not only result in a modification of the eventual response to the event, but will also affect the eventual emotional charge, if any, that will be emitted in conjunction with that response. This modification of the initial emotional response prior to its public display could be achieved through private imagery, in which images having a different emotional charge are used to offset that which may have been initially associated with the event. Similarly, private self-directed speech can modulate emotional reactions by eliciting contrasting emotions, relative to the prepotent emotional reaction. Such use of private action to countermand or counterbalance the initial emotional charge of external events contributes to the development of *emotional self-control* (Kopp, 1989).

Levenson (1994) and Scherer (1994) have both discussed how emotions may have initially evolved to serve as a form of communication to others, particularly regarding the nature of one's intentions to act, and thus probably have a controlling function over others' behavior. Much earlier, Darwin (1871/1992) likewise described a similar evolutionary function of the human emotions. But just as language may have originally evolved as a means of communicating with others in an effort to control their behavior and later evolved to become a form of communicating with and controlling oneself, so also may the development of emotional self-control have proceeded in a similar manner. We may start out in childhood emitting emotions purely as public forms of communicative behavior with others, but come to emit them to ourselves in an initially public form as well. Such self-directed emotions may become progressively more private or covert in form over development, eventually becoming internalized and having little or no publicly observable manifestations. But, like self-speech, self-emotion may become public once again as a function of the level of difficulty of a problem situation and the level of emotional charge it has associated with it.

Among the variety of human emotions, it may be the negative array of emotions that will be most in need of such self-control (Kopp, 1989). This is because negative affect may prove more socially unacceptable, thereby producing more salient, long-term negative social consequences for the individual relative to positive emotions, such as laughter or affection. Such negative displays may achieve in the immediate context positive reinforcement or, more likely, escape or avoidance of aversive events (Patterson, 1982, 1986). But in the long run, they produce a variety of negative consequences for the individual, detracting from the net maximization of future outcomes (Patterson, Dishion, & Reid, 1992). For this reason, negative prepotent emotions are more likely to be in need of inhibition and self-regulation than are positive emotional reactions to events.

Objectivity

As Bronowski (1967/1977) noted, such a process permits the original affective charge of an event to be separated and modified during the period of delayed responding, so that not only is the eventual response made by the individual more deliberate, conscious, and reasoned, but so is the eventual emotional tone that will be associated with it. Impulsive prepotent responses are often charged with far more emotion than are those responses that are emitted after a delay and period of self-regulation. That is to say, internally guided behavior, such as that being governed by rules, is often associated with significantly less emotion than behavior that is impulsive and contingency-shaped (Skinner, 1969). The delay in the emotional response and the self-regulation of that response would seem to permit individuals the capacity for *objectivity* (Bronowski, 1967/1977) and even the ability to consider the perspective of another (*social perspective taking*) in determining the eventual response to an event. Social perspective taking arises in conjunction with the assistance of working memory; the individual is now able to delay and even defer his or her initial affects regarding selfishness or self-interest, and his or her own immediate gratification. The person is then able to hold the event in mind and consider it from the perspective of another, freed from or at least more independent of these immediate, prepotent, self-serving affective reactions.

Motivation, Arousal, and Goal-Directed Action

Also included in the affect/motivation/arousal component is the *self-regulation of* drive or *motivational and arousal states* that support the execution of goal-directed actions and persistence toward the goal. This combination of emotional self-control with that of motivational self-control into a single component makes sense. Lang (1995) has cogently argued that the array of human emotions can be reduced to a two-dimensional grid, of which one dimension is *motivation* (reinforcement and punishment) and the other is level of *arousal*. Other researchers in the field of emotion likewise associate it with motivational properties, even defining an emotion as a motivational state (see Ekman & Davidson, 1994, for reviews). Emotions are the result of continual appraisals that take place as the individual moves about and interacts with the external world; they inform the individual about the significance of events for his or her concerns (Clore, 1994; Frijda, 1994; Gray, 1994; Lazarus, 1994). The emotions have motivational or reinforcement significance; they motivate action in response to an event that elicits them and may induce adjustments to energy resources or level of activation as a consequence (Frijda, 1994). This analysis suggests that the ability to self-regulate and even *induce* emotional states as needed in the service of goal-directed behavior also brings with it the ability to regulate and even induce motivation, drive, and arousal states in support of such behavior.

Self-Regulation of Affect/Arousal

Children may learn to create more positive affective and motivational states in themselves when angered, frustrated, disappointed, saddened, anxious, or bored, by learning to manipulate the variables of which such negative states and their positive alternatives are a function (Cole et al., 1994; Eisenberg et al., 1993; Kopp, 1989). These self-directed forms of manipulation may be public in form initially, yet, like private self-speech, come to be more covert or internal in form across development. Such self-directed actions may involve efforts at self-comforting, self-directed speech, visual imagery, and self-encouragement and self-reinforcement, among other means (Kopp, 1989). This process of self-regulating motivation and affect may begin as early as 5–10 months of age (Stifter & Braungart, 1995). It seems to be assisted by parental motivating statements during task performance that serve both to model self-directed encouragement statements for the child and probably to directly reinforce self-control and task persistence, as Berk (1992) has shown.

It is also conceivable that children may learn to *self-regulate arousal levels* by means similar to those used to self-regulate emotion *for the purposes of goal accomplishment.* This would be expected from the fact that arousal states are clearly affected by motivational and emotional states (Ekman & Davidson, 1994).

Summary

The affect/motivation/arousal component of the model, therefore, includes the following subfunctions: (1) the self-regulation of affect, (2) a capacity for objectivity and social perspective, (3) the self-regulation of drive and motivational states, and (4) the self-regulation of arousal, all of which are carried out in the service of goal-directed actions.

The executive functions are believed to be interactive in nature. Therefore, the interaction of a function or mental module for the regulation of affect and motivation, when coupled with a module for representing past and future and anticipating and preparing for future events (working memory), should result in an increase in anticipatory affect and motivation ahead of the arrival of events conjectured to lie in the future. This may even provide the means by which motivation is initiated in support of behaviors directed toward that future event or goal. Whether that is the case or not, this model suggests that those with a well-developed module for working memory should also demonstrate greater anticipatory emotion for future events or, more likely, demonstrate such anticipatory affect/motivation farther in advance of those events than would others less endowed with these functions.

RECONSTITUTION

The reconstitution component of the hybrid model is obviously based upon Bronowski's (1967/1977) concept of the same name and is shown in Figure 7.6. It represents two important interrelated activities, namely, analysis and synthesis of behavior. Analysis represents the ability to take the units of behavioral sequences apart, as might be seen in the capacity to break a sentence down into its component elements (words), to divide words into their syllables, or to separate syllables into their phonological units.

But what is meant by a unit of behavior? For my purposes, a unit of behavior can be defined as similar to a gene of DNA. Dawkins (1982) has defined a gene as "that which segregates and recombines with appreciable frequency" or "any hereditary information for which there is a favorable or unfavorable selection bias equal to several or many

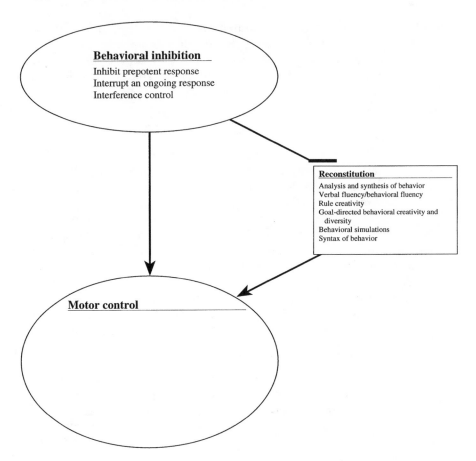

FIGURE 7.6. The functions of the verbal working memory system and its relationship to the behavioral inhibition and motor control systems.

times its rate of endogenous change" (p. 287). Like genes, a unit of behavior is a unit of information or even a sequence of such units that segregates and recombines with appreciable frequency. A twitch of a small muscle in my finger would not be considered a unit of behavior because it does not segregate or recombine with any frequency in behavioral performances, but a finger tap could be considered such a unit, as could the gesture used for pulling a lever, turning a knob, shifting a car's gearshift, or writing or speaking a word.

As Fuster (1989) described this process, units of behavior are built into sequences, and these behavioral structures can be combined into more complex sequences, which can be hierarchically organized into more complex sequences having subroutines of sequences within them, and so on, giving human behavior its complex and hierarchically organized nature. Complex hierarchies can be broken down into the subhierarchies of which they are comprised, which in turn can be divided into behavioral units and subunits in this process of analysis.

These behavioral units can then be recombined to create novel behaviors and sequences of behaviors out of previously learned responses, in a process Bronowski called synthesis. While Bronowski (1967/1977) was focusing his remarks upon the nature and uniqueness of human language, I extend this concept to all forms of human behavior so as to capture the synthetic function of the prefrontal cortex so often noted by researchers in neuropsychology (Fuster, 1989; Stuss & Benson, 1986). The analytic and synthetic functions are not just evident in human speech, but in nonverbal forms of fine and gross motor behavior.

The point is easily made by drawing attention to the human capacity to play the piano. The rapid assembling of such fine motor gestures by an accomplished pianist into such extraordinarily complex sequences of the simultaneous movements of digits on both hands when playing a concerto is a marvel of human ability, unduplicated in any other animal species. While this nicely demonstrates the synthetic function of behavior, the capacity to reduce these same gestures to their component parts illustrates the analytic function just as nicely. The recombination of these dismembered units (synthesis) once again results in a novel sequence of fine motor actions, not to mention a new melody from the sounds those gestures create on the keyboard. Many examples of other forms of complex human motor responses and their reconstitution so as to provide new behavioral structures could be used to illustrate this process (e.g., ballet, modern dance, gymnastics, drawing, handwriting, etc.), but the point should be evident.

Bronowski (1967/1977) mentioned *verbal fluency* as one manifestation of this reconstitutive function. This would be evident in the person's capacity to rapidly and effectively assemble the units of language to create a diversity of verbal responses. But it would also be evident in nonverbal, or *behavioral, fluency* in keeping with my extension of Bronowski's concept to other forms of motor behavior besides that of speech. Fine or gross motor fluency, written fluency, musical or vocal fluency, and even design fluency ought to be manifestations of this process of reconstitution. Whenever a goal must be accomplished, regardless of the form of behavior that may be required to attain it, the reconstitutive function will be available to act upon the archive of previously acquired structures of those forms of behavior to generate a range of novel, complex structures that may be of value in the attainment of that goal. Reconstitution, then, is the source or generator of behavioral diversity and novelty not only in language and the rules that language can be used to formulate, but in nonverbal behavior as well.

The *diversity of rules* or strategies that may be generated by the function of reconstitution need not be in verbal form, though many are or can be so communicated to others. Rules comprise any form of contingency-specifying stimuli (Skinner, 1953, 1969): A sheet of music or pictorial diagrams arranged in a sequence are sets of rules as much as is a written recipe or manual for performing some mechanical procedure. Rules specify patterns in event sequences—the contingent "if–then" relations among these events—and such specifications can be represented in many forms. This clarification is important so as to understand that the function of reconstitution is the analysis of previously experienced sequences and the synthesis of new arrangements of such sequences arising from that analysis.

Behavioral inhibition and the delay in responding it creates permits these analytic and synthetic functions to operate on the archive of previously learned behavioral contingencies so as to result in the creation of novel, complex, and hierarchically organized sequences of goal-directed actions. In a sense then, the reconstitutive function contributes to *goal-directed behavioral flexibility and creativity*—the power to assemble multiple potential responses for the resolution of a problem or the attainment of a future goal. Such new response assemblies are, in a way, *simulations of behaviors* that can be covertly constructed and tested out before one is eventually selected for performance (Dehaene & Changeux, 1995). They are probably selected, in part, as a function of the somatic markers or affective/motivational features associated with them that help to constrain decision making and signal the likely outcomes of such response options (Damasio, 1994, 1995).

It is very likely that the reconstitution function I have identified can be subdivided into both a verbal and nonverbal form, consistent with the separation of nonverbal from verbal working memory in the model, and with the more well-recognized distinction between verbal and nonverbal (visual–spatial–constructional) intelligence. For the time being, I have set up this function as a single component within the hybrid model developed here, because I am uncertain as to whether its processes are domain specific, even though the goals, problems, or tasks to which it is applied may well be domain or content specific. Thus, one may find that measures of verbal analysis, fluency, and synthesis comprise separate factors from those which assess design analysis, fluency, and synthesis, for example. But the metaprocesses at work on both of these domains may turn out to be rather similar or even identical, operating as relatively random processes, with some constraints in their parsing and reconstituting of units of behavioral information, in much the same way that meiosis parses and then recombines sequences of DNA.

The analogy to the creative mechanisms in genetics is not coincidental. Dawkins (1974) has hypothesized that behavioral (even cultural) evolution may operate much like biological evolution, with the basic unit of cultural information being the *meme* instead of the gene. The meme can be conceptualized as the smallest unit of behavioral information that is capable of transmission to and replication by others. Vicarious learning, imitation, and especially language may well be some of the means by which memes are transmitted by brains (meme vehicles) to other brains and so spread throughout the population—the behavioral equivalent of biological reproduction. The function of memes is a selfish one—survival within the cultural meme pool—much as, in Dawkins's view, genes are selfish, in that they function to get themselves replicated into the next generation.

I have come to think of memes as the smallest units of information concerning a behavioral contingency. Consequently, the reconstitutive function in this model could be thought of as the mechanism or process whereby memes of various lengths (sequences of information concerning behavioral contingencies) are parsed and reconstituted to create new memes. And so the brain may not just be a meme vehicle, but, like the reproductive organs of the gene vehicle (the body), may serve also as a generator of new memes reconstituted from those in the existing repertoire. The heuristic analogy between genetic creativity and the analytic/synthetic activities of the prefrontal cortex may, if nothing else, serve to focus research attention in psychology on the metaprocesses (non-content specific) by which sequences of behaviors (contingencies, actually) within the individual's existing repertoire are parsed, sorted, and recombined to constitute novel behavioral sequences. Obviously, extant research on ideational creativity in psychology may be instructive in these regards.

Syntax of Behavior

A problem arises, however, when such analytic and synthetic functions are operative. The combination of units of behavior must be based upon a syntax or set of rules governing the temporal sequencing of such units and especially their contingent "if–then" relations. Just as many recombinations of genes are harmful or even deadly, so, too, many potential recombinations of behavior may prove themselves to be utterly useless or even life-threatening (e.g., squeezing the trigger *before* aiming the gun). A *syntax for assembling units of behavior* into potentially useful sequences undoubtedly exists, just as one exists for the composition of words into sentences. Therefore, the syntax of behavior, little understood as it seems to be at the moment, is placed within this component. Such a syntax probably has much to do with aspects of causality or event contingencies in the external world as the individual has previously encountered them. This formulation seems logical, given that the novel behaviors being created by this executive function are intended to operate upon that world so as to derive a certain outcome or attain a particular goal. I have, therefore, included the formulation of the syntax of behavior in this component, while adding the actual execution of that syntax to the title of the motor control component in Figure 7.7.

There is ample evidence in the neuropsychological literature (see the section on working memory in this chapter) that lesions to the prefrontal cortex disrupt this capacity to properly sequence behavior (Fuster, 1980, 1989; Godbout & Doyon, 1995; Milner, 1995; Sirigu et al., 1995; Stuss & Benson, 1986). Developmental psychological research also demonstrates that there exists a dimension of motor performance related to sequencing that is separate from those related to balance and coordination (Dewey & Kaplan, 1994). That form of motor sequencing may involve this concept of behavioral reconstitution.

Summary

In summary, reconstitution represents the capacity to dismantle and reassemble behavioral sequences. It probably arises from the capacity to covertly manipulate, act upon, and experiment or play with previously learned contingency arrangements that are being held in mind (working memory) so as to specify new ones and create new behavioral sequences in accordance with those contingency arrangements. This function is the generator of behavioral diversity and novelty; it creates new and original contingency-specifying arrangements of information (verbal and nonverbal), otherwise known as rules, that serve to guide the formation of complex, hierarchically organized, goal-directed behavioral structures.

The complexity of organisms created by evolution are founded upon the biological principles of fecundity (proliferation of offspring), fidelity (the relative preservation of characteristics of the previous generation), mutation (the opportunity for small changes), and competition for resources (Dawkins, 1982). Is behavioral diversity and complexity founded on similar concepts at the level of the analysis and synthesis of the units of behavior? Just as biological diversity can be

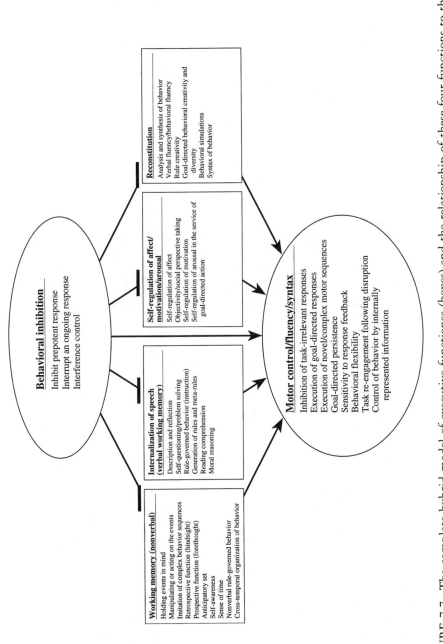

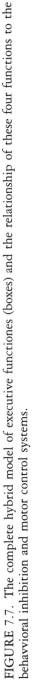

FIGURE 7.7. The complete hybrid model of executive functiones (boxes) and the relationship of these four functions to the behavvioral inhibition and motor control systems.

traced to a simple algorithm that repeats itself over long spans of time, could not behavioral diversity arise from a similar process? Our fecundity rests in our power to repeat behaviors and their sequences endlessly and with reasonable fidelity; however, each performance is not identical to the last, as small mutations may occur in the performance that may be retained into the next performance. Despite our relative ignorance of the particular mechanisms involved in the analytic and synthetic processes associated with reconstitution, there seems little doubt that some such function exists with the domain of executive activities.

MOTOR CONTROL/FLUENCY/SYNTAX

Internal, covert forms of self-directed behavior and the information they generate increasingly come to control the actions of the behavioral programming and execution systems across child development, giving behavior not only an increasingly deliberate, reasoned, and dispassionate nature, but also a more purposive, intentional, and future-oriented one as well. These executive functions produce observable effects on behavioral responding and motor control. Many of these were either directly mentioned or implied in the discussion of each executive function. I will reiterate those effects on motor control here so as to complete the model. That completed model of executive functioning is now shown in Figure 7.7.

As a result of the internal regulation of behavior, both sensory input and motor behavior that are unrelated to the goal and its internally represented behavioral structures become minimized or even suppressed during task or goal-directed performances. This occurs not only during the operation of these executive functions but also during the execution of the complex, goal-directed motor responses they generate. Once goal-directed actions have been formulated and prepared for transfer to the motor execution system, the motivation or drive necessary to maintain this sequence of goal-directed behavioral structures must be recruited or self-induced. This may happen automatically, as Damasio (1994, 1995) suggests, by the affective and motivational states that are associated with the internally represented information held in working memory and used to formulate the goal-directed behavior. Regardless of precisely how it arises, such a recruitment of motivation in the service of goal-directed behavior, when combined with working memory and interference control, serve to drive that behavior toward its intended destination. This creates goal-directed persistence, characterized by will-power, self-discipline, determination, single-mindedness of purpose, and a drivenness or intentional quality.

Throughout the execution of goal-directed behaviors, working memory permits the feedback from the last response(s) to be held in mind (retrospective function) so as to feed forward (prospective function) in modifying subsequent responding, thereby creating a sensitivity to errors, and behavioral flexibility. Just as important, when interruptions in this chain of goal-directed behaviors occur, the individual is able to disengage, respond to the interruption, and then reengage the original goal-directed sequence because the plan for that goal-directed activity has been held in mind despite interruption. Thus, inhibition sets the occasion for the engagement of the four executive functions, which then provide considerably greater control over behavior by the internally represented information they generate.

COMPARISONS TO OTHER MODELS

It is important to recognize that several of the executive functions probably entail feedback effects that assist with further behavioral inhibition, thereby creating an interactive reciprocity between the executive functions and the component of behavioral inhibition in the model. Such a reciprocity was inherent in Fuster's (1989) and Goldman-Rakic's (1995a, 1995b) views of the working memory system and its relationship to inhibition, and it has been more recently reiterated by Roberts and Pennington (1996) in discussing that system. Therefore, behavioral inhibition sets the occasion for the executive functions to occur. They not only provide the internal guidance over motor behavior, but may reciprocally influence the behavioral inhibition system as well by further increasing activity within that system as needed to support the goal-directed behavioral structures the executive functions are controlling. For instance, internalized speech may contain language and rules that are inhibitory or suppressive of behavior in nature. These would be expected to produce additional inhibitory effects on motor behavior, probably through feedback effects on the behavioral inhibition system. Moreover, private sensing, such as in visual imagery, may also yield information of an inhibitory nature, producing a similar feedback effect.

The critical reader by now may have recognized an apparent oversight of mine in the construction of this model, particularly if one is familiar with Gray's (1982, 1987, 1994) neuropsychological model of anxiety. Gray, and many others, have identified both a behavioral inhibition system and a behavioral activation system as being critical to understanding emotion. Some mechanism for basic nonspecific arousal would also seem to be a critical element of any attempt to model functions of the brain. I have identified only a behavioral inhibition system in this model. Moreover, linkage of emotional self-control with that of drive and arousal or activation in this model would also beg the same question, namely, where in the model are the constructs of arousal and activation to be found?

I confess to having intentionally omitted these two systems because I was attempting to develop a model solely of the executive functions. I am not trying to develop a model of the entire array of functions of the human brain that may be involved in emotion, as Gray was trying to do. While I admit that both a unit for generating nonspecific arousal and one for behavioral activation are necessary to any affective, drive, or motivational state, I would not consider arousal or activation to be executive functions in themselves. That is because they do not meet the definition of self-control I set out in Chapter 3 as being instrumental to defining a function as being executive; the arousal and behavioral activation systems do not seem to me to be self-directed forms of behavior that are designed to alter subsequent responses so as to maximize long-term outcomes.

Such components, particularly the behavioral activation system, are activated by the short-term reinforcers and other consequences that are signaled as being available in the immediate context. Those consequences serve to activate prepotent responses toward the production of those immediate consequences. It is precisely those prepotent behaviors that the behavioral inhibition system must inhibit if self-regulation is to occur. The prepotent responses must be so inhibited if the future rewards and other consequences for behavior are to receive adequate deliberation and so stand any chance of taking control over behavior and away from that control exerted by the immediate environment. I believe that these nonspecific arousal and behavioral activation systems must be harnessed or enslaved by the executive functions so as to employ them, when needed, in support of future-directed behavior.

This is why I do not recognize the brain arousal and behavioral activation systems as being executive in nature and thus do not include them in this model. Yet I readily accept their supportive role behind the scenes and their enslavement by the executive system in the service of its intentions. If I were pressed to include them in a model solely for the sake of completeness, I would cast these "ghost" components by way of gray outlines and arrows/footplates, as I have done in Figure 7.8. In doing so, however, I do not want to suggest that they should be taken to represent executive functions. I will not extend them to

ADHD in Chapter 9, as I am much less certain of what, if any, involvement they may have in explaining that disorder.

This more complete model as shown in Figure 7.8 bears a resemblance to that of Gray (1987), as adapted by Newman and Wallace (1993), which I reprint here in Figure 7.9. These two figures are quite similar in specifying components for nonspecific arousal, behavioral activation, and behavioral inhibition. Both also specify a level at which self-monitoring, evaluation, and motor control by that evaluation may be taking place. But they clearly differ in that Gray (and Newman and Wallace) sets forth in the middle of his diagram an appraisal and decision-making component that is quite ambiguous in its nature and its specific contents.

In contrast, the model developed in this chapter goes so far as to specify what the elements of that decision-making component may be, elevates them to the status of the executive system, and links them as being critical to the development of human self-control. It further specifies the critical role that time, timing, and timeliness play in self-regulation by articulating the concepts of hindsight and fore-thought and the sense of time they permit. These forms of temporal awareness play a critical role in determining the calculation of risk–benefit ratios associated with various response options under considera-tion by way of the system for self-regulated affect/motivation/arousal

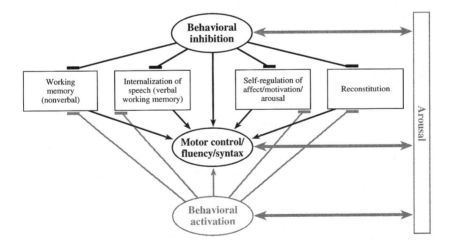

FIGURE 7.8. The relationship of the behavioral activation system and a nonspecific arousal system to the hybrid model of executive functions (Figure 7.7).

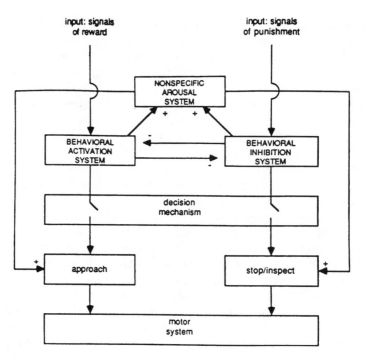

FIGURE 7.9. Gray's neuropsychological model of approach–avoidance learning. Reprinted from Newman and Wallace (1993, p. 702). Copyright 1993 by Pergamon Press. Reprinted by permission. Adapted from Gray (1987). Copyright 1987 by Cambridge University Press. Adapted by permission.

(Damasio's [1994, 1995] somatic marker system). I have also stipulated the critical role that internalized language plays in vastly expanding the individual's repertoire for rule-governed behavior in the service of goal-directed, future-oriented responding and the bridging of time such rules permit. Moreover, I have specified a unit of executive function that is capable of creating novel, complex sequences of goal-directed actions and hierarchies of such actions via the function of reconstitution. Thus, I am far more concerned here with the nature of the executive functions themselves rather than the arousal and activation systems that I fully recognize must exist to support them. I acknowledge, however, that my own model can be easily integrated within Gray's model to yield a more complete picture of brain functions, particularly as they may be related to human emotions and especially their self-regulation.

Newman and Wallace (1993) have used Gray's theory in attempting to understand the nature of disinhibitory psychopathology in children and psychopathy in adults. They, likewise, recognize the role that disinhibition probably plays in ADHD by its disruption of self-regulation. While they do attempt to define self-regulation as the effortful monitoring, evaluating, and, if need be, altering of behavior, they do not recognize the larger purpose self-regulation serves, which is the net maximization of long-term outcomes for the individual. Nor do they specify the precise executive functions that participate in self-regulation and why they are disrupted by disinhibition, as I have tried to do in this model.

Newman and Wallace (1993) do recognize, however, the importance of delayed responding in permitting the analysis of patterns of feedback and the regulation such feedback exerts over continued responding. They refer to this as response modulation and argue that this is what is deficient in children with disinhibitory forms of psychopathology. This response modulation process sounds very similar to that accomplished within the working memory system in its interaction with the behavioral inhibition system as described earlier, for it gives rise to a sensitivity to errors in performance. But the nature of this response modulation system is not specified by Newman and Wallace (1993).

Those authors further stipulate that disinhibitory forms of psychopathology in children, particularly the three forms of conduct disorder (CD)—socialized, neurotic, and psychopathic—may arise from three different disturbances in the arousal, activation, and inhibition components of Gray's model. The socialized type arises from overactivity in the behavioral activation system that also increases nonspecific arousal, both of which serve to overwhelm the decision-making component of the model. In doing so, these components create an individual whose behavior is dominated by reward-seeking activities in the immediate context that are unchecked by the monitoring and decision-making component. The neurotic form arises from activity in the behavioral inhibition system which increases nonspecific arousal and thus overwhelms the decision-making mechanism. Note that both of these pathways to CD specify a higher than normal state of nonspecific arousal, but that state is achieved by two different pathways (overactive behavioral activation system vs. overactive behavioral inhibition system). Such overarousal in response to environmental signals of either immediate reward or impending punishment overwhelms the decision-making component, leading to more rapid responding and reduced opportunities for self-regulation.

The psychopathic type arises out of poor response modulation, which is an intrinsic deficit in the decision-making system itself. The individual is less able to shift attention from ongoing, more automatic forms of goal-directed behavior to more self-regulated (modulated) forms of goal-directed behavior that have been properly evaluated for their long-term outcomes. The interested reader is referred to the review paper by Newman and Wallace (1993) for the evidence they marshal in favor of this tripartite distinction in CD and psychopathy.

More important to my purposes here, Newman and Wallace suggest that ADHD, like psychopathy, may arise out of a defective response modulation system. They are quick to recognize, however, that many differences exist between them, and that the subtype of ADHD most closely resembling psychopathy is that which is comorbid with CD or aggression.

I concur with Newman and Wallace up to a point on this extrapolation of their response modulation hypothesis to ADHD. Individuals with ADHD do appear to have difficulties with self-regulation, and such difficulties do arise from difficulties with monitoring, evaluating, and altering ongoing behavior, given feedback for performance. But rather than arising directly out of a defect in those executive functions that I believe permit such response modulation (nonverbal working memory, internalized speech, self-regulated affect/motivation/arousal, and reconstitution), ADHD arises from a deficit "upstream" from this executive system, in the behavioral inhibition system itself as I have argued in Chapter 4.

Like Quay (1988a, 1988b, 1997), who has also extended Gray's model to CD and ADHD, I believe the latter arises from underactivity within the behavioral inhibition system. It is less clear to me how that underactivation or underfunctioning arises and whether or not Gray's model can account for it, given that he posits anxiety disorders to arise from overactivity of that same system. If that is true, then Quay's use of Gray's theory to explain ADHD would imply that children with ADHD cannot demonstrate an anxiety disorder because ADHD arises from underactivity and anxiety from overactivity within the same system. However, research has certainly shown that children with ADHD can have anxiety disorders, or higher than normal levels of internalizing symptoms (Biederman et al., 1992; Tannock, in press). They still manifest greater impulsiveness than normal, though less than that evident in ADHD children without high levels of internalizing symptoms (Tannock, in press). This would seem to contradict Quay's assertion about ADHD.

I believe that this coexistence of ADHD with anxiety implies that some forms of anxiety are arising out of a different brain system than that which gives rise to behavioral inhibition. Perhaps it is the system in Gray's model, not shown in Figure 7.9, that he refers to as the fight-or-flight appraisal system. This system automatically evaluates the potentially threatening nature of stimuli. It imparts to them an affective bias early in their midbrain unconscious processing, before they undergo further higher level and more conscious information processing, perhaps at the cortical level. Such an appraisal/affective bias (i.e., threat, anxiety) placed on events early in their unconscious information processing, before they even impact upon the behavioral activation and inhibition systems, would serve to increase activity in the behavioral inhibition system that is downstream from this early event appraisal system. Thus, ADHD children, whom I hypothesize are deficient in behavioral inhibition, if possessed of an appraisal/affect system that imparts such a threat and anxiety bias to events early in their processing, could display findings identical to those seen in the extant, albeit limited, literature on those having both ADHD and high anxiety levels. ADHD children would still be less inhibited than normal but more inhibited than ADHD children without high levels of anxiety. This is because the early appraisal of threat and anxiety can serve to increase activity within an inhibitory system that is underfunctioning relative to normal. Moreover, such an explanation would clearly permit the two disorders to coexist without being theoretical contradictions to each other, as in the Quay/Gray model of ADHD. In short, some forms of anxiety arise out of an affective bias imparted early on in the processing of information that serves to increase activity in the BIS that is downstream from that event/affect appraisal system, whatever and wherever it may be. This would account for those with high anxiety levels without ADHD having increased levels of behavioral inhibition as well as for individuals with ADHD who also have higher than normal levels of anxiety.

In any case, previous attempts to use Gray's model to explain ADHD converge with the present model along a number of avenues of thought, including concerning the nature of inhibitory problems, their importance to self-regulation, and their utility in understanding ADHD.

THE PLACE OF SUSTAINED ATTENTION IN THE MODEL

If the proposed model of self-control and executive functions is to be at all applicable to ADHD, it must identify the nature not only of the inhibitory deficiencies known to be associated with this disorder but also the difficulties with inattention, particularly poor sustained attention, involved in this disorder. This relationship can now be readily understood as resulting from the interaction of the behavioral inhibition system with those executive functions that provide for the control of behavior by internally represented information (especially covert imagery, rules, and self-motivation). Interference control seems particularly critical to the persistence of goal-directed behavior, which I believe represents a special form of sustained attention. When responses that are under the control and guidance of internally represented information must be sustained over long periods of time, the individual must resist responding to distractions that may arise both internally and externally during task performance or in pursuit of a goal. This resistance is provided by the interference control functions of the behavioral inhibition system. The individual must also formulate and hold in mind the goal of the task and the plan for attaining that goal so that it serves as a template for constructing the necessary behavioral structures to that end. Thus, the working memory functions may be involved in goal-directed persistence as well. But most importantly, the individual must also kindle, sustain, and renew internally represented sources of drive and motivation that continuously support behavior toward the goal in the absence of external sources of reinforcement or motivation for doing so.

These covert, self-controlling functions are not necessary in situations or tasks where the individual's pattern of responding is simply being maintained by the prevailing schedule of immediate reinforcement. That form of sustained responding is not being internally guided, but is a function of the motivational factors in the immediate task and context; it is, in a sense, externally maintained attention or sustained responding.

The internally guided sustained attention is better termed goal-directed persistence, and its origin lies in self-regulation and the interaction of the executive functions, especially self-regulation of motivation and effort. The other type of sustained attention is contingency-shaped or context-dependent, and its origins lie in the nature of those immediate contingencies operating within the task or setting and the individual's contact with them. Both of these forms of sustained attention will appear as sustained responding to the casual observer. Their differences in origins and the variables maintaining them, however, can be readily detected by removing any source of immediate reinforcement that may be provided by the task or external context. This should have little or no effect on goal-directed persistence that is being internally (covertly) mediated or guided, while resulting in a significant decline in or extinction of the sustained responding that is contingency-shaped and maintained by the external consequences prevailing in the task.

Skinner (1969) made a similar distinction concerning the nature of contingency-shaped versus rule-governed forms of human behavior, and it is a useful distinction to make in the construct of sustained attention as well. Contingency-shaped behavior is likely to be more variable, associated with emotion, impulsive, less conscious or even unconscious or automatic, more prone to superstitious conditioning (control by spurious or coincidental consequences), and likely to extinguish as the immediate consequences become weak or nonexistent (Skinner, 1969). As I will discuss in Chapter 9, it is the goal-directed, self-regulated form of sustained attention or persistence and not the contingency-shaped, externally regulated kind that is disrupted in ADHD.

As noted in Chapter 6, most measures of sustained attention in psychological and neuropsychological research on this construct are actually assessing goal-directed persistence rather than contingency-shaped sustained attention. Neuroimaging and other neuropsychological studies have found that the right prefrontal region is more likely than the left to be involved in the performance of tasks that involve the type of behavioral or motor persistence I have described here (Goldman & Podell, 1995; Kertesz, Nicholson, Cancelliere, Kassa, & Black, 1985; Knight et al., 1995; Pardo, Fox, & Raichle, 1991; Rueckert & Grafman, 1996). Other neuroimaging research has shown that this region seems to be smaller in those with ADHD (Castellanos et al., 1996; Filipek et al., 1997) perhaps explaining why those with ADHD may have difficulties on such tasks.

The involvement of the prefrontal cortex is probably not necessary for the contingency-shaped type of sustained attention. The goal-directed form, however, is dependent on the prefrontal cortex and the executive functions that cortex and its networks permit.

ON THE NATURE OF THE "CENTRAL EXECUTIVE"

Neuropsychologists have debated the nature of "the central executive" among the executive functions for decades. In other words, what process is it that determines which goals will be selected, which plans, rules, and other sources of information will be considered in support of them, and what forms of private self-directed actions are necessary to generate that information? That process has been labeled the central executive (Baddeley, 1986; Goldman-Rakic, 1995a; Pennington, Bennetto, McAleer, & Roberts, 1996), yet its specification has been left ambiguous. It has, alas, become the black box within the black box (brain) that information-processing models of cognition have been attempting to explain; another homunculus placed within the brain like a reductive series of Russian dolls housed within a larger doll. The central executive is presumed to be that mechanism used to account for why decisions about responding are made the way they are by an individual (Hayes et al., 1996). Who or what decides in what service the executive functions and self-regulation will be put, and for what purpose?

The nature of this central executive, if such an entity must be specified, now seems clear to me—it is time. More specifically, it is the conjecturing of the future that arises out of reconstruction of the past and the goal-directed behaviors that are predicated on these activities. Such activities, along with the other executive functions, permit self-regulation relative to time. The goal in support of which these private behaviors are undertaken becomes the central executive, that goal has been based on an analysis where time becomes the critical factor. Goals seem to arise as a result of a computation, often outside of awareness, of those risks–benefits associated with various response options to an event or situation (Damasio, 1994, 1995). That computation is certainly assisted by the motivational and affective tone or markers associated with those response options (Clore, 1994; Damasio, 1994, 1995). Important yet often left unspecified in such discussions of a risk–benefit appraisal system is the time span or temporal horizon over which such response options are evaluated. Individuals who consider risk–benefit calculations across short temporal foreperiods (future time horizons) are likely to make very different decisions concerning responses to events than are those whose temporal foreperiods, or windows on the future, contain a much longer time horizon into that future. The selection of the goal and of the response options for the attainment of that goal, therefore, are very much a function of time and the future interval over which forethought is operative. *Time, or the individual's sense of the future, is ultimately the central executive.* As Green et al. (1996) have commented, differences among individuals in the future time periods (delays to rewards) over which they come to discount future rewards (their preference for delayed over immediate rewards) make a significant contribution to the decision making of those individuals in their selection of responses to events. Those individual differences in future time horizons thereby come to have a substantial impact on the long-term successes and failures those individuals are likely to experience in their adaptive functioning. That preference for delayed rewards must be predicated on a span of time over which those delayed consequences are evaluated; they are based on a sense of the future.

HUMAN VOLITION AND WILL

The hybrid model presented in this chapter is intended to capture those executive functions that provide for self-regulation, that is, the transfer of behavior from external control by the immediate environment to internal control by mentally represented information and the goals which it subserves—from control by the moment to control by the hypothetical future. Such a transfer in behavioral control results in a shift from the maximization of merely immediate consequences to a net maximization of long-term consequences relative to those immediate consequences.

As Bastian (1892/1992) and James (1890) both noted, behavior that is being internally guided gives the appearance of the organism possessing a will. The organism could be said to have a free will. But that will is free only in the sense that behavior has been freed of its control by immediate, momentary, and external sources of control. It is still being controlled by other sources, which are the result of internal, self-directed actions and the information that they yield. That information contributes to decision making about response options.

Control over behavior has not been removed by such a process of internal self-regulation, nor has behavior become totally free. The control of behavior merely has been transferred. It has been shifted from the present to the hypothetical future, from the immediate consequence of a response to conjectures regarding its delayed or more distant ones, from the immediate three-dimensional spatial environment to a four-dimensional environment in which time is a more salient dimension in the control of behavior.

From this perspective, a person's will is not truly free, or uncontrolled by external sources. The executive functions and the self-regulation they permit do not free the individual's behavior from control by the environment—far from it. They actually allow the person's behavior to be more effectively controlled by that environment. This apparent paradox can be explained as follows. Where the executive functions may become impaired, as through a brain injury, the individual appears to be *more* controlled by the environment, not less so. But the facts available seem to indicate that the person has simply become more controlled by the immediate three-dimensional setting and less controlled by the actual four-dimensional reality of space combined with time, or what physicists refer to as space–time (Davies, 1995). The change in sources controlling behavior has actually been a reduction from a more realistic four-dimensional context to the more obvious one of the immediate three-dimensional setting. In the latter setting, time as a factor of behavioral control has been diminished. To attend to time, individuals must reallocate their attentional resources away from the immediate spatial environment and toward the analysis of event sequences or sequences of moments (J. W. Brown, 1990; Zakay, 1992). The more that spatial information must be processed within the immediate context, the less capable is the individual of accurately attending to time. Thus, individuals whose behavior has become more governed by the spatial context of the moment are less able to be governed by time.

Time is an integral, inseparable part of the physical world. To fail to be affected or controlled by this dimension of the physical world is analogous to the brain-injured patient having a neglect syndrome failing to be affected or controlled by visual–spatial information. From this perspective, prefrontal lobe lesions create a form of temporal neglect, or time blindness, resulting not only in the most obvious shift in the control over behavior from internal to external guidance, but in a more subtle yet socially devastating reduction in the control over behavior from four dimensions to three in such individuals. In a very real sense, then, disturbances to the prefrontal lobes that disrupt self-regulation result in a reduction in the effective control of the individual's behavior by the physical world rather than an increase in environmental dependence. It is no longer space within time, or space–time, that is effectively regulating the individual's behavior but space within the temporal moment that is doing so.

Self-regulation and the executive functions permitting it may create the illusion of freedom from external control because of three factors inherent in self-regulation. One of these is the more immediately and palpably discerned shift from control by external sources to control by internal self-generated sources of information. We experience the information being represented within ourselves. The second is that we experience these executive functions as our own actions being directed at our self; we experience the effects of those functions on our own behavior. This gives us a feeling of agency in the process and in ultimately affecting the world around us. The third is that such self-generated activity is simply a means of increasing the control over the individual's behavior by time, a far more subtle dimension or source of control to detect than other external sources. We can, therefore, be forgiven in overlooking its important influence in this process; time seems invisible, while events within each temporal moment do not.

These three factors, I believe, conspire to give the individual the illusion of being free. The freedom, however, is simply one of being less controlled by the moment; the control over the individual's behavior by the temporal dimension of the world has actually increased in this process. If freedom is really an absolute reduction in the sources of control that affect the individual's behavior, then the brain-injured patient with a prefrontal injury and the individual with ADHD are probably more free of such control, given that time has lost its grip upon them. The irony in all of this, of course, is that individuals who demonstrate greater self-regulation are far more under the control of their environment than are those with less self-regulation, that is why the former individual benefits far more in the long run than does the latter. *Self-regulation increases the effectiveness of control of the individual by the physical world, a world in which time is an inherent feature.*

This further explains why I concluded, indeed had no choice but to conclude, that time is the central executive. The ghost of such an executive mechanism of agency may haunt the study of prefrontal brain functions because the subtlety of time haunts the physical world. As any self-respecting, self-regulating adult comes to realize with age, we progressively become a slave to time. The controller of our decisions, the determiner of the object of self-regulation is time. This may be why, as we mature, we experience time as a new burden to bear. From this perspective, the young child is more free from, more innocent of, and less burdened by time than is the adult. If we pine for the days of our childhood, in part what we long for is this innocence from the awareness of time, as James Carroll so eloquently stated in the quotation accompanying the dedication of this book.

Our will, therefore, is not free. It is at time's beck and call. A person capable of self-regulation can no more help but use that self-regulation in response to the siren's call of time than he or she can help seeing, hearing, or sensing in general. We not only have an instinct for self-control, as I will argue in the next chapter; we have a compulsion to employ it in the service of our own self-interests.

This view of the functions of the prefrontal cortex and the executive control that it affords us in regulating behavior relative to space and time has a significant implication for testing these functions. It suggests that the neuropsychological tests that are most likely to elicit the executive functions are those that set up competing sources of control between the immediate three-dimensional world and that world with time included as a factor in the task. The ultimate competition here is not so much between rules and other sources of behavioral control, as Hayes et al. (1996) suggested, though that is true in a sense. That competition is between space in the temporal moment and space–time in the regulation of behavior. Rules are simply one means through which time exerts its control over behavior. The conflict set up by a test of executive functions is between the future and the present, between time and the temporal now.

As is evident from Chapters 5–7, this shift in control is directly attributable to the prefrontal cortex. This makes the prefrontal cortex of the human brain, in a sense, a time machine. More accurately, it is a space–time machine. It acts to perceive sequences of events and uses those sequences to regulate behavior. Thus, time comes to control behavior. The perception of events in sequences makes the sense of time seem to flow or have a direction, as a consequence. Patterns are discerned in those event sequences, which will be used to make educated guesses concerning future events. As Fuster (1989) said, this brain region thus organizes behavior across time on the basis of internally conjectured future events. Such behavior appears intentional, purposive, future-oriented, self-disciplined, and having a single-mindedness of purpose, as Skinner (1953, 1969) and others (Bastian, 1892; Fuster, 1980) have noted. But the future cannot actually control behavior because it has not yet happened to that individual. What controls behavior is an internal representation of the expected future—a hypothetical conjecture of the likely sequence of events that may unfold—which has been derived from a resensing of past event sequences and our experiences with them (Bastian, 1892; James, 1890/1992; Fuster, 1980, 1989; Goldman-Rakic, 1995a). In other words, the present elicits a past from which is conjectured a future, the anticipation of which controls our behavior. As James (1890/1992) stated in describing human will, "The essential achievement of the will, in short, when it is most 'voluntary,' is to ATTEND to a difficult object and hold it fast before the mind. The so-doing is the fiat; and it is a mere physiological incident that when the object is thus attended to, immediate motor consequences ensue" (pp. 815–816).

While few neuropsychologists have acknowledged it, any efforts to develop a model of the functions of the prefrontal lobes—to construct theories of executive functions—are efforts, in a way, to specify the nature of human volition and will. This makes Crick's (1994) recent declaration of the Astonishing Hypothesis—the novelty of which seems to be the localization of free will to the prefrontal cortex—seem to me to be not so astonishing nor novel after all. It has been anticipated all along by past theorists working on the nature of the functions of the prefrontal cortex. It was anticipated by Still (1902), as discussed in Chapter 1, in his description of ADHD children as being deficient in volitional inhibition and the moral control of behavior (i.e., regulation by internally represented information). But as even Bastian (1892) commented, such a conceptualization of human volition and will means that it is not capable of discrete localization within any explicit region of the brain. These concepts of volition and will are multidimensional because the executive system that gives rise to them is multidimensional. Injuries to one region and the function it affords will create a different impairment of volition than will injuries to the other regions and the functions they permit. Nor is it necessarily true that these concepts of volition and will could be localized entirely to the prefrontal regions. As neuroimaging studies have shown, these executive functions organize and orchestrate a variety of functions of the posterior hemispheres in support of goal-directed behavior. It seems fair to say, however, that the prefrontal cortex is most important in these concepts of volition and will. It provides the executive functions that permit human self-regulation, and those functions go about their business at the behest of time, in the service of goals, and in the individual's long-term self-interest.

CONCLUSION

In this chapter I have attempted to construct a hybrid model of executive functions out of prior theories of the nature of such functions. Greatest emphasis was placed on Bronowski's (1967/1977) model because of its greater comprehensiveness in capturing the diversity of these executive functions. Concepts from the more recent and empirically derived theories of prefrontal lobe functions were then used to provide greater detail concerning the nature of each executive function and the linkages among them.

The model developed here and shown in Figure 7.7 contains six components. The first component is that of behavioral inhibition, which provides the foundation on which the other four executive functions are dependent. These four functions are nonverbal working memory, verbal working memory, the self-regulation of affect/motivation/arousal, and reconstitution. They are covert, self-directed forms of behavior which yield information that is internally represented and that will exert a controlling influence over the sixth component of the model, the motor control and execution system. Although I have resorted to the more common neuropsychological terms used for these four executive functions, they could be redefined in terms of their behavioral equivalents as (1) covert, self-directed sensing (nonverbal working memory), (2) covert, self-directed speech (verbal working memory), (3) covert, self-directed affect/motivation/arousal, or emoting to oneself, and (4) covert, self-directed behavioral manipulation, experimentation, and play (reconstitution). Each is believed to be derived from its more public, outer-directed and observable counterparts in human behavior that have become turned on the self and that have been made progressively more private, covert, or unobservable (internalized) in form.

These executive functions permit outer behavior to be guided by forms of inner behavior that serve to effectively bridge cross-temporal contingencies and direct behavior toward hypothetical future events (outcomes, goals, etc.). They also give rise to a new form of sustained responding (attention), apart from that form controlled by the immediate prevailing contingencies, that arises out of such internally guided forms of behavior directed toward a goal.

Time, timing, and timeliness, then, become important concepts in understanding such goal-directed behavior and in determining it, thereby making time, in a way, the "central executive." These forms of covert executive behaviors and the future-directed behavior they permit comprise the human will or volition. They provide a means for greater prediction and control over one's own behavior relative to the environment, and resulting in greater prediction over that environment and hence more effective control of behavior by it. The environment is not simply physical space, but physical space–time. The ultimate utility function of these executive actions and the self-regulation relative to time they provide is the net maximization of long-term consequences or outcomes for the benefit of the individual's self-interests.

I fully recognize that I have painted this model with large strokes and that many of the finer details of each executive function and their linkages need to be specified. At this stage of theory development, however, it seems to me that all that can be achieved is a relatively crude approximation of what a theory of self-regulation and executive functions may eventually be. But even that rough approximation of a theory created here brings with it a substantial number of implications, many profound, for the nature of human self-regulation and, especially, for the nature of ADHD. Before examining these implications in Chapters 9 and 11, the rough model of executive functioning needs to be placed within a developmental context. That is the goal of the next chapter.

CHAPTER 8

———•———

Developmental Considerations: Self-Control as an Instinct

THIS CHAPTER CONSIDERS some of the developmental implications that derive from the model of executive functions and self-control constructed in the previous chapter. The executive functions schematically represented in Figure 7.7 probably follow a developmental course similar to that of the development of private speech (Berk, 1992). They originate from their external, more public and outer/other-directed counterparts, which probably functioned initially to sense and to control the external world and especially to sense, inform, and control the behavior of others within it. The executive forms of these public behaviors, I believe, eventually became turned on the self as a means of informing and controlling one's own behavior so that the individual becomes more effective in the prediction and control of the external environment for his or her long-term benefit. Once turned on the self, these executive forms of behavior come to lose the outward, publicly observable musculoskeletal manifestations of their occurrence and are said to be internalized. This does not mean that they have moved to some higher, internalized, metaphysical plane, but only that their more public manifestations have become suppressed, as Dennett (1995) has suggested.

DEVELOPMENT OF THE EXECUTIVE FUNCTIONS

Undoubtedly, these executive functions and the future-directed forms of behavior they permit do not all arise suddenly nor simultaneously in human development. There are likely to be phases or stages to their

209

development, arising as they probably do in some staggered sequence during maturation.

Inhibition and Nonverbal Working Memory

Research in developmental psychology suggests that the capacity to delay a response and to privately (mentally) represent visual information during the delay is present as early as the first 5–12 months of life (Diamond et al., 1994; Hofstadter & Reznick, 1996). Both working memory and response inhibition have been shown to be separate yet important elements in performing delayed response tasks even at this age (Diamond et al., 1994). Over the next 6–18 months, improvements in both response inhibition (Vaughn et al., 1984) and representational memory (Zelazo, Kearsley, & Stack, 1995) will occur. One determinant is the subject's level of general development (Vaughn et al., 1984). However, individual differences in inhibition appear to be an even greater determinant of performance in delayed-response tasks than is age or general developmental level (Lee, Vaughn, & Kopp, 1983). By age 3–4 years, children are quite proficient at such memory-for-location tasks, implying that both response inhibition and working or representational memory are well developed by this age (Daehler, Bukato, Benson, & Myers, 1976; Loughton & Daehler, 1973).

Not only is inhibition of prepotent responses important in the development of working memory, but so is interference control. As Bjorklund and Harnishfeger (1990) have argued, children demonstrate an increasing ability to protect working memory from interference by intrusions or irrelevant information from nursery school age through sixth grade. This results in increased proficiency in the performance of tasks that place greater demands on working memory and attention (Higgins & Turnure, 1984). It is not clear from research on this issue whether the problem of interference control is one of inefficient inhibition of information entering working memory (intrusions) or of competing response choices that may be represented in working memory. In either case, the development of efficient inhibition appears to assist with the development of more effective working memory.

It would appear from such research that the behavioral inhibition and nonverbal working memory systems arise earliest in child development. Given what is known about the development of internalized speech (Berk, 1992), it would be difficult to argue that verbal working memory is also underway or is contributing to the performance of delayed-response or working memory tasks below age 3 years. The internalization of speech, which I believe forms the articulatory loop or verbal working memory, comes later, as a separate developmental stage of the executive functions.

Self-Regulation of Affect/Motivation/Arousal

Bronowski (1967/1977) suggested that the self-regulation of affect probably begins next in the developmental sequence of the executive functions. As noted in Chapter 5, theorists of executive functions believe that sensory representations held in working memory are likely to elicit their associated somatic markers (affect/motivation/arousal properties). This provides a rudimentary form of covert emoting to oneself that automatically occurs in concert with holding mental representations on-line. But apart from such inferences, is there evidence of the early emergence of self-directed affective or motivational behaviors in developmental psychology? Apparently so.

Kopp (1989), in reviewing the development of emotional self-regulation, particularly as it is used by children to manage distress, discomfort, and negative emotion, notes that rudimentary forms of self-directed emotion regulation are evident between 3 and 9 months of life. Children at this age seem to use gaze aversion and fussing more than self-soothing and self-distraction methods as a means of emotion regulation (Mangelsdorf, Shapiro, & Marzolf, 1995). In a few months, these public forms of emotion regulation may take the form of self-distraction toward pleasurable toys when children experience periods of discomfort or distress, or become self-comforting behaviors, such as touching one's body, grasping at one's body parts, manipulating those parts, and sucking on one's fingers or other body parts (Stifter & Braungart, 1995). By the end of the first year of life, as infants' motor abilities are developing, they increasingly use self-directed motor actions as a means of coping with periods of distress or negative emotional arousal (Kopp, 1989). These gestures may include rocking, stroking oneself, rubbing the genitals, or chewing on fingers and thumbs. As mobility increases between 12 and 18 months of age, the young child now has the capacity to locomote so as to distract him- or herself with available toys and objects in the vicinity during periods of distress (Kopp, 1989; Mangelsdorf et al., 1995). Throughout development to this point, an infant becomes increasingly adept at manipulating caregivers with facial expressions, vocalizations, and gestures to enlist the caregivers in the reduction of the child's distress and negative emotional states.

According to Kopp (1989), by the second to third year young children have begun to develop self-awareness, bringing with it the sense that they not only feel emotions but can do something to themselves to cope with them. They have also developed the capacity to identify some causes of their emotional distress, and so may use various means of eliminating or reducing such causes. The young child's use of transitional objects, such as favorite toys or blankets, as means of reducing emotional distress is one such coping mechanism at this stage of development. More sophisticated enlistment of caregivers to assist with eliminating the causes of emotional distress is another way such coping may be evident at this age. Kopp (1989) attributes these developments to the further growth of the representational memory system (working memory), which permits holding representations of one's own behavior and eventually one's identity in mind.

The development of language provides another important means of emotional self-regulation. Young children seem to improve markedly in their talking about emotions between 18 and 30 months of age, in concert with their growth in language during this period. Such language becomes another means of enlisting others, such as caregivers, in assisting the child with emotional self-regulation as well as a means by which caregivers can encourage and teach the child forms of emotional self-control (Kopp, 1989; Raver, 1996). Eventually, as speech becomes turned on the self at approximately 3 years of age, such self-speech provides a means of reassurance and other means of emotional control through self-directed dialogic commentary and instruction (Gottman, 1986; Kopp, 1989). As discussed in Chapter 3, preschool-age children have already developed a repertoire of self-directed verbal as well as motor strategies for coping with frustration and self-motivation during delay of gratification tasks (Mischel, 1983; Mischel et al., 1988, 1989). Self-speech in the preschool years is one means by which children are regulating not only their emotions, but their motivation and task persistence as well (Masters & Santrock, 1976). Of course, throughout this preschool age parents are teaching children means of emotional self-regulation and acceptance of responsibility for one's own behavior (Kopp, 1989).

By 3–5 years of age, the peer group becomes another source of teaching the child about emotional self-regulation. How children come to control their emotions in the presence of peers seems to have a great deal to do with their status with their peers. Eisenberg and colleagues (1993) have shown that preschool teacher's ratings of children's use of constructive emotional coping and attentional control (distractibility) were positively related to boys' social skills and peer status, whereas displays of negative affect were negatively related to social skills and status with peers. For girls, their use of avoidant coping methods was positively related to their social skills.

At what point in development emotional self-regulation becomes private or covert in form has not been well-studied. Self-speech becomes more covert in form in the later elementary grades (see Diaz & Berk, 1992), so this form of emotional self-regulation becomes internalized as speech progressively does so. But what about the nonverbal forms of emotional self-regulation witnessed earlier in child development? At what age are children able to emote to themselves privately without public manifestations? As nonverbal working memory or self-directed sensing becomes more developed, does private emoting correspondingly develop? What then becomes of the aforementioned association of somatic markers with such private representations? These are difficult questions to answer at this time. But apparently, as Kopp (1989) has suggested, the self-regulation of emotional states, and of their implicit motivational and arousal states, is well underway before self-directed speech becomes evident. This implies that self-regulation of affect/motivation/arousal as an executive function may follow self-directed sensing (nonverbal working memory) in the developmental stages of executive functions. Thus, by the time speech is acquired and turned on the self, the young child is already capable of three executive functions: behavioral inhibition, nonverbal working or representational memory, and the self-regulation of affect/motivation/arousal states.

Not mentioned to any appreciable extent in developmental psychology is the prospect that as these executive functions develop and interact, they should give rise to anticipatory affect/motivation in advance of future events. With maturation, such anticipatory affect may be generated further ahead of the anticipated events than is seen in younger children. It may be this development of anticipatory motivation that underlies the capacity for motivating and persisting in future-oriented behavior.

Internalization of Speech

The development of private, internalized speech was described in some detail in Chapter 5, which will not be reiterated here. It would appear from that discussion that the internalization of speech is the next executive function to arise in development, and a highly important one at that. Suffice it to say that by 3–5 years of age, self-speech has emerged in children and is publicly observable at this stage. It becomes increasingly covert across the early elementary grades until it is predominantly internalized by ages 9–12 years (see Berk, 1992, and other chapters in Diaz & Berk, 1992, for more details). It also becomes increasingly powerful as a means of controlling motor responding. As it does so, I believe that it becomes the basis for verbal working memory, as I have stated earlier. Further, the privatization of language and the rule-governed behavior it permits certainly provides a substantial contribution to the development of deferred gratification (Berkowitz, 1982; Mischel et al., 1989), self-control (Kopp, 1982), and moral conduct (Blasi, 1980; Kochanska, Aksan, & Koenig, 1995;

Kochanska, Murray, Jacques, Koenig, & Vandegeest, 1996; Peterson, 1982). Yet while the publicly observable manifestations of the oral musculature associated with speech become increasingly inhibited, as inner, covert speech develops, some micromovements of the oral musculature may still be detectable, even in adults, during silent or "inner" speech (Livesay, Liebke, Samaras, & Stanley, 1996). This further supports the point that inner speech or internalized language is based on public speech but with its public manifestations mainly, though not entirely, suppressed.

Children's awareness of their own private, covert speech may lag somewhat behind their actual development of such speech. Flavell and colleagues (Flavell, Green, Flavell, & Grossman, 1997) have recently shown in two studies that 4-year-olds appear not to realize that others can and are engaging in silent self-speech, as might be used in reading to oneself, counting, or recalling items via covert private speech. Nor are such 4-year-olds cognizant of their own capability for silent or inner speech. In contrast, 6- to 7-year-olds do have such knowledge about the possibility of inner speech by others and come to be aware of their own ability to engage in it. Such knowledge about others and self-awareness of inner speech continues to develop into the adult years, according to the results of these studies.

Under 3 years of age, the capacity of a child to follow rules given by caregivers and the social community is present (Vaughn et al., 1984) but not well formed (Goodwin, 1981; Kopp, 1982; Luria, 1961; Zelazo, Reznick, & Pinon, 1995). As with behavioral inhibition and working memory, individual differences in compliance to rules is partly a function of developmental level, with more advanced children demonstrating greater compliance (Vaughn et al., 1984). Children below 3 years of age appear to follow instructions that initiate a behavior better than they follow instructions that are designed to prevent a behavior from occurring or to stop an ongoing response (Luria, 1961; Skotko, 1992). By the end of the third year of life, rules appear to be considerably more effective in controlling a child's motor behavior (Luria, 1961; Skotko, 1992; Zelazo & Reznick, 1991). Consistent with the model developed in Chapter 7, Zelazo, Reznick, and Pinon (1995) have shown that this shift in the capacity of rules to govern behavior may be dependent on the development of the capacity to inhibit prepotent responses more than to the development of representational or working memory. For instance, below 3 years of age, young children seem to make more perseverative errors on sorting tasks where rules for sorting are being changed periodically during the task (Zelazo & Reznick, 1991; Zelazo, Kearsley, & Stack, 1995). Knowledge of the rule, reminders to use the rule, and working memory during the task do not seem to account for such perseveration. Such tasks resemble the WCST and imply that performance on that task by older individuals reflects behavioral inhibition as well as rule formulation and rule-guided behavior, as discussed in Chapter 7. From 18–30 months of age, the forms of self-control children use become more coherent or more closely associated with each other. For instance, Vaughn et al. (1984) showed that the capacity to delay a response is not significantly associated with compliance to maternal rules at ages 18 and 24 months but is so by 30 months of age.

It seems, then, that by the time that rules given by others are coming to exert some control over behavior, speech is becoming turned on the self as a means of self-control. This private but not yet covert speech appears to function not only as a means of self-guidance (Luria, 1961), but apparently as much or more a means of problem solving (Berk, 1992; Goodwin, 1981). The self-speech that children emit seems much less designed to control their immediate behavior than to improve later performance of similar tasks through verbal problem solving, such as self-questioning, problem clarification, and conjecturing about possible rules. As Berk (1992), Azmitia (1992), and others (Goodwin, 1981) have noted, private (though audible) speech appears most likely to occur in young children during problem-solving tasks and especially following failure experiences. Such self-speech correlates highly and positively with the subsequent performance of such tasks, whereas it may correlate negatively or not at all with current task performance (Azmitia, 1992; Frauenglas & Diaz, 1985).

Reconstitution

It is not clear at what age children develop the capacity to act upon and manipulate mental representations of events, such as visual imagery or self-directed speech, and their behavioral or prospective counterparts. In other words, when might reconstitution begin as an executive function? Berkowitz (1982) argues from developmental research at the time that the manipulation of visual imagery may not develop until 5 years of age even though younger children have the capacity to engage in such visual imagery. Given my thesis in this volume that reconstitution is a form of self-directed manipulation, experimentation, and play, the answer to this question might be found in the developmental psychology literature on the stages of children's play development, particularly that dealing with imaginative or fantasy play. Reconstitution as discussed here may reflect a means of conducting behavioral simulations covertly and testing them for their probable outcomes before choosing one to perform. Alternatively, perhaps the study of verbal and design fluency may shed some light on this developmental process, given that, in the previous chapter, such measures were argued to reflect this process of analysis and synthesis of verbal and motor units of behavior. Measures of fluency appear to be highly associated with creativity, so the development of children's creativity may, likewise, offer clues as to the developmental course of the executive function of reconstitution. This would seem to be particularly so for the development of ideational or "usage" creativity, as this ability may directly reflect the power to analyze and synthesize behavioral contingency arrangements.

Planning Ability

Although the development of reconstitution does not seem to have received a great deal of attention in the neuropsychological or developmental literatures, the problem-solving aspect of planning incorporates reconstitution. Planning has been repeatedly emphasized as a major aspect of human executive functions. However, as discussed in the previous chapter, planning is not a single function but the result of the interaction of several, if not all, of the executive functions in the model. As Fuster (1989) has argued, the cross-temporal organization of behavior is, after all, the ultimate over-arching function of the prefrontal cortex, and that organization represents planning.

Developmental researchers on the subject would seem to agree with this assessment of planning as involving multiple components of executive functioning. Scholnick and Friedman (1993) have defined planning as "the use of knowledge for a purpose, the construction of an effective way to meet a goal" (p. 145). It is said to comprise at least five major processes. The first of these is "using past knowledge to build a representation of the environment that will provide information relevant for action" (p. 147). It requires constructing and then integrating representations about the task, including both its current state and the desired end point. Clearly, this requires the use of working memory, both verbal and nonverbal, so as to hold this information on-line in the formulation and control of a response. The second process in planning is the selection of goals, which is evaluative in nature and refers not only to the desired end state but also the reason for undertaking the plan to begin with; this evaluative phase is inherently a motivational and not just a cognitive activity. It likely involves the executive function of self-regulation of affect/motivation/arousal, akin to Damasio's (1994, 1995) somatic marker theory that serves to assist with and constrain decision-making. The third process is "the decision about whether it is realistic and worthwhile to formulate a plan in advance" (p. 147). This latter stage requires the ability to delay responding, defer gratification, and engage in self-reflection. The need for behavioral inhibition, internalized language, retrospective and prospective functions of working memory, and self-motivation would seem to be key executive functions involved at this stage. The fourth stage flows from this decision; it is the formulation of the plan. This involves the capacity to generate a variety of possible options for meeting the goal and to evaluate their likelihood of achieving the goal. It would seem to me that the reconstitutive executive function would be involved at this stage of strategy development. Last, the individual must be capable of executing the plan and monitoring its execution, revising the plan and its execution along the way as feedback for performance of the plan occurs. Once more, the interaction of behavioral inhibition (interference control), the prospective function of working memory, and motor control would be critical executive elements necessary for this stage of planning.

Scholnick and Friedman (1993) argue persuasively that context, personal beliefs, and socialization play a significant role in the ecology of planning, rather than just cognitive abilities alone. While I could not disagree with that assertion, I do not believe that their developmental perspective on planning sufficiently emphasizes the fundamental importance of behavioral inhibition as a necessary precondition for and important determinant throughout these stages of planning. Planning, as just illustrated, would seem to require the healthy development of all of the executive functions in the hybrid model and their interaction. But priority of place must be given to behavioral inhibition as the lead function in this chain of events.

Supporting the critical role of inhibition and working memory in the development of planning is Hudson and Fivush's (1991) study of preschool children's ability to plan a shopping trip for breakfast materials. The 3-year-old children made significant mistakes in the development of the script by failing to discriminate breakfast items from other foods. The 4- to 5-year-olds were able to accomplish this scripting of the task with greater success, but despite their development of adequate shopping lists they were poor in executing their plan. They were more likely to forget what they wanted on their lists and had difficulties ignoring distracting events. Such research suggests that while some of the executive functions necessary for planning are present in rudimentary form during the preschool years, successful planning requires further maturation and coordinated interaction among these functions that will transpire over the years of later childhood and adolescence.

Studies of Developmental Changes in Executive Functions

Studies of the development of executive functions in children illustrate the probable differential timing for the maturation of these functions. For instance, Levin et al. (1991) found significant increases as a function of age on a number of executive function measures. To illustrate the findings of this study, I have selected from Levin's results, several of the measures of executive function I have most commonly cited in this volume: the go/no-go test (behavioral inhibition), the Tower of London (TOL) test (planning and working memory), the WCST (persistence, rule generation, and response flexibility), and verbal fluency (reconstitution or behavioral creativity).

The results of the go/no-go task are shown in Figure 8.1. They illustrate a steep decline in impulsive errors (false alarms) and errors of omission (missed responses) in normal children between ages 7 to 8 and 9 to 12 but with little further improvement, if any, beyond the latter age level.

In Figure 8.2 are some of the results from the Levin et al. (1991) study for the TOL test. As I discussed in Chapter 6, this measure is often used to evaluate planning ability. It probably involves several

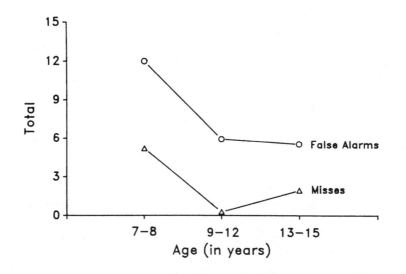

FIGURE 8.1. Total number of false positive responses and number of misses on the go/no-go task as a function of age. From Levin et al. (1991, p. 391). Copyright 1991 by Lawrence Erlbaum Associates, Inc. Reprinted by permission.

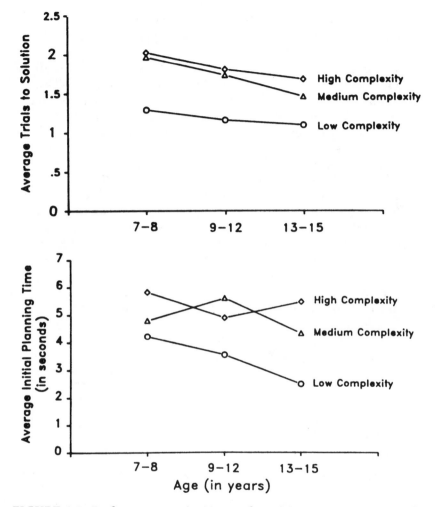

FIGURE 8.2. Performance on the Tower of London plotted against age for problems of varying complexity. Average number of trials to solution (top) and initial planning time (bottom) are shown. From Levin et al. (1991, p. 387). Copyright 1991 by Lawrence Erlbaum Associates, Inc. Reprinted by permission.

different executive functions acting in concert, including response inhibition, nonverbal working memory, rule formulation and reconstitution, and, certainly, persistence of effort. In the top graph are shown the results for the average number of trials needed to solve the design construction problem, which illustrate a developmental trend to improved efficiency of performance with age. The differences between the youngest and oldest age groups were significant for both the high and medium complexity design constructions, supporting this conclusion for those scores.

Factor-analytic and neuroimaging studies that employed the WCST were discussed in depth in Chapter 6. As with the TOL, the WCST was found to involve several executive functions acting in concert rather than to represent the performance of any single such function. Inhibition of perseverative responses, sensitivity to feedback about errors (working memory), rule generation and response flexibility (reconstitution), as well as persistence of effort were thought to be reflected in the performance of this task. The age-related changes on this measure found in the Levin et al. (1991) study are shown in Figure 8.3. They indicate improvements with age in the measures reflecting response flexibility (categories obtained) and rule formulation (conceptual level) measures as well as declines in the tendency to perseverate in outmoded response patterns (perseverative errors).

Finally, from this study, I selected the graph representing a measure of verbal fluency as I have discussed this concept several times

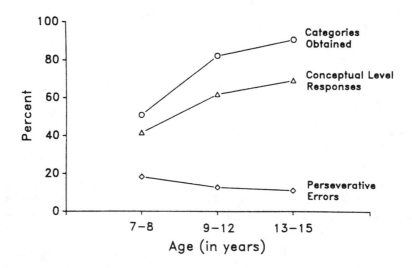

FIGURE 8.3. Performance on the Wisconsin Card Sort Test plotted against age group. The number of categories obtained (expressed as a percentage of total categories), the percentage of conceptual level responses, and the percentage of perseverative errors are shown. From Levin et al. (1991, p. 385). Copyright 1991 by Lawrence Erlbaum Associates, Inc. Reprinted by permission.

throughout this volume, that is, as probably reflecting Bronowski's concept of reconstitution within certain age ranges of children. The results for this measure are shown in Figure 8.4. These results indicate not only significant age-related increases in fluency, but also significant gender differences in these increases. Females appear to show a larger improvement than males in verbal fluency over the age ranges studied. The authors also reported significant age-related improvements in design (nonverbal) fluency as well. Gender effects were not found to significantly interact with age on the latter measure. These findings intimate that the function of reconstitution continues to show improvements with age into the adolescent years, long after response inhibition appears to have leveled off in its development.

To summarize the results of the Levin et al. (1991) study, significant age-related changes were noted on measures of sensitivity to feedback, problem solving, concept formation, and impulse control between 7- to 8-year-old and 9- to 12-year-old age groups of normal children. Further significant developmental advances were noted in memory strategies, memory efficiency, planning time, problem solving, and hypothesis seeking between 9- to 12-year-old and 13- to 15-year-old age groups of normal children.

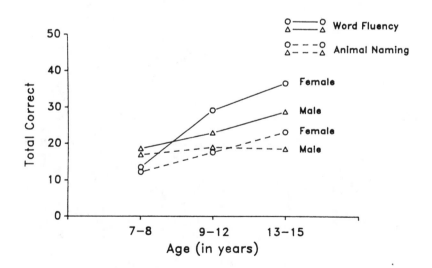

FIGURE 8.4. Total number of correct responses plotted separately for girls and boys against age for two measures of verbal fluency including Controlled Oral Word Fluency and Animal Naming. From Levin et al. (1991, p. 389). Copyright 1991 by Lawrence Erlbaum Associates, Inc. Reprinted by permission.

The study by Levin et al. (1996) did not take specific measures of verbal or nonverbal working memory and so the developmental pattern of these executive functions is not well represented in their results. A recent study by Hale, Bronik, and Fry (1997), however, helps to illustrate the development of nonverbal and verbal working memory in tandem with the development of interference control, a form of inhibition that protects the contents of working memory from disruption. In this study, children of ages 8, 10, and 19 years were given spatial and verbal working memory tasks. The former consisted of recalling a series of visually presented digits while the latter involved recalling the locations of X's within a series of grids or matrices. While performing these tasks, subjects also had to perform a secondary task of reporting on the color of the stimuli as they were presented, with the report consisting of a verbal or spatial response. The results are graphically depicted in Figure 8.5.

All of the age groups studied showed domain-specific interference from the secondary task. That is, the verbal secondary task was more likely to disrupt the primary verbal working memory performance, and the spatial secondary task was more likely to disrupt the primary spatial working memory task. This supports Fuster's (1989) point that the closer the content of the source of disruption to that in working

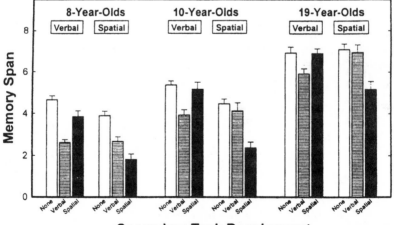

Secondary Task Requirement

FIGURE 8.5. Memory spans for the two primary tasks (verbal and spatial) as a function of the secondary task requirement (none, verbal, spatial) for 8-, 10-, and 19-year-olds. From Hale, Bronik, and Fry (1997, p. 368). Copyright 1997 by the American Psychological Association. Reprinted by permission.

memory, the more difficult it will be to provide interference control over working memory from that form of disruption. For the youngest age group studied here (8-year-olds), there is also evidence of nonspecific interference, in that both types of secondary tasks produced significant interference with the opposite domain of the primary task (i.e., verbal secondary response disrupted primary spatial working memory and vice versa). Such results intimate that at this early stage of the maturation of working memory, interference control is also relatively primitive in its development, such that forms of interference less related to the content or form of working memory may be more disruptive than they will be later in development. These results also indicate that as the ability to hold information in mind over time improves (working memory) the interference control also improves, consistent with Dempster's (1992) hypothesis that the development of working memory requires the development of a process that inhibits interference from irrelevant information.

In other studies of developmental changes in executive functions, Welsh et al. (1991) and Passler, Isaac, and Hynd (1985) found that organized strategic and planful behavior was detected as early as 6 years of age in normal children, more complex search behavior and hypothesis testing matured by age 10 years, and verbal fluency, motor sequencing, and complex planning abilities had not reached adult level performances by age 12 years. It would not be difficult to redefine the measures used in these studies and their findings into the executive functions presented in the model developed in Chapter 7. All of these studies indicate significant improvements with age in the executive functions discussed throughout this volume, and support the assertion advanced here that the timing of these developmental trends is probably different for the different executive functions in the hybrid model.

Developmental Speculations: The Interactive Impact of the Executive Functions

The foregoing discussion suggests that most of the executive functions are well underway in their development by the early school-age years. All of these forms of self-regulation are not fully covert or internalized as yet and may not be so until early adolescence. Their publicly observable counterparts, however, seem to have emerged by entry into formal schooling. The availability of these diverse executive functions appears to give rise to a marked increase in self-regulation between ages 5 and 7 years (Berkowitz, 1982).

Although the precise timetables for, developmental trajectories of, and relative order of development of the various executive functions represented in the hybrid model require much more research to establish with precision, it is interesting to speculate about some of the developmental implications of this model. It assumes that there is a progressive increase in the efficiency of the processes representing behavioral inhibition across development, in parallel with the development of the prefrontal regions of the brain, and particularly the orbital–prefrontal cortex and its interconnections with the striatum. As children mature, they are increasingly able to inhibit prepotent responses, delay their responses, and interrupt responses that are underway as feedback about performance becomes available. They also are able to protect working or representational memory from interference not only during delays in responding, but also during the execution of goal-directed responses governed by the executive functions.

This progressive increase in the power of behavioral inhibition is associated with an increase in the various forms of working memory or private sensing to the self in all forms of sensory–motor behavior. Undoubtedly, the various forms of private sensing may not emerge simultaneously, but may follow a course similar to the development of the publicly observable expressions of the primary senses. Regardless, these forms of sensing to the self probably occur initially as the capacity to simply sustain or prolong mental sensory representations and their associated motor actions on-line during delays. Children eventually develop the capacity to manipulate these internally represented forms of information.

Along with this ability to hold events on-line and even manipulate them comes the increasing developmental capacity for imitative behavior, especially of complex, novel sequences of behavior. Such imitative behavior is related to the performance of behaviors and the contextual contingency arrangements acquired through vicarious learning. This would imply that the power to apply behaviors acquired through observational or vicarious learning rather than experientially should also increase as representational (working) memory matures.

As discussed earlier, nonverbal working memory provides the means by which hindsight (retrospective function) and forethought (prospective function) can develop. With them comes the emergence of a mental window on time, the breadth of which appears to open increasingly wider with age, pushing the future time horizon being used to consider options and outcomes ever farther into the future. Events moving into this temporal window initiate preparatory behaviors directed toward the anticipated arrival of such events. With development, such preparatory behaviors will occur at increasingly earlier periods in the chain of events leading up to the anticipated event. That is to say, children, as they mature, will show an increasing ability to begin preparations for events more distant in future time than was characteristic of them when younger. The power to organize behavior across time toward goals and the future becomes increasingly sophisticated and complex over development, involving time periods of increasingly longer durations and behavioral structures of increasing complexity and hierarchical organization. In this process emerges the psychological sense of time itself. Also emerging in concert with the progressive development of working memory is self-awareness (Kopp, 1982).

As these developmental processes occur, control of behavior increasingly shifts from being context-dependent and contingency-shaped (externally governed) to being increasingly regulated by internally represented information. Along with this shift from external to internal forms of information comes a shift away from the control of behavior by the moment and toward increasing control of behavior by future events (via their conjecturing). The behavior of the developing child is shifting away from regulation by the temporal now and toward governance by hypothetical futures. Increasingly longer and complex forms of goal-directed behavior and persistence of effort therefore should be evident as inhibition and working memory develop.

As discussed earlier, the development of internalized speech begins in the later preschool years, succeeding the emergence of behavioral inhibition, working memory, and the self-control of affect/motivation/arousal. Covert speech provides another means of mentally representing information so as to guide behavior and vastly expands the child's repertoire for rule-governed behavior. In so doing, covert speech provides yet another means by which control over behavior is being shifted away from the immediate, external environment and toward internally represented sources of control.

When combined with the retrospective and prospective functions of working memory and the sense of time associated with them, the capacity for internalized speech provides the means for children not only to talk to others and themselves about time, but to employ the sense of time in their own self-regulation. Time should therefore become an increasingly occurring feature in the content of children's speech to self and others and in the plans that they formulate and follow. It should also allow children to develop the capacity to comply with instructions that involve a delayed behavioral performance. The more mature the child is neurologically, the greater should be the span of time over which an instruction can make reference to such a deferred performance and still be successfully complied with by the child. This combination of the executive mental modules represented by the two forms of working memory would also give rise to greater powers of reading comprehension with the progression in the development of working memory, given that material read to oneself must be temporarily held in mind so as to derive the maximal semantic and inferential content from it. As I have noted previously, this same combination probably contributes to the development of moral reasoning and the moral regulation of behavior with maturation.

Over development, there should be in evidence a decreasing reliance on the need for immediate and frequent reinforcement so as to sustain a child's persistence in an activity or task. Increasingly, children should become capable of effectively mediating delays to reinforcers not only through the private sensing afforded by the development of working memory and through private speech, but through the affective and motivational markers that are associated with such private events. Not only self-motivation but emotional self-regulation as well should become increasingly obvious as this domain of psychological development becomes increasingly private and covert in form. As Bronowski (1967/1977) noted, the separation of affect from events and one's initial reactions to them affords one a greater capacity for objectivity and social perspicacity. These elements of self-control should also increase with the development of the executive functions. Given that this mental module for the self-control of affect and motivation is developing in the midst of an already developing mental module for working memory, their interaction should produce a progressive increase, as development proceeds, in the expression of anticipatory affect and motivation increasingly in advance of future events.

I share Bronowski's contention that the last stage in the development of these executive functions is probably that of reconstitution, requiring, it seems, the preexisting development, at least in rudimentary forms, of the nonverbal and verbal working memory systems. With maturation across childhood, an increasing ability to take apart and recombine behavioral structures so as to create novel and more complex behavior, chains of behavior, and hierarchies among these behavioral sequences should become evident within the child's repertoire of responding. These should not only serve to bridge increasingly longer delays to future outcomes, but should also give rise to a growing complexity of children's behavior as hierarchies and their goals come to be units of larger hierarchies and longer-term goals. The purposive, intentional, and future-oriented quality of behavior should likewise be increasingly evident in children's behavior.

The results of these progressively improving executive functions should be a vastly greater power of internally represented information to take over the management of behavior from that of the immediate external environment. Task-irrelevant activity should become increasingly restrained, while goal-directed persistence becomes more evident and more prolonged. A growing sensitivity to feedback and errors in the performance of goal-directed behaviors should also be evident across development. This, along with the increasing capacity for reconstitution, or behavioral creativity, should contribute to both a greater flexibility of responding and a greater efficiency in task accomplishment. Unnecessary behavioral components are evaluated and discarded and more efficient strategies are increasingly deployed. Should the goal-directed actions become interrupted by events, children should demonstrate a growing capability both to resist responding to such distractions and to return to their goal-directed activities should they need to temporarily interrupt those activities to deal with the distracting event. A sense of time, timing, and timeliness in behavior should be progressively more evident across development as the capacity to organize behavior across time grows.

SELF-CONTROL AS AN INSTINCT

It is my contention that the basic cognitive or neuropsychological mechanisms that form the executive functions in this hybrid model create a virtual instinct for self-control. More than 120 years ago, Charles Darwin (1871/1992) recognized this possibility: "It is possible, or as we shall see later, even probable, that the habit of self-command may, like other habits, be inherited" (p. 314). This is not to say that socialization has no part to play in the development of children's self-control, as it surely seems to do and as even Darwin recognized. But it is to say that the basic capacities that permit humans to engage in self-regulation are neurogenetic in origin. In other words, the capacity for self-regulation is not taught but emerges as a result of an interaction between the child's maturing neurological capabilities for self-regulation (the executive functions) and his or her interactions with a social environment that stimulates, encourages, and places a premium on such behavior.

Just as language is an instinct (Pinker, 1995) that is not actually taught to children but is wired into the brain's development, so, too, does there appear to be an instinct for self-control that is likewise a feature of neurological development. In both cases, this instinct emerges out of an interaction between the child's neurological capacity for the instinct and a social environment that stimulates that instinct. The precise content of self-control may well arise out of socialization and the child's unique experiences with the particular culture. The type of language children speak to themselves, the sensory impressions which they are capable of resensing and representing on-line during delays in motor behavior, the events and outcomes they find to be motivating, and even the future goals that self-regulation will subserve may all derive from this interaction with a specific culture of self-control. No psychological ability can develop normally devoid of an environment that stimulates that ability, and self-control appears to be no exception. But that children are able to develop behavioral inhibition, self-control, and the executive functions associated with them results, I believe, from a neurological instinct having substantial genetic contributions. No amount of environmental stimulation will be able to completely make up for genetic contributions that are lacking or are delayed or impaired by neurogenetic aberrations. I will present two lines of argument for the proposition that self-control or executive functioning is a developmental instinct, one logical, and the other empirical.

Logical Argument

The executive functions I have identified in the hybrid model are forms of public, outer/other-directed behavior that have become turned on the self. Those public behaviors evolved as means to sense, respond to, and generally attempt to control that environment, and their turning toward the self serves much the same purpose—to sense, respond to, and control one's own behavior. The overt forms of sensory perception on which the covert forms are based arise in development chiefly out of biological factors, albeit interacting with a stimulating environment that affects them. Seeing, for instance, unlike reading, is not taught, and neither are the other senses. The content of what I see is mostly environmentally and culturally determined, but that I see at all is not a social invention. If working memory is, as I suspect it to be, the covert resensing of events, then there is every reason to suspect that, like the public counterparts on which it is founded, this capacity to resense and reperceive events covertly is largely biologically determined.

   A similar argument can be used for the other executive functions. Although Vygotsky (1978) and others (Azmitia, 1992; Berk, 1992) have argued that covert self-speech originates in an earlier stage of social interactions with others, particularly caregivers, this may not be quite correct. Internalized speech or verbal working memory has its obvious public counterpart in language toward others. That language, unlike the reading which will be based upon it, is not taught (Pinker, 1995). It is acquired rapidly by a linguistically thirsty organism that absorbs the linguistic stimulation and its content provided by its cultural and familial environment. Just as the individual, if normally developing, cannot help but speak given such an environment, I would contend that this individual, if normally developing, cannot help but use self-speech for self-control, given exposure to a social environment that manifests self-control. A person cannot help that such privatized speech develops and thereby forms the very means for his or her verbal thought. The self-control that self-speech affords, and the welding of that self-speech to the control of motor behavior, are, like the language capacity upon which they are based, largely instinctive.

Likewise, so is the capacity for covert emoting and motivating to oneself. The capacity to experience affect, motivation, and arousal are not taught by the social environment, although once more the content of them may well be. As with language, exposure to a social environment may shape or mold this capacity to some degree. But who would foolishly argue that the capacity for affect, motivation, and arousal originates in that social environment? Thus, how could one argue that the covert or private forms of these affective/motivational/arousal states also originate in and are purely taught by that social environment? That the social environment encourages and provides consequences for affective/motivational self-control, as Kopp (1989) so well describes that process, is unquestioned here. However, that the child even develops the capacity to covertly self-regulate those affective/motivational states, like the publicly observable states upon which they are based, is not a cultural invention that must be taught to each generation. How could the social community achieve such instruction when, as Damasio (1994, 1995) has argued, much of this emoting and motivating to the self may be taking place at a largely unconscious level? If the contents of working memory largely and automatically trigger their affective/motivational associations contributing to this covert emoting to the self, how could this ever be taught by a social community?

This same line of argument would seem to apply in the case of reconstitution as well. For if reconstitution (behavioral analysis/synthesis) is the covert form of earlier stages of play, experimentation, and manipulation of the environment by children, as I believe it to be, then this also does not seem to originate purely in the social environment. Once more, the content of that play and experimentation, its shape, form, and substance, and the objects, actions, and properties of the environment that it takes as its focus may all be largely environmentally or socially influenced. But that such play and experimentation occurs and that it eventually becomes private to form imaginative, fantasy, or symbolic play, giving rise to a capacity for covert simulations of behavioral contingencies, does not seem to me to be taught. Anyone who has raised a child through toddlerhood and the preschool years knows full well that this age group of our species lives to disassemble its environment, almost ceaselessly exploring that environment, attempting to take it apart and recombine it, and playing with it without much concern for its parents' approval of such conduct. If this is the basis for the executive function of reconstitution, then this function is largely untaught because the capacity for its public counterpart is largely untaught. The instinct to play with the environment and with our behavior relative to that environment, I believe, also forms the instinct to covertly or "mentally" play with those same features as well.

But not only are the executive functions likely to arise more from instinct than training because their public, outer/other-directed counterparts appear to exist for much the same reason, but the very process by which these public counterparts become turned on the self and then undergo a developmental progression of "internalization" would itself be difficult to explain by some process of socialization. Formal training of this privatizing process does not seem to occur in the preschool years when it is becoming evident in the executive functions, nor does there seem to be any proposed socializing mechanism that can credibly explain it. The mechanism, instead, appears to be a neural one, influenced more by the timing of neuromaturational development than by any recognized course of formal teaching or socialization.

The issue under discussion here is not the overly simplistic one of nature versus nurture. It *is* a discussion, however, of the relative weight that should be given to one side versus the other in the naturally occurring reciprocal interaction of these sources of influence on development. *The phenotype for self-control, like that for language, is undoubtedly shaped by the environment, but it arises out of a genotype that constructs a brain that contains the innate capacity for language and self-control. Much of the variance in that phenotype appears to be influenced by genetic rather than environmental factors. What the latter factors may contribute seem to fall more within the realm of unique (nonshared) environmental sources than common (shared) environmental sources.*

Empirical Argument

The second line of argument for a self-control instinct is the empirical one. I believe there are several forms of evidence available, undoubtedly limited as each may be. One such source of empirical evidence is that pertaining to the heritability of some of the components of this model of self-control. Admittedly, this issue has not been well studied. But a few of these executive functions have received some preliminary scrutiny in large-scale twin studies, and the evidence suggests a large genetic contribution to them. For instance, consider the construct of behavioral inhibition. This, I believe, represents the dimension that underlies the hyperactive–impulsive–inattentive behavior studied using rating scales of such behavior. Twin studies, as discussed in Chapter 2, are reasonably consistent in demonstrating a ratio of genetic to environmental contributions to individual differences of 3:1 to 4:1. The average heritability for this trait across studies is on the order of approximately .80, with common environment contributing .00 to .06 and unique environment contributing .15 to .20 to the variance in these studies. Thus, individual differences in the bedrock executive function of behavioral inhibition, which supports the performance of the others built upon it, seem to be largely genetically determined. For working memory, studies have found that the ratio of genetic to environmental contributions to individual differences is approximately 2: 1 to 3:1 (Cardon et al., 1992; Luo et al., 1994; Pedersen et al., 1994). Such genetic contributions appear to exist apart from those associated with general cognitive ability, or *g*. *Further, environmental contributions to this executive function seem to be more in the realm of unique (nongenetic) environmental factors than common environmental factors.*

This finding certainly fits with the conclusion that individual differences in the capacities that subserve and permit self-regulation are largely biologically (genetically) determined. I am unaware of studies that have examined the heritability of the other two executive functions, namely, the self-regulation of affect/motivation/arousal and reconstitution (behavioral creativity and flexibility). Consequently, empirical support for the claim that they are largely instinctive cannot be marshaled here, but there seems little logical reason to expect them to be otherwise. This is especially so for the function of reconstitution, which seems to depend quite heavily on the development of the working memory functions on which it will operate.

The second source of evidence comes from the neuropsychological and neuroimaging literatures discussed in the previous two chapters. This evidence not only points to the likely existence of the executive functions described in the model, but suggests that there are specialized regions of the human prefrontal cortex that support most of them. The exception, as noted in those chapters, may be the function of reconstitution, which may simply be a more complex activity occurring within the working memory systems rather than a function entirely distinct from them. The role of these specialized regions that give rise to such relatively specialized executive functions is difficult to reconcile with any view other than that those functions are, in a sense, intended for development and will unfold as their underlying neural structures mature.

Further evidence for this position is that several of the executive functions—behavioral inhibition and representational memory—are also present in primates, albeit in more rudimentary forms (Fuster, 1989; Goldman-Rakic, 1995a, 1995b). These functions appear to be subserved by regions of the prefrontal cortex similar to those in humans, arguing for their evolutionary continuity across primate species most closely related to humans. Moreover, these more rudimentary forms of executive functioning are found to exist in infants as young as 5–6 months of age. By 12–24 months, the young human far surpasses its primate relatives in these executive capacities. Such findings are more consistent with a view of these executive functions as primarily instinctive rather than as being primarily culturally entrained.

The foregoing assertions that self-control is largely instinctive and that individual differences in this set of traits are largely heritable should not be taken to mean that such traits are immutable, as is so often mistakenly done. As noted emphatically earlier, the content of the executive functions, the environmental conditions that may serve to activate or increase activity in them, and even the goals which they select and subserve for the individual may well be largely culturally determined, and, to some degree, proficiency in these executive functions may be influenced by environmental factors as well. As a result, changes in social environmental factors may well result in large shifts in the level and proficiency of self-control in the population or among individuals within it. But individual differences within that population or subgroup so improved will still largely be accounted for by genetic factors. Human height serves as a fine analogy for this lesson. The heritability of human height has been determined to be very close to that for hyperactive–impulsive–inattentive behavior, approximately .81. Yet human height has also been increasing over the past few generations of children, a trend that speaks to the mutability of this trait. Even so, differences among individuals in height despite its overall increase largely remain accounted for by genetic factors. The same may well be true for behavioral inhibition and the executive functions subserving self-regulation.

I do not wish to appear overly confident in this assertion. As a scientist I remain a skeptic on most things and am open to empirical information that contradicts the tentative conclusions reached here. But I am also not blind to the trends in the extant literature on these functions, on the regional prefrontal lobe substrates that seem to mediate them, and on the findings of behavioral genetic studies concerning the preponderance of heritable influence that seems to account for a large proportion of individual differences in some of the more critical functions. Even assuming, however, that the evidence is not as supportive of this assertion of self-control as an instinct as I perceive it to be, that circumstance would not automatically confirm the alternative assertion—that self-control is a largely social invention, individual differences in which are primarily environmentally determined. This alternative interpretation, which has come to be termed the social science model of psychological abilities (Pinker, 1995), must muster its own supportive evidence to reject its own version of the null hypothesis. That will not be easy, in my opinion, in view of the evidence accumulated to date.

CONCLUSION

This chapter has reviewed findings that pertain to the developmental course of some of the executive functions stipulated in the hybrid model of those functions described in Chapter 7. It has also considered some speculations that seemed to be implied from this model about the developmental processes that may occur across maturation in these executive functions. I then asserted that, in view of the totality of information available to date on these neuropsychological functions, the human capacity for self-regulation appears to be largely instinctive. I based this assertion on several lines of evidence. One was the apparent localization within the prefrontal cortex of relatively separable regions for each of the executive functions. Another was the existence of some rudimentary forms of these executive functions in some primates as well as their early onset in infancy, suggesting that social teaching of these functions is much less likely to be their point of origin. A third was the large contribution of hereditary influences to individual differences in some of those functions studied to date. But I also advanced a logical reason why these executive functions may be largely instinctive: the public, outer/other-directed counterparts of these same functions, on which I believe their covert forms are based, are themselves presumed to be relatively instinctive. Sensing, speaking, emoting, and playing do not originate in the teachings of a social community, as much as that community may shape their content and form as well as the larger purposes (goals) to which they are put. In short, I have posited here that humans do not so much acquire self-control through formal social indoctrination or education but develop it largely as a result of the unfolding maturation of the neural structures of the prefrontal cortex that subserve it. The social stimulation and encouragement provided by a self-controlling culture to the executive functions arising from this maturational process is sufficient to see to their development. Formal education and socialization in the content of these

functions is surely important, but it does not account for their existence. Just as language arises in the course of neural maturation
occurring within a speaking community, so, too, does self-regulation
arise from a neuromaturational source existing within a self-controlling
community.

   In the next chapter, I will turn my attention to extending the
hybrid model of executive functions developed in Chapter 7 and these
developmental considerations to a better understanding of attention-
deficit/hyperactivity disorder.

CHAPTER 9

———•———

Extending the Hybrid Model of Executive Functions to ADHD

COMPELLING EVIDENCE EXISTS that ADHD comprises a deficit in the development of behavioral inhibition (see Chapter 4). The hybrid model of executive functions developed in Chapter 7 posits that behavioral inhibition makes a fundamental contribution to the effective performance of four other executive functions—(1) nonverbal working memory, (2) internalization of speech (verbal working memory), (3) the self-regulation of affect/motivation/arousal, and (4) reconstitution—because it permits the internalization of behavior that goes into the formation of these executive functions. The inhibitory deficit that characterizes ADHD disrupts the control of goal-directed motor behavior by its detrimental effects on these executive functions and the internally represented information they generate. In short, ADHD delays the internalization of behavior that forms the executive functions and thereby delays the self-regulation they afford to the individual.

I will discuss in this chapter the predictions of the hybrid model for those with ADHD. In the next chapter, I will review the evidence that may exist for these predicted deficits. Some comments on terminology are necessary at the outset of this task. I will use the terms "deficit" or "deficiency" interchangeably to refer to relative delays in the development of the abilities under discussion. To some, the term deficiency implies that a function or ability once existed at its normal level and then was lost or impaired through some pathological process. This is not the meaning I wish to imply for that term. Those with ADHD are behind in the proficiency of the executive abilities because they are behind their peers in their development of behavioral inhibition. Further, in using or implying the term "delay" here, I do not wish to connote that the ability under discussion is expected to eventually catch up with that of the normal peer group, as in some temporary delay in a developmental process that will bloom later on. Just as mental retardation is taken to imply a chronic developmental delay in general cognitive ability that is not outgrown with time or maturation, so do I wish to impart a similar meaning when I state that ADHD represents a developmental delay in behavioral inhibition.

The depiction of the hybrid model in Figure 7.7 is reprinted in this chapter as Figure 9.1. However, I have rephrased each executive function and its subfunctions into their negatives so as to directly state the deficiencies expected to arise from the impairment in each that is secondary to the primary delay in behavioral inhibition. The evidence reviewed in Chapter 4 already supports the existence of deficits in the first component of the model specifically, the delay in the three processes comprising behavioral inhibition, in those with ADHD. That evidence need not be reiterated here.

Before proceeding to the main task, however, it deserves mention that I am not the first to conjecture that ADHD may involve a deficit in working or representational memory and response flexibility. Pontius (1973) reviewed her clinical experience with approximately 100 patients having minimal brain dysfunction (MBD; a historical precursor to ADHD, although not diagnosed precisely the same way). She found that 85% of these cases had symptoms that were analogous to those of patients having frontal lobe and caudate damage. She advocated conceptualizing MBD as a disorder comparable to injuries to these regions, basing this conclusion on finding individuals with MBD had an inability to construct a plan and a goal of action, keep it in mind, and follow it through under the guidance of planning. These patients were also observed to be less able than normal to shift the principle of their actions during an ongoing activity when given verbal commands to do so. Pontius further cited an unpublished study of hyperactive children by Clarkson and Hayden showing that these children had greater difficulties on the Trail Making Test, Part B. This, she felt, was further evidence of the inability of MBD children to shift their responding according to task demands. She further speculated that the WCST may be another means of detecting this inflexibility in responding in MBD children. While other researchers have speculated previously that ADHD may involve deficient frontal lobe functioning (see Chapter 2), Pontius's work is one of the earliest attempts to specify the types of executive function deficiencies in such children that would be consistent with a frontal lobe syndrome.

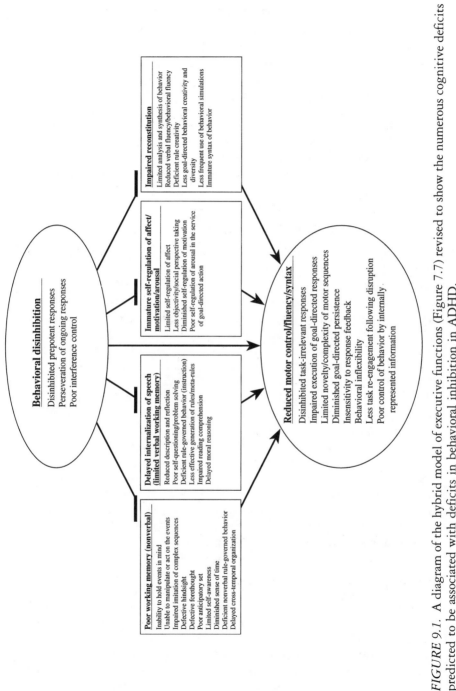

FIGURE 9.1. A diagram of the hybrid model of executive functions (Figure 7.7) revised to show the numerous cognitive deficits predicted to be associated with deficits in behavioral inhibition in ADHD.

PREDICTIONS OF THE HYBRID MODEL

A general prediction of the model is that ADHD results in a developmental delay in the critical neuropsychological process of the internalization of behavior. That process not only has received little or no research attention in contemporary neuropsychology, it has received almost none in the study of ADHD as well, with the exception of Berk's (1992; Berk & Potts, 1991) superb program of research. One of the major research agendas that awaits the fields of ADHD and developmental neuropsychology is the study of how behavior comes to be turned on the self and internalized so as to give rise to these executive functions.

Nonverbal Working Memory and ADHD

The hybrid model in Figure 9.1 predicts that a delay in behavioral inhibition, as in ADHD, should lead to secondary deficiencies in nonverbal working memory and its subfunctions. Such deficits should be evident not just in the more obvious forms of working memory, such as covert visual imagery or covert audition, but also in the representational activities for the lesser senses of taste, smell, touch, and kinesthesia–proprioception and the combinations among them. Specifically, those with ADHD should be more influenced by context and less controlled by internally represented information than normal same-age peers. They should not be able to hold information in mind as well as others, in large part, because they do not inhibit prepotent responses to ongoing events. Therefore, the delay in responding that is a prerequisite to working memory would be insufficient. They also should be just as unable to protect the activities of working memory and its informational contents from being disrupted by competing sources of interference or behavioral control. As normal children come to be able to act upon and manipulate the contents being represented in working memory, those with ADHD should be found to be less able to do so for much the same reasons.

Diminished Imitation and Application of Vicarious Learning

The relative deficiency in the power to mentally represent information should interfere with the ADHD child's capacity to imitate novel, complex behaviors demonstrated by others because the template required for imitation resides in the capacity for representational memory that is disrupted by ADHD. Working memory is not just providing the template for imitation; it provides the means by which past information about behavioral contingencies that was acquired through vicarious or observational learning comes to be applied to the formulation and execution of a response to an event. Those with ADHD should not just be found to have a diminished capacity for complex imitative behavior, specifically. More generally, they should be found to be less effective in the deployment of information derived from prior observational learning about the experiences of others in the formulation and execution of their own behavior. Recall that I stressed in Chapter 7 that it is not the acquisition of information from vicarious learning that so much requires working memory but the *application of information from vicarious learning* in the formulation and execution of current and future directed behavior. To apply past vicariously acquired information to the preparation of current behavior, it must be recalled into working memory (resensed) *before* the individual's response to an event is prepared and released.

Diminished Hindsight, Forethought, Anticipatory Set, and Self-Awareness

The deficiency in working memory should leave those with ADHD more influenced by immediately surrounding events and their immediate consequences than by those events and consequences more distant in time. The behavior of such individuals should be characterized more as "live for the moment" and "damn the torpedoes, full speed ahead" than as prudent, deliberate, and having due regard for the temporally distal consequences of one's conduct. Information about the past should be less likely to be recalled and held in mind (hindsight) by those with ADHD before they emit a response to an event. If those with ADHD cannot engage in the retrospective function of working memory effectively, then they should also be less able to conjecture the possible futures that may be related to events and to formulate their response options and select one for deployment. This is forethought, or the prospective function of working memory.

As Fuster (1989) has stated, the retrospective and prospective functions of working memory give rise to an *anticipatory set,* or preparatory behaviors founded upon them. This model would predict that such anticipatory or preparatory behaviors should be less evident in those with ADHD. Also, the motor presetting that takes place in anticipation of the arrival of future events should be deficient. This suggests that not only are those with ADHD less prepared to meet the arrival of future events that others would have anticipated and prepared for, but that even the timing of those preparatory behaviors they initiate may itself be deficient. Working memory does nothing if it does not impart time, timing, and timeliness to behavior and its cross-temporal organization.

I would expect, then, that ADHD is associated with a form of *temporal myopia* concerning the direction of behavior toward conjectured future events. Deficits in hindsight, forethought, and preparatory action result in a life that is more chaotic than that lived by others. The activities of those with ADHD career from one momentary event to another and the spurious changes that may arise along the way. Life for those with ADHD is more one of living from crisis to crisis. It is a lifestyle, however, for which others have little sympathy or patience because the crises were generally avoidable with even average amounts of forethought and preparation. Such neglect of the future could easily result in others judging those with ADHD as being willfully irresponsible in their ill-preparedness, because anyone else would have done the things needed to be prepared for the readily predictable event.

Further, as I noted in Chapter 7, representational or working memory and the hindsight and forethought of which it is comprised give rise to self-awareness. If this is so, then those with ADHD should show a diminished capacity for self-awareness relative to normal individuals. Further, if self-awareness evolved in part to predict the intentions, motives, and behavior of others, perhaps so as to control it more effectively, as Humphrey (1984) has speculated, then those with ADHD should be less adept at these activities, given that they are predicted to be less aware of themselves and their own motives, intentions, and actions.

Diminished Sense of Time

As the nonverbal working memory component of Figure 9.1 suggests, those with ADHD should show a developmental delay in the psychological sense of time. As one adult with ADHD said, "time escapes me and I have never been able to effectively deal with it" (Barkley, 1994b). Those with ADHD are adrift and disorganized within time. As I described in Chapters 5 and 7, the psychological sense of time derives from the capacity to hold sequences of events in mind and to make comparisons among the elements of those sequences. To sense time one must be able to sense changes in the relative positions of things. What makes the next instant different from the last one is that things have changed. To perceive that change, these moments must be held in a sequence and comparisons made among them. Out of such comparisons among temporally represented sequences of moments comes the sense that time has a direction and flow and that durations among the elements can be estimated (J. W. Brown, 1990).

Those with ADHD should be deficient in their sense of time, giving both estimations and productions of temporal durations that are more inconsistent and less accurate than is seen in their normal peers. If sense of time is delayed, it should appear to be experienced by those with ADHD as it appears to be experienced by younger individuals. Young children appear to perceive time as moving more slowly than do older children or than it does in actuality (i.e., as measured by a time-keeping device). When asked to do something within a time period, they act as if they have more time available to do the work than they do. When asked to be at a certain place at a certain time, they are less likely than older individuals to be punctual for the appointment. When asked to wait during a delay period, they should perceive it as lasting longer than others, display greater impatience or frustration with the delay, and even act to escape from or terminate the delay. This is because they perceived the delay as boring and mildly aversive, and thus escape behaviors will be difficult for them to inhibit. As Sonuga-Barke (1995) has described them, these individuals should be "delay averse," behaving in ways that seek to terminate delays as early as possible. Contexts requiring waiting in line, taking turns, delaying responses, and waiting patiently for promised outcomes should prove less tolerable for those with ADHD, given their sense that time is playing out more slowly than it seems to do for others.

All of this suggests that the performance of those with ADHD under cross-temporal (if–then) contingencies will be less effective. They cannot bridge the delays in the contingencies using internally represented information as well as others. The longer the delays in time that separate the components of a behavioral contingency, the less successful ADHD individuals will be in effectively managing those tasks.

Poorer Cross-Temporal Organization of Behavior. As discussed in Chapter 8, the increasing temporal span of hindsight and forethought over development expands the arc of experience over which one can deliberate, creating a cognitive window on time, in a sense, that opens wider with age. This window onto the future results in a future time horizon that will serve several purposes. First, it will serve to initiate preparatory actions for conjectured future events that have now moved to within that time horizon from the once distant future. Given that this temporal span over which future events are being conjectured is hypothesized here to be deficient in those with ADHD, such future events will not serve to initiate preparatory actions until the event is considerably closer in time than would have been the case for others. In short, those with ADHD will appear to wait until the last minute before initiating preparations for upcoming events. Such reliance on

11th-hour preparations to deal with anticipated future events may suffice under some conditions for which minimal preparation is needed to respond adequately to the event's arrival into the temporal now. But for many of life's events it will not suffice, and the individual with ADHD will be found, once more, to be poorly organized and ill prepared for the arrival of an event that peers have long since been prepared to handle.

Second, this future time horizon will be used in the deliberation of risk–benefit ratios with regard to various response options when individuals contemplate current events and their likely sequences and outcomes. The time span over which response options are being evaluated for their consequences by those with ADHD should be found to be far shorter than those spans employed by normal peers. As a result, the delayed consequences of such options become even more steeply discounted as a function of time than is the case in the normal peer group. The individual with ADHD is then seen to be making seemingly impulsive choices that are governed by more temporally proximal outcomes than would have been chosen by those relying upon a much longer future time span or a more distant time horizon to deliberate the outcomes of their options.

Recall that these temporally proximal outcomes involve both positive and negative forms of reinforcement. That the person with ADHD is observed to attempt to maximize the former type of consequences is easily appreciated. Overlooked in such an analysis, however, is the prediction that those with ADHD will act equally as impulsively to terminate, escape from, and avoid in the future those situations that impose immediate unpleasantness yet which would yield a richer vein of delayed consequences for the individual, if tolerated or undertaken. Inhibiting behavior that is under the control of negative reinforcement involves the capacity not just to delay gratification but to enter into states of self-imposed hardship and deprivation or even states of aversive or psychologically painful experiences that, if successfully negotiated or tolerated, will result in greater long-term gains for the individual. Such persistence in the face of hardship and adversity so as to attain a later and greater outcome should be more difficult for those with ADHD, not only because they cannot inhibit these prepotent tendencies to escape and avoid immediate aversiveness, but also because their difficulties with working memory may lead to a steep discounting of the value of those delayed, rewarding outcomes. Such delayed outcomes are simply not sufficient to serve to motivate the individual with ADHD to persist in such goal-directed behaviors.

Therefore, those with ADHD should have less ability than normal individuals to successfully persist in goal-directed behavior, given that such goal-directed persistence is predicated on and being guided by information being internally represented in working memory. Even when goal-directed behavior is being undertaken by those with ADHD, it should be subject to greater interference by sources of disruption in both the external and internal environments, resulting in less success at attaining goals. Such distractions should not interfere with non-goal-directed behavior or with tasks in which self-control and the executive functions are less necessary for adequate performance. But the more self-regulation a task demands, or the heavier the load it places on these executive functions and especially working memory, the more likely are such sources of interference to disrupt that task.

Diminished Temporal Sequencing of Events and Responses to Them. Inherent in conceptualizations of working memory is the capacity to represent events in their proper temporal order (Fuster, 1989). Those with ADHD should not only show difficulties with retaining information in working memory, but have as much or more difficulty sequencing this information in its proper temporal order. Like patients with frontal lobe injuries (Godbout & Doyon, 1995; McAndrews & Milner, 1991; Sirigu et al., 1995), those with ADHD should demonstrate difficulties with sequencing information recalled from long-term memory, as well as with incoming new information that must be retained in a proper temporal sequence.

The latter has been studied in brain-injured populations using analysis of behavioral scripts (McAndrews & Milner, 1991; Sirigu et al., 1995). Patients are asked to generate a list of 10–20 actions in their proper order that must be performed in completing a familiar activity, avoiding idiosyncratic activities based on their personal behavior (e.g., getting up in the morning, going to a movie; going to a wedding or doctor's appointment, etc.). It would be of considerable interest to see how children and adults with ADHD perform such tasks relative to normal control subjects, given the prediction here that such a syntax to the ordering of actions would be impaired in those with ADHD.

This problem with temporal sequencing might create problems with the syntax of motor planning and execution, making it disorganized as well. Not only should the timing of motor responses in anticipation of events be impaired in those with ADHD, but the *sequencing* of those responses may be as well if that sequence is novel, complex, and not already overlearned (automatic).

Diminished Thinking and Talking about Time. As Bronowski (1967/1977) noted, the capacity to think about time creates the capacity to talk about time—to make temporal references in language, given that outer language reflects cognitive content. If deficient working memory creates a greater impoverishment in considerations about time in those with ADHD, then this impoverishment should be evident in the ADHD individual's discourse with others. There should be fewer references to time, the past, and especially the future. Along these lines, it could be argued that those with ADHD should demonstrate a delay in the development of a sense of one's own mortality, or the universality concept of death given their diminished capacity for forethought (see Chapter 7).

Reduced Consideration of Time in Social Interactions. A large proportion of proper social conduct is predicated on a sense of the future. If so, then those with ADHD are likely to manifest significant deficiencies in the performance of those social skills (i.e., sharing, cooperation, etc.) as well as other adaptive behaviors (i.e., concern for safety, health consciousness, etc.) predicated on the valuation of future personal and social consequences over immediate ones. The knowledge of those social and adaptive skills or behaviors is not at issue here; that knowledge should not be as deficient in those with ADHD. It is the *application* of that knowledge in day-to-day functioning that should be so impaired because the reason for its application is a delay in responding that allows a sense of the future to occur. *The problem, then, for those with ADHD is not one of knowing what to do, but one of doing what they know* when *it would be most adaptive to do so.* This same problem is typical of patients with injuries to the prefrontal cortex (Dellis, Squire, Bihrle, & Massman, 1992; Stuss & Benson, 1986). It could be predicted, as a consequence, that not only will certain social skills, etiquette, and moral conduct be less evident in those with ADHD, but there should exist a greater probability for their social opposites—lying, stealing, selfishness, boorishness, and, possibly even impulsive social aggression to attain immediate gains.

Nonverbal Rule-Governed Behavior

In Chapter 7, I introduced the notion that nonverbal information can function as a rule, in that it can provide contingency-specifying information (Skinner, 1953, 1969), such as a line on a map. Information that is held in nonverbal working memory probably serves just such a function. Mental representations of past events initiate and regulate motor responses associated with those events, taking on the power of rules in the control of behavior. I describe later in this chapter the deficits likely to accrue to those with ADHD who have poor verbal rule-governed behavior, as predicted by my theory. Similar characteristic deficits, as described in that later section, are just as likely to be found in those with ADHD whose behavior is ineffectively guided by nonverbal working memory.

Internalization of Speech (Verbal Working Memory) and ADHD

The model portrayed in Figure 9.1 predicts a delay in the internalization of speech or verbal working memory in those with ADHD that creates widespread difficulties for them in the use of self-speech for self-regulation. Because of their delay in behavioral inhibition, those with ADHD should show evidence of a delay in the developmental course over which speech becomes turned on the self and internalized. It will be recalled that the internalization of speech may occur in roughly three stages. The first is the occasion in development when speech is turned from being directed toward others to being directed at the self. This typically occurs during the late preschool years (ages 3–5 years). The model predicts, then, that preschool children with ADHD should not be turning their speech upon themselves at the same time that normal children come to do so. The second stage of internalization is the increasing power such self-speech seems to have in regulating behavior. This model therefore predicts that those with ADHD will demonstrate less ability of their speech to regulate behavior; assist with problem solving and, especially, task failures; and improve later task performance, as self-speech has been shown to do in normal young children. The last stage of internalization occurs when self-speech progresses to becoming quieter, more telegraphic in nature, and eventually fully covert (unobservable). Those with ADHD should be found to have remained behind their normal peers in this progression to covert speech, manifesting more public self-speech characteristic of younger normal children. Ultimately, those with ADHD should be found to eventually internalize speech to its primarily covert stage at an age that is later than that seen in normal children.

Given this deficiency in the progression to internalized speech, those with ADHD would be predicted to rely less on description and reflection to themselves through covert speech before responding to events. Since self-speech is becoming wedded to motor control, welding verbal thought to action across development, children with ADHD should find their own self-speech less effective in controlling their motor behavior. The control of motor action by verbal thought is weakened by the deficiency in inhibition characterizing ADHD, such that knowing what to do is not so much the problem as doing what one knows.

ADHD also would be expected to make it more difficult to follow through on the rules and instructions given by others, particularly in the absence of the individual establishing the rule, when retention of the rule in mind and its periodic restatement may be necessary to stay the course and complete the assigned activities or continue compliance with the rule. Consequently, a deficiency in rule-governed behavior should exist, as that normal process was described in Chapter 7.

Deficient Rule-Governed Behavior

As discussed in Chapter 7, Skinner (1953) hypothesized that this influence of language over behavior occurs in three stages. Those with ADHD should be delayed in their advancement through these stages. They will remain less compliant with the rules and instructions of others longer into development, finally making the transition to the use of self-speech later than do normal children, and such self-speech should prove less effective at regulating their behavior. They should also be slow to move to the stage wherein self-speech assists with problem solving and the self-creation of rules achieved via self-questioning. Normal children of the same age should be found to be more deliberate and effective problem solvers and rule constructors than are those with ADHD.

The capacity to sustain behavior across large delays in time among the elements of a behavioral contingency is greatly assisted by the use of rules. I hypothesize that ADHD diminishes the capacity for rules to bridge temporal gaps. Those with ADHD should be less able to formulate and especially less able to apply the novel rules that must be constructed in situations involving temporal delays. And even if they are initially applied, it is unlikely that an individual can sustain adherence to such rules for very long, given his or her diminished capacity to retain such rules on-line in verbal working memory. Thus the very basis for constructing and sustaining lengthy and hierarchically complex chains of behavior toward distant goals is handicapped in those with ADHD by virtue of their secondary deficiency in rule-governed behavior.

Rules are strategies that, once formulated, can be used to guide behavior more efficiently and effectively. Such strategies are often critical to managing complex work or problem-solving tasks, particularly where subsets of strategy-guided behavior must be organized into a larger hierarchy to accomplish the task or goal. This would lead me to predict that those with ADHD are less likely to formulate such strategies and, even if formulated, are less able to apply them effectively in their own task performance. Like patients with frontal lobe injuries who are often found to be deficient in task performances due to poor utilization of strategies (Gershberg & Shimamura, 1995; Mangels, Gershberg, Shimamura, & Knight, 1996; Stuss et al., 1994), those with ADHD should likewise be found to be deficient in the formulation and application of strategies.

Internalized speech, along with the sense of past and future afforded by working memory, combine to give the individual the capacity to understand and comply with commands or rules that have prolonged references. That is, such instructions or rules make reference to a behavioral performance at a place and time temporally distant from the temporal now in which the command or direction is given. If working memory is deficient and rule-governed behavior is also weak in those with ADHD, then instructions that make prolonged references concerning future behavioral performances should be less effective at initiating the later performance of that behavior in those with ADHD than would instructions concerning performance in the temporal now, contiguous with the instruction. The farther into the future the behavioral performance is to be made, the more difficult it should be for those with ADHD to comply with this temporally prolonged instruction. Granted, a similar pattern to this decrement in performance as a function of time to the future performance should be seen in normal individuals, but the model would predict that the decline would be greater and occur at earlier temporal distances from the time period of the instruction than would be characteristic of normal individuals.

The interaction of nonverbal working memory with that of verbal working memory or private speech was also predicted to contribute to the capacity for reading comprehension; for meaning to be derived, the internalized speech of silent reading must also be held in mind. The deficits predicted to exist in both of these executive functions due to ADHD would be predicted to create a diminution in the power of reading comprehension in those with the disorder.

Specific Characteristics of Rule-Governed Behavior in ADHD. Characteristics associated with rule-governed behavior should be less evident in those with ADHD. Recall that rule-governed behavior would be typified by a number of features that contrast with more contingency-shaped (context-dependent) behavior (Cerutti, 1989; Hayes, 1989). Those with ADHD would be expected to display fewer of these features. ADHD would result in the following characteristics. (1) The variability of responses to a task will be much greater because behavior is more contingency-shaped (developed and maintained by the environmental contingencies alone). (2) Behavior will be more affected by the immediate contingencies operating in a situation or by momentary and potentially spurious changes in those contingencies. (3) Where rules and immediate contingencies compete in a given situation, the contingencies should "win out" over the rule and gain control over behavior, and should do so longer into development than in normal individuals. (4) Responding under some conditions may be less rigid or more flexible when the rule in effect is later shown to have been incorrect, since ADHD individuals are not governed by the rule as much in the first place. (5) Self-directed rules are less likely to assist them with persisting in responding under conditions of very low levels of immediate reinforcement or the absence of reward, or during extreme delays in the consequences for responding. To this list might be added deficits in some of the additional characteristics of rule-governed behavior cited earlier (Skinner, 1969). (6) Their behavior is likely to be associated with more emotion or passion, given that the individuals with ADHD are being exposed more often to the actual contingencies in the setting, which would give rise to greater affect associated with responding. (7) Their behavior is likely to appear less conscious, intentional, deliberate, and purposive than normal and so would be characterized as more automatic, thoughtless, unintentional, ill considered, random, and impulsive.

Development of Rule-Governed Behavior in ADHD. In the model formulated in Chapter 7, I noted three levels in the development of rule-governed behavior identified by Hayes et al. (1996), which these researchers hypothesized might also represent corresponding stages of moral development. Individuals with ADHD would be delayed in their development, leading to the following problems:

1. Impaired pliance. This involves difficulty complying with rules even though one has been previously socially rewarded for doing so.
2. Defective tracking. The ADHD individual is less able to follow rules that have a history of agreement with the actual contingencies to which they pertain. In other words, just because the individual has followed rules in the past that succeeded in predicting the actual contingencies will not result in an increase in rule-following behavior.
3. Diminished augmenting. This refers to an inability of rules to alter the capacity of particular events to function as consequences. Motivative augmentals increase or decrease the degree to which previously established consequences operate as rewards and punishments, while formative augmentals establish new consequences as being rewarding or punitive. Neither form of augmenting will be as effective in those with ADHD as they are in same-age normal children.

Delayed Moral Reasoning

The control of behavior by the sense of past and future, as well as by the more general rules or metarules formulated from them or acquired via socialization, contributes to the development of conscience and moral reasoning (see Chapter 7). If this is so, then this hybrid model predicts that those with ADHD will be found to be delayed in the stages of moral development.

Diminished and Disorganized Verbal Thought

Covert, self-directed speech along with the nonverbal forms of working memory greatly enrich the mental life of the individual. Therefore, it seems reasonable to conclude that the mental lives of those with ADHD would have to be more "externalized" than "internalized," that is, more public in nature. The boldness, clarity, and organization of the content of thinking might also be diminished as well, particularly under circumstances wherein goal-directed activities must be performed, given the previously hypothesized deficiency in temporal sequencing and organization associated with ADHD.

When combined with deficits in the nonverbal forms of working memory, these deficits in internalized language associated with ADHD result in a general diminution in the regulation of behavior by internally represented information. Similarly, lesions to the prefrontal lobes, particularly the dorsolateral regions that subserve these forms of representational memory, have been shown to result in a release in the control over behavior by such internally represented information. Not only is there likely to be greater perseveration of responding in such individuals, but their behavior seems to become more environmentally dependent. A result of this is often an increase in utilization behavior (Goldberg & Podell, 1995; Lhermitte, 1983; Lhermitte, Pillion, & Sraru, 1985), that is, utilizing objects within the visual field and larger immediate context without regard for the appropriateness of such behavior for that context. The manner in which the object is used is not impaired; the individual utilizes it properly. But that utilization is out of place in that particular setting or context. Behavior seems to be driven more by incidental objects in the surrounding context than is normal (Goldberg & Podell, 1995). For instance, if the individual encounters an umbrella in a clinic examining room, he or she may begin opening and closing the umbrella, demonstrating its proper mechanical use but clearly violating the rules for that social context. The present model predicts that such utilization behavior should be more apparent in those with ADHD than in normal individuals of the same age group. Is this the source of much of the fidgeting behavior

and increased inappropriate playing with objects during work assignments that is often displayed in observational studies of ADHD
children (see Barkley, 1990; Barkley, DuPaul, & McMurray, 1990; Luk,
1985)? It would seem to be quite promising to evaluate this prediction
using paradigms similar to those used in studying utilization behavior
in patients with prefrontal injuries.

Impaired Self-Regulation of Affect/Motivation/Arousal

An integral aspect of private, self-directed sensing and speech is the
associations such mentally represented forms of information will have
with affective, motivational, and even arousal states.By being less
capable of mentally representing and sustaining internal information
about prior contingencies, those with ADHD are less able to reawaken
their associated affective and motivational states. This should create a
condition in which those with ADHD are unable to covertly emote to
and motivate themselves. They should also be less capable of bridging
delays in contingencies and especially delays to reinforcers. They cannot
self-motivate, and so remain dependent on external forms of immediate
reinforcement in order to persist at tasks and activities and to defer
gratification. They are not developing the capacity to motivate themselves as readily or effectively as normal children.

Diminished Emotional Self-Control

If those with ADHD are less able to inhibit their prepotent responses
to events and to delay those responses, then we should also witness in
them a diminished capacity to inhibit prepotent emotional responses
as well. The affect that is engendered in the individual with ADHD
by a particular event is much less likely to undergo a period of
contemplation, modification, and even reformulation by the executive
functions if a delay in emotional responding is deficient in them
relative to normal individuals. The use of internalized imagery, private
speech, reconstitution, and their related forms of covert behavior stand
little or no chance to act upon the initial emotional reactions an
individual has to an event, as there is little or no delay in these
dominant emotional expressions, and thus cannot make them more
socially acceptable before their eventual expression. Contrasting emotions that might be voluntarily created so as to countermand the initial
prepotent reaction are also less able or even unable to be induced
because the delay in emotional responding they require is abnormally
shortened in those with ADHD. Consequently, the maturation of

emotional self-control so well described by Kopp (1989), will be delayed in those with ADHD.

Diminished Objectivity and Social Perspective Taking

The aforementioned difficulties with emotional self-control cannot help but render those with ADHD less objective in their reactions to events. That objectivity requires the individual to set aside for the moment his or her personal feelings and the immediate, often selfish, prepotent reactions elicited by an event, and to consider the content of the event apart from the emotional valence it may carry for that individual. The content cannot be sanitized of its initial emotional valence when a delay in responding is diminished or even absent. Delays in responding permit the eventual behavior of an individual to an event to be internally guided, often by rules, giving it a more reasoned, objective, and purposive quality (Skinner, 1969). Given that those with ADHD are less able to delay their responses, to develop forms of internal information such as rules to guide their behavior, and then to actually apply those rules in the service of behavioral control, their behavior will be less reasoned, more emotional and immediately self-serving, and more reactive or ill-intentioned in its nature. Consequently, in their reactions to events, they will be less able to take the perspective of another or to consider another's feelings apart from their own.

Diminished Self-Generation of Motivation, Arousal, and Goal-Directed Action

The covert self-generation of motivational (drive) and arousal states in support of the execution of goal-directed actions and persistence toward the goal is critical to self-regulation. ADHD diminishes the individual's capacity to regulate and even induce motivation and arousal states in support of such behavior. The covert resensing of past events and their associated motivational states cannot give rise to the construction of future plans with corresponding motivational states in those with ADHD as well as in others, leaving their motivational states at the mercy of the surrounding context.

Diminished Self-Regulation of Affect/Arousal

Negative affective or motivational states, such as anger, frustration, disappointment, sadness, anxiety, and boredom are more problematic for ADHD children than others because it is harder for the former to manipulate the variables that would create more positive states. The self-directed forms of manipulation, such as efforts at self-comforting, self-directed speech, visual imagery, and self-reinforcement, among other means, that normal children are developing and deploying should be less developed and deployed in those with ADHD. The developmental progression in the internalization of emotion (see Chapter 8) is likely to be delayed in those with ADHD, leaving them to manifest their emotions impulsively and publicly far longer into their development than normal children, most surely to their social detriment.

Recollect that I suggested that among the variety of human emotions, it may be the negative array of emotions that will be most in need of such emotional self-regulation. Negative affect is likely to be less socially acceptable and so will elicit more salient, long-term negative social consequences from others relative to positive emotions, such as laughter or affection. Yet because such negative displays seem to achieve immediate positive reinforcement or, more likely, escape or avoidance of aversive social events, such as the imposition of demands by parents and teachers (Patterson, 1982, 1986), they will be more difficult to inhibit because of their prepotent nature in those with ADHD. Over the long haul, however, these negative displays serve to produce a variety of negative consequences for the individual with ADHD, detracting from the net maximization of future social outcomes.

To summarize, those with ADHD should be more impulsively emotional and less able to self-regulate their emotional states than are their normal peers. They should be similarly less able to motivate themselves to delay gratification and persist in goal-directed responses. They should also be less capable of self-imposed states of immediate hardship, deprivation, and other aversive conditions that may be required to maximize longer-term gains. Since the self-regulation of both emotion and motivation are likely to be associated with corresponding changes in states of nonspecific arousal as well, it seems fair to say that ADHD should result in difficulties in the self-regulation of these arousal states when they are needed in the service of goal-directed activity.

The interaction of the function for self-regulation of emotion and motivation with those of working memory (both nonverbal and verbal) leads to some additional predictions about the affective and motivational behavior likely to be evident in those with ADHD. The recall of the past and the construction of hypothetical futures based upon it should give rise not only to anticipatory motor behavior, but anticipatory affect and motivation as well. Therefore, those with ADHD should show far less anticipatory affect and motivation with regards to events that lie in the future than would others of the same age who do not have ADHD. Coupled with the prediction made earlier, one might expect that those with ADHD should demonstrate greater emotion in the moment, because of their poor inhibition of emotional responses, but should demonstrate less anticipatory emotion in advance of future events.

Reconstitution

Reconstitution involves behavioral analysis and synthesis, and it depends on behavioral inhibition to support it. If those with ADHD cannot inhibit responding as well as others, they should be found less able to take the units of previously acquired behavioral sequences in their repertoire apart (analysis). As a result, they are less able to recombine such units to create novel behaviors and sequences of behaviors out of previously learned responses (synthesis). This problem should be evident in those with ADHD not only in their speech, but in nonverbal forms of fine and gross motor behavior as well.

One of the most obvious signs of reconstitution in verbal behavior noted by Bronowski (1977) was verbal fluency, or the capacity to rapidly and accurately assemble diverse units of language into messages for others. Given that such fluency is dependent on behavioral inhibition and that inhibition is deficient in those with ADHD, verbal fluency should likewise be deficient as a consequence of having ADHD. And given my extension of Bronowski's idea of reconstitution to the realm of nonverbal behavior, I would also argue that those with ADHD should have a diminished ability to perform tasks involving nonverbal fluency, such as design, vocal, musical, fine, and gross motor fluency. In short, whenever a task demands the construction of a novel, complex sequence of nonverbal responses, those with ADHD will be less capable of quickly and accurately assembling such novel responses from their past repertoire of behavior others who are unaffected by this disorder. Research on patients with frontal lobe lesions indicates that they are impaired in the spontaneous flexibility of generating ideas (ideational fluency), as well as in verbal and figural fluency (Crowe, 1992; Eslinger & Grattan, 1993; Lee, Strauss, McCloskey, Loring, & Drane, 1996). Using similar tasks with patients with ADHD is likely to reveal similar dysfluencies, according to the predictions of this theory of ADHD.

More generally, those with ADHD should be less adept in situations that demand the formation of novel, complex, and hierarchically organized sequences of behavior, so as to attain a future goal. This results from the impairment that ADHD is hypothesized to render in the reconstitutive executive function. Those with ADHD cannot delay the prepotent response to an event as effectively as others can, thus reducing or even eliminating the delay in responding, which is crucial to the individual's ability to reflect upon, dismember, and recombine the units of past behaviors within his or her repertoire and then construct the required response to the event. The range of novelty and diversity of behaviors in those with ADHD should be more constricted as a consequence of this impairment, not only in language and the rules that language can be used to formulate, but just as much in nonverbal forms of behavioral fluency and creativity. Thus, ADHD exacts a toll on the behavioral flexibility and creativity of the individual, which is needed in the service of future goals. In a sense, these assemblies of novel responses provided by the reconstitutive function are a form of behavioral simulation that permits covert creation and testing out of various response options before one is selected for performance in the setting (Dehaene & Changeux, 1995). And so those with ADHD would be less likely to engage in such covert simulations of behavior than individuals without the disorder.

The combining of units of behavior must be based upon a syntax or set of rules governing the temporal sequencing of such units, especially their contingent "if–then" relations. Those with ADHD therefore should have more difficulties with that syntax, making them more disorganized in their attempts to assemble complex, hierarchically arranged, goal-directed behavioral structures. It has been suggested that the syntax of language may be more disrupted by lesions to the left than right prefrontal cortex, while those to the right prefrontal cortex may have more of an impact on the syntax of nonverbal, visual–spatial–construction tasks (Goldberg & Podell, 1995). As those with ADHD have smaller brain regions in this right prefrontal area, they may also have greater difficulties with the syntax of nonverbal behavioral organization than with that of language, though this notion is more speculative than are the other predictions made here.

Motor Control/Fluency/Syntax

As a result of the inhibitory deficits associated with ADHD, the observable products of the executive functions as they contribute to the execution of behavior should be less evident in those with ADHD.

As Figure 9.1 indicates, those with ADHD will be found to display greater task-irrelevant activity than normal, as they cannot suppress prepotent responses that may be elicited during the performance of goal-directed tasks. The diminution in the control of their behavior by internally represented information results in a partial release of behavior to control by the immediate environment, which would predict an increase in utilization behavior. Those with ADHD should be found exploring, touching, manipulating, and utilizing objects that enter their sensory fields in the immediate context more than should others of the same chronological age. Such effects would greatly disrupt the ability to successfully execute goal-directed responses, as they would be repeatedly interrupted by ongoing environmental events.

Those with ADHD should also evidence an impairment in the ability to execute complex, novel, and hierarchically organized goal-directed behavioral structures. The formulation of such response options and their temporal sequencing arises from the working memory and reconstitutive functions but must be translated into motor behavior. Goal-directed behavior will be less flexible, less diverse, less complex, and more poorly temporally organized in those with ADHD.

Given the deficiency predicted in the function related to the self-control of affect and motivation, those with ADHD should be found to put less effort into goal-directed responses, especially those that must be sustained over long periods of time with minimal or no ongoing reinforcement. Goal-directed persistence should be less evident because goal-directed motivation is less forthcoming and because the information needed to guide such behavior over extended periods of time is not being internally represented as well in working memory as it is in others.

I have mentioned previously (Chapters 3 and 7) that the interaction of working memory with behavioral inhibition gives rise to a sensitivity to errors in motor responding as well as to increased flexibility of behavior during tasks. The poor inhibition associated with ADHD will disrupt this process, leading to patterns of perseverative responding in tasks that require greater flexibility, such as the WCST, and to a diminished likelihood of benefiting from feedback about errors in performance during repeated trials involving motor responding.

The behavioral performance of those with ADHD during goal-directed activities should also give evidence of a diminished ability to return to those activities if they are temporally disrupted by the need to attend to another activity. Interruptions of goal-directed work will lead ADHD individuals to be less likely to return to that work, in part because of a deficit in the capacity to retain the goal in mind (working memory). Thus, without reminders, those with ADHD would be slower to reengage the task and even less likely to do so when interruptions occur.

I discussed earlier in this chapter and in Chapter 7 how the syntax that is an inherent part of working memory permits past events to be held in mind in proper temporal, sequential order (retrospective function). This should inform the prospective or response-planning function of working memory as well giving the proper syntax to the temporal ordering of responses that will be executed based upon the represented information. If ADHD disrupts the syntax of this retrospective–prospective process, then it should be evident in the syntax of observable behavior as well. Those with ADHD should be far more temporally disorganized in their behavior, performing the subunits of goal-directed activities out of their proper temporal sequence more than would others of their chronological age. The time, timing, and timeliness increasingly evident in the motor behavior of children as they mature should be delayed in those with ADHD.

THE NATURE OF INATTENTION IN ADHD

The executive function deficits discussed earlier can now be used to account for the appearance of inattention seen in ADHD. Recall from Chapter 1 that such inattention was characterized by difficulty in sustaining attention as well as in resisting distraction. The poor sustained attention that apparently characterizes those with ADHD probably represents an impairment in goal- or task-directed persistence arising from poor inhibition and the toll it takes on self-regulation (the executive functions). The distractibility ascribed to those with ADHD most likely arises from poor interference control, which allows other external and internal events to disrupt the executive functions that provide for self-control and task persistence. The net effect is an individual who cannot persist in effort toward tasks that provide little immediate reward and who flits from one uncompleted activity to another as disrupting events occur. Thus, "inattention" in ADHD can now be seen as not so much a primary symptom but a secondary one; it is a consequence of the impairment that poor behavioral inhibition and interference control create in the executive control of behavior.

This line of reasoning supports the critical distinction I made in Chapter 1 between two forms of sustained attention (persistence): that which is *contingency-shaped* and that which is *self-regulated and goal-directed*. The former is largely a function of motivational and other factors operating in the immediate environment. The second type of sustained attention arises as *an emergent property out of the interactions of the executive functions that permit self-regulation and control over the motor system by internally represented information*. This latter form of persistence is controlled by covert, self-directed actions that permit much longer, more complex, and more novel chains of responses to be created and executed toward achieving later goals. These goal-directed behavioral structures do not require immediate reward for execution, as the motivation driving them is self-created. It is this self-regulatory type of sustained attention that is developmentally delayed in ADHD children, not the type that is contingency-shaped.

The model also explains the rather dramatic fluctuation in such symptoms across settings and tasks, given that the behavior of those with ADHD is more contingency-shaped than rule-governed—more context dependent than internally guided. So long as immediate and frequent reinforcement is available in the context for persisting in performing responses, those with ADHD should be less or even not distinguishable from normal. They should become increasingly distinct from normal as immediate consequences are reduced or removed entirely from tasks because their persistence is dependent on those consequences. Those with ADHD should also be increasingly distinct from normal when tasks and settings demand that longer chains of behaviors must be strung together to achieve more temporally distant consequences in the absence of immediate consequences for doing so.

This explanation clarifies why the "inattentive" symptoms are found to form a separate but only semi-independent dimension from hyperactive–impulsive behavior in ratings by parents and teachers. The inattention (impersistence) is at least one step (or more) removed from the problems with behavioral inhibition via the intermediary constructs of working memory and the other executive functions. It is this self-regulated form of attention that should prove to be qualitatively distinct from the type of inattention seen in children with the predominantly inattentive type of ADHD. These children, as discussed in Chapter 1, likely have a deficiency in focused or selective attention that is not related to problems with behavioral inhibition and self-regulation.

Some evidence already exists to support a distinction between goal-directed persistence (internally or self-dependent) and contingency-shaped (context-dependent) sustained attention, as well as to support the association of the former with poor inhibitory control. Shoda et al. (1990) found that normal preschool children's ability to inhibit responding in a resistance-to-temptation task significantly predicted parent ratings of those subjects' concentration, sustained attention, and distractibility at adolescence. Measures of working memory, such as delayed spatial memory, mental arithmetic, digit span, and reproduction of hand movement sequences, have been found to correlate with tests and behavioral observations frequently interpreted as measuring sustained attention and behavioral persistence in preschool ADHD children (Mariani & Barkley, 1997). Levy and Hobbes (1989), likewise, found that measures of vigilance (a CPT) loaded on the same factor as a measure of working memory (related to spelling ability) and that this factor significantly distinguished their ADHD and control groups. These studies suggest links between inhibition, working memory, and persistence or sustained attention.

CONCLUSION

This chapter extended the hybrid model of executive functions and self-regulation to an understanding of ADHD. Numerous predictions were made about what should be expected to be observed in those with ADHD if this model of that disorder is correct. In essence, this model states that the behavioral inhibition that is deficient in ADHD should give rise to secondary deficits in the four executive functions, thereby resulting in behavior that is less internally guided, less purposive and goal-directed, less governed by and oriented to time, and less likely to be aimed at maximizing net future outcomes over immediate ones. The model was also shown to provide a potential explanation for the attention deficits said to characterize ADHD, in the process making a critical distinction between two forms of sustained attention not previously distinguished in research on this disorder. This theoretical model predicts that contingency-shaped, context-dependent sustained responding will not be deficient in those with ADHD, while goal-directed persistence, arising as it does from the executive functions and guided by their internally represented information, will be deficient relative to normal peers.

Important to appreciate here is that this model of ADHD does not arise out of the scientific literature on ADHD. It originates in theories of executive functions developed independent of that experimental literature on ADHD. Such theories were either efforts to explain the unique properties of human language (Bronowski, 1967/1977) or the functions of the prefrontal lobes (Damasio, 1994, 1995; Fuster, 1980, 1989, 1995; Goldman-Rakic, 1995a, 1995b). Understanding these origins is critical to addressing any criticism of this model of ADHD as being circular; that criticism could claim that the model was developed out of the literature on the cognitive deficits seen in ADHD and, therefore, ought to account for those deficits. Fortunately for this model, this was not the case. The predictions about ADHD derived from this hybrid model can, therefore, be construed as valid theoretical predictions to be tested out by comparison to the literature on cognitive deficits in ADHD. Those predictions and the theory giving rise to them can potentially be falsified by an analysis of the literature on ADHD in comparison to the model. Where no evidence yet exists concerning these predictions, they can come to serve as valid experimental hypotheses that are also a means of testing and falsifying this model of ADHD. The model, thus, becomes not only a means of better organizing the existing literature on cognitive deficits associated with ADHD but, more importantly, a means of supporting future theory-driven research into the nature of ADHD. In the next chapter, I will evaluate the literature on cognitive deficits found in those with ADHD for its consistency with these predictions.

CHAPTER 10

———•———

Evidence Supporting Executive
Function Deficits in ADHD

IN THIS CHAPTER I examine the empirical literature on ADHD for its consistency with the predictions advanced in Chapter 9, based on the hybrid model of executive functioning. In many instances, however, evidence is simply unavailable. There is a great need for more research into the executive functions in ADHD individuals. Further, the relevance of some existing research findings on ADHD to these executive functions is sometimes difficult to determine, given that the researchers did not set out to intentionally test the predictions derived from this model. Even so, there is enough literature on the executive functions to permit an initial evaluation of some of the predictions about ADHD associated with them. First, however, I will consider some important issues about research methods in the study of executive functioning.

IMPORTANT METHODOLOGICAL CAVEATS

There are at least six key issues of methodology involved in casting the model of executive functions (Chapter 7) and extending it to ADHD (Chapter 9), as I have done in this text. *The first is that the deficits predicted to exist in the four executive functions as a consequence of the impairment in inhibition in ADHD will not be as severe as the impairment in inhibition.* These deficits will be of a smaller magnitude than is the inhibitory deficit because they are, in fact, secondary to that deficit. Further, the deficit in inhibition will not translate automatically into a deficit of comparable degree in each of the executive functions. For example, if the correlation between measures of behavioral inhibition and those of nonverbal working memory is .35 (only a conjecture), then the degree of impairment in inhibition will not automatically result in the same amount of deficiency in nonverbal working memory. In addition, because the executive functions are not likely to be related to behavioral inhibition to the same degrees, the secondary impairments created in the executive functions may not be equivalent. This could mean that some studies may not find deficits in the executive functions to be statistically significant if they employ samples of relatively mild cases of ADHD. Such cases might be found in samples derived from community or school screenings and chosen merely for having high levels of hyperactive–impulsive–inattentive symptoms, as opposed to clinically referred samples meeting formal clinical diagnostic criteria.

The relationships between measures of behavioral inhibition and those of each executive function may appear to be of low to moderate degree in studies employing statistical correlation methods. Therefore, the second methodological point in testing this model is that *the relationships expressed in the model are not completely bidirectional, but are conditional.* The conditional nature of the relationship can make simple correlations between measures of inhibition, and measures of any one of the other executive functions appear to be rather modest, and hence unimportant or unsupportive of this model, when that may not actually be the case. Bayesian conditional probabilities may prove more informative about these relationships.

For instance, an excellent measure of the inhibition of prepotent responses (see Chapter 4) in research on ADHD has proven to be the stop-signal paradigm used with great effectiveness by Schachar and colleagues (1993) and, more recently, Oosterlaan and Sergeant (1995). Let us suppose this measure were to be found to correlate with a measure of reconstitution at a magnitude of .30, for example. This would suggest a rather modest relationship that might be statistically significant if the sample size were sufficiently large. However, less than 10% of the variance in one construct (reconstitution) is shared with or explained by the other (response inhibition), which is not very impressive evidence for the model. However, in a conditional relationship such as the one I have hypothesized in the model between these two functions, inhibition does not cause reconstitution to occur per se, but only permits the occasion for its occurrence. Other factors in the task at hand will determine whether or to what extent reconstitution may be required to assist with problem solving. Thus, reconstitution depends on inhibition but does not cause inhibition to occur, while, conversely, inhibition sets the occasion for reconstitution to occur but does not necessarily ensure that it will be needed in the task nor that one will be proficient in it. To put it another way, an individual may be very proficient at inhibiting prepotent responses on the stop-signal task but demonstrate merely low average scores on measures of reconstitution. In contrast, an individual demonstrating exceptional talents in reconstitution would also need to have at least average or better proficiency at inhibition to support such an achievement of reconstitution.

In short, specifying relationships as conditional and even unidirectional in their dependencies often makes them appear relatively weakly associated in statistical correlations when their true relationship to each other is a far more important one. Future research on the hybrid model of executive functions as well as on its extension to understanding ADHD will need to give due consideration to such conditional relationships and how they might best be demonstrated apart from merely calculating statistical correlations among measures of each construct specified in the model.

A third methodological consideration in research on executive functions and on their application to ADHD is the requirement that such *research must use sample sizes for ADHD and various control groups that are sufficiently large to permit the study to have satisfactory statistical power.* The effect sizes (magnitude of group differences) that may exist in the executive functions are probably going to be at least in the medium range. Depending on the nature of the measure, the number of times it is given to each subject, and the number of groups being compared in the study, such sample sizes will need to be in the range of 52–64 per group (three and two groups, respectively) or more if the probability value for the statistical test is set at $p < .05$, and in the range of 76–95 subjects per group if the probability level is set at $p < .01$ (Cohen, 1992). The vast majority of studies that will be discussed in this chapter did not employ samples of nearly this size, and many used samples only half of this level or less. That being the case, it is quite possible that a failure to find the predicted group differences on measures of these executive functions result from the inadequate power of some studies to detect such differences, rather than from the fact that those differences do not exist. This limitation, in conjunction with the first methodological issue, suggests that a research study may have just enough power to detect group differences in a measure of behavioral inhibition but not in a measure of one of the other executive functions, such as working memory. Too often, investigators tend to interpret their lack of findings as confirming or disconfirming particular hypotheses rather than as reflecting the extraordinarily low power of the study to detect the finding predicted by the hypothesis (Cohen, 1992).

I am as guilty of this methodological sin as any investigator in the field of ADHD. This problem is due in large part to the exigencies of conducting research in clinical settings, and particularly of assisting one's students with their research obligations. In such instances, samples of relatively pure cases of ADHD are difficult to come by, the expense of doing so is great, money may be tight or nonexistent, and time to complete the project is often a major limiting factor. While these are not reasons to forgo research in clinical settings, they provide all the more reason for striving to use sample sizes as close to the ideal as possible or, more likely, for exercising due caution in the interpretation of negative findings when samples are small.

Another important methodological issue involves *the ghost of comorbidity, which haunts much of the research on ADHD and particularly on cognitive deficits*. Many, if not most, people with ADHD seen in clinical settings are likely to have at least one if not two or more additional disorders. Oppositional and conduct disorders are probably the most common disorders that coexist with ADHD, with learning disabilities running a close second. Mood and anxiety disorders also affect a sizable minority of ADHD subjects recruited from clinical settings. In such cases of comorbidity, differences between the ADHD and control groups could possibly be the result of the coexisting disorder(s) rather than of ADHD itself. A few recent studies of executive functions in ADHD have controlled for such coexisting disorders, but the majority of studies discussed here did not. The former suggest that deficits in inhibition and the executive functions are much more likely to be associated with ADHD than with other disorders. Despite these encouraging conclusions, there is still reason to be cautious in interpreting all of the findings discussed in this chapter as resulting from ADHD in these samples.

A fifth methodological issue for consideration by researchers intending to evaluate executive functions in children as well as their deficiency in those with ADHD is that of *the developmental sensitivity of the measures being used to assess these executive functions at particular ages*. The deficits predicted by the model are actually delays, as discussed in Chapter 9. This means that children with ADHD are likely to be behind other children in the development of inhibition and these other functions by a modest but significant degree for their age group. If measures are chosen that are too easy for this particular age group, then no group differences between ADHD and control children will be evident. The conclusion would be that no executive function deficits exist in such a case would be false, however. The inverse can also occur. The measure chosen can be so difficult for children of a particular age that even normal children have not mastered such tasks or attained their prerequisite psychological abilities. This results, once more, in no group differences being found between normal and ADHD children. All of this suggests that at any given age at which ADHD and normal children are being compared, the tests of inhibition and executive functions must be chosen such that most normal children have only recently mastered this level of difficulty or are well in the midst of doing so. One is then likely to find that ADHD children are lagging behind in their mastery of this level of difficulty of the task.

The span of such a developmental "window of sensitivity" to group differences for a measure could be fairly narrow. For instance, suppose that children with ADHD tend to place approximately 30% behind their normal peers on measures of verbal working memory. If the age of children in the study is 10 years, then the developmental sensitivity of the task should be aimed at 9- to 11-year-olds. If the task is too easy, such that even 5- or 6-year-olds can perform it well, then 10-year-old ADHD children can also do so, as they are likely to be at least at the 7-year-old mastery level of difficulty on that task. The result is a finding of no group differences between ADHD and normal children on the task. Conversely, if the task chosen is typically sensitive to children 14 years of age or older, then both groups of children will fail the test, resulting, again, in no group differences appearing on the measure.

This leads to the sixth and final methodological issue that researchers must consider in studying the development of executive functions and/or their delay in those with ADHD: that *measures that reflect executive functioning at one particular age may not do so at another*. I made this point at the outset of Chapter 6, when discussing the possible changes that can occur in factor loadings of tests of executive function as a consequence of age, but it demands reiteration here. Ignoring this issue could result not only in failure to find executive function deficits in studies of ADHD, but also failure to find a measure loading on any dimension reflecting the executive function of interest in ADHD children of a given age, even if the measure did so at an earlier stage of the children's development.

With these precautionary remarks in mind, then, let us turn to a review of the evidence for deficits in executive functions in people having ADHD. Future studies of executive functioning and its development in normal and/or ADHD children and adults, including those studies which set out to test some of the predictions of this model, will need to take the preceding methodological concerns into account.

EVIDENCE FOR WORKING
MEMORY DEFICITS IN ADHD

I have argued throughout this volume that the executive functions, particularly nonverbal and verbal working memory, arise as a result of the internalization of self-directed sensory–motor behavior and self-directed speech. No research has directly addressed this prediction in the field of ADHD, but there is ample indirect evidence to support the prediction of a delay in the internalization of behavior in ADHD. Evidence of delays in both realms of working memory will be reviewed here.

Working memory has been assessed in neuropsychological research using a variety of tasks. Nonverbal working memory has been less studied than verbal working memory (see Becker, 1994, for reviews). Tasks assessing nonverbal working memory typically involve memory for objects, and particularly for their spatial location (see factor-analytic and neuroimaging studies in Chapter 6). Measures assessing nonverbal planning ability as well as sense of time are also considered to fall within this domain, though such measures rarely reflect pure assessments of nonverbal abilities. I will first review evidence, sparse as it is, relating to nonverbal working memory deficits associated with ADHD, before turning to the evidence pertaining to verbal working memory and internalized speech, which is far more substantial.

Nonverbal Working Memory

The limited evidence for impaired nonverbal working memory associated with ADHD includes findings of impaired memory for spatial location (Mariani & Barkley, 1997). However, Weyandt and Willis (1994) were unable to find deficits associated with ADHD in an apparently related task requiring visual search of a display for a target item.

The use of nonverbal working memory might seem to be involved in the organization and reproduction of complex designs, such as in the Rey–Osterrieth Complex Figure Drawing Test. A number of studies have identified organizational deficits in ADHD children on this task (Douglas & Benezra, 1990; Grodzinsky & Diamond, 1992; Sadeh, Ariel, & Inbar, 1996; Seidman et al., 1996). Two studies have not found such group differences (Moffitt & Silva, 1988; Reader et al., 1994), and another found deficits only in ADHD children with reading disorders (McGee, Williams, Moffitt, & Anderson, 1989). Two of the three studies finding nonsignificant results for ADHD children employed samples drawn from community screenings of children, whereas most of those studies finding differences used clinic-referred samples. As I mentioned at the beginning of this chapter, community-derived samples may not be as severe in their symptoms of ADHD as those referred to clinics, which perhaps explains these inconsistent results.

Hindsight, Forethought, and Planning

The retrospective and prospective functions defined by both Fuster (1989) and Goldman-Rakic (1995a, 1995b), also known as hindsight and forethought (Bronowski, 1967/1977), are crucial to understanding working memory. These constructs have not been well studied in those with ADHD, except as they are likely to pertain to measures of planning, such as the TOL or Tower of Hanoi test (Glosser & Goodglass, 1990) and maze performances. However, if in its most elementary form hindsight can be taken to mean the ability to alter subsequent responses based upon immediately past mistakes, then research findings imply a deficit in hindsight in ADHD. ADHD children, like adults with prefrontal lobe injuries (Milner, 1995), are less likely to adjust their subsequent responses based on an immediately past incorrect response in an information-processing task (Sergeant & van der Meere, 1988). The findings of perseveration on the WCST also suggest such a problem.

Research using complex reaction time tasks with warning stimuli and preparation intervals may be relevant to the construct of forethought. Findings reveal ADHD children often fail to use the warning stimulus to prepare for the upcoming response trial (Douglas, 1983), with longer preparatory intervals making the performance of ADHD children worse than in control children (Chee et al., 1989; van der Meere et al., 1992; Zahn et al., 1991). The capacity to create and maintain anticipatory set for an impending event also has been shown to be impaired by ADHD (van der Meere, Vreeling, & Sergeant, 1992).

The TOL was discussed in Chapters 6 and 8 as placing heavy emphasis on working memory, particularly, though not exclusively, on the nonverbal form. Forethought and planning were discussed as being instrumental to the performance of the TOL, which was shown (in both the factor-analytic and neuroimaging studies) to probably involve several executive functions besides working memory, given its demands for response inhibition and interference control, reconstitution, and sustained motivation. Recall that this task requires that individuals be able to mentally represent and test out various ways of removing and replacing disks on a set of pegs or spindles to match a design presented by the experimenter. This involves substantial mental planning that must occur before and while undertaking the actual motor execution of the rearrangement. Studies of ADHD using the TOL and a related task, the Tower of Hanoi (TOH), have consistently found ADHD children to perform more poorly than normal children (Brady & Denckla, 1994; Pennington, Grossier, & Welsh, 1993; Weyandt & Willis, 1994).

Like the TOL and TOH, maze performance probably reflects aspects of planning ability as well, though perhaps not as much as the former tests. After all, the solution to the maze is obviously within the maze design that sits before the child and simply must be discovered, while the solution to the TOL design problem is not so readily apparent. Perhaps this explains why some studies have found ADHD children to perform poorly on maze tasks (Weyandt & Willis, 1994), while many others have not (Barkley, Grodzinsky, & DuPaul, 1992; Grodzinsky & Diamond, 1992; Mariani & Barkley, 1997; McGee et al., 1989; Milich & Kramer, 1985; Moffitt & Silva, 1988). The young age of the subjects may be a factor in some of the negative findings (Mariani & Barkley, 1997), as may be the low power associated with the use of small samples ($n < 20$ per group) (Barkley, Grodzinsky, & DuPaul, 1992; McGee et al., 1989; Moffitt & Silva, 1988). The TOL and TOH tasks may better reflect the capacity to plan or "look ahead" (Pennington et al., 1993) than do mazes, and children with ADHD perform poorly on these tasks. While hardly definitive, the findings reviewed here are at least suggestive of deficiencies in hindsight, forethought, and planning ability, which depend on working memory.

I had predicted in Chapter 9 that the diminution in forethought hypothesized to be associated with ADHD should result in a delay in the development of a child's concept of the universality of death—one's personal mortality. I know of no research that has examined this issue, though it seems to be worthy of study.

Imitation and Vicarious Learning

The predicted incapacity of ADHD individuals to hold information in mind should create difficulty with imitating the complex and lengthy behavioral sequences performed by others that may be novel to the subject. It should also result in a more general delay in the ability to apply information acquired through vicarious learning to the formulation and execution of current behavior. No studies of ADHD were found that expressly tested these predictions. However, several studies have employed more rudimentary imitation tasks that could be taken to suggest a deficit in imitative behavior. These studies found that

children with ADHD are less proficient at imitating increasingly
lengthy and novel sequences of simple motor gestures than are normal
children, such as those required on the K-ABC Hand Movements Test
(Breen, 1989; Grodzinsky & Diamond, 1992; Mariani & Barkley,
1997). Adults with ADHD have also been shown to be less able to
replicate increasingly longer sequences involving pointing to locations
than are non-ADHD adults (Barkley et al., 1996b). Though hardly
definitive, such findings suggest that this prediction is worth testing
in future studies in ADHD.

Sense of Time and Cross-Temporal Organization of Behavior

Nonverbal working memory was described as being integral to the
development of psychological awareness of time and the organization
of behavior relative to time. The hybrid model discussed in Chapter 7
would, therefore, predict an impaired sense of time in those with
ADHD. Gerbing et al. (1987) also argued that the impairments in the
performance of time estimation/production tasks may be related to
impulsiveness, and White et al. (1994) found some evidence supporting that argument. But more direct evidence for an impairment in
sense of time in children with ADHD has been found in several studies.

Cappella, Gentile, and Juliano (1977) conducted two studies using
hyperactive and normal children. In the first study, subjects were
required to estimate time by indicating when they thought intervals
of 15, 30, and 60 seconds had elapsed. Despite using only 12 subjects
each in their hyperactive and control group, results indicated that the
hyperactive children made significantly larger errors of estimation than
the control subjects. The ADHD children demonstrated a significantly
greater increase in the magnitude of such errors as the length of the
duration increased than did the controls, who also showed such an
increase in time estimation as duration increased. In a second study
reported in this same paper, the authors compared 25 hyperactive and
75 normal subjects using a similar task. In this case, the time durations
(7, 15, and 30 seconds) had to be produced by the child by pressing a
button to indicate the beginning and end of the trial. Such a change
in procedure may seem minor, but even minor variations in testing
procedures can produce significantly different results in studies of
children's sense of time (Zakay, 1992). Nevertheless, the hyperactive
group once again made larger errors of time estimation than did
controls and showed a significantly greater increase in these errors as
the time durations increased than did the control subjects.

In a more recent study, Grskovic, Zentall, and Stormont-Spurgin
(1995) compared children rated by their teachers as having high levels

of ADHD symptoms with control subjects on a measure of retrospective time estimation, known as recall estimation. In this procedure, subjects are asked to recall routine life experiences they have had and to estimate how long a future activity should take based on this recollection. This is a very different form of time estimation than that used by Cappella et al. (1977) and my colleagues and me (Barkley et al., in press) in our research on time estimation, which I will describe later in this section. Such retrospective accounts of the temporal durations of routine activities constitute a very interesting and unique way of evaluating sense of time. Unfortunately, it is unlikely to purely reflect working memory ability, as would prospective time paradigms, wherein subjects estimate durations experienced at the time of their laboratory evaluation. The retrospective accounts used by Grskovic et al. (1995) may be partially confounded by difficulties with the storage, retention, and retrieval of information placed in long-term memory (Zakay, 1992). As a result, they cannot be interpreted as being comparable to the prospective methods of time estimations, productions, and reproductions used by the other studies described here.

Nevertheless, Grskovic et al. found that ADHD children who also had cooccurring emotional handicaps, as well as LD children, performed significantly less well on this measure than did control children. Children with ADHD but without emotional handicaps and children having only emotional handicaps and no ADHD did not differ significantly from the remaining groups in this regard. However, the group differences that were found became nonsignificant when IQ was statistically controlled in the reanalysis of these data. The authors question whether other research findings on differences in sense of time in inattentive children actually confound this construct with differences in intelligence.

At least three problems with the methodology of this study render this conclusion doubtful. First, the sample sizes of the groups were extraordinarily small, ranging from 6 to 13 in each and resulting in substantially deficient power to detect actual group differences on this measure. Second, the retrospective recall procedure used here to evaluate time estimation abilities is simply not comparable to the methods used by others to evaluate the capacity to estimate ongoing temporal intervals (prospective methods). Even if removing the differences in IQ among the groups resulted in the originally significant differences among groups becoming nonsignificant, this would not necessarily imply that IQ accounts for the differences found in other studies using very different time estimation procedures.

The final problem is the questionable value of statistically controlling for IQ differences in the analyses of measures of executive functions, in this case, time estimation. I have elsewhere challenged the wisdom of such practices in group comparisons between ADHD and control groups (Barkley, 1996; Mariani & Barkley, 1997) and will address the issue again later in this chapter. These deficits in IQ in children with ADHD may be directly related to ADHD and the toll that disorder takes on executive functioning. Thus, to control for IQ in studies of ADHD is to remove part of the influence of the very independent variable (ADHD) one is attempting to study. Grskovic et al. (1995) are not the first investigators to find their differences between ADHD and control groups disappearing when IQ has been used as a covariate in statistical analyses of these comparisons. Consequently, I am far less convinced than they were that differences among groups in time estimation may merely reflect group differences in general cognitive ability.

In a recent series of studies, my colleagues and I evaluated the ability of ADHD children to reproduce prospectively presented time intervals (Barkley et al., in press). Time reproduction tasks are some of the most difficult for subjects to perform and therefore may·be a more rigorous means of testing this construct than are studies that merely employ time estimation methods ("How long was that interval just presented?") or time production procedures ("Show me a duration of 10 seconds"). In time reproduction, the subject is presented with a sample duration but is not told its length. The subject then uses some device (e.g., a flashlight) to signal the beginning and end of an interval to demonstrate that duration.

In a preliminary study of 32 ADHD and 32 control children, we had the children reproduce 6- and 10-second durations with no distraction present. We then had them reproduce intervals of 10 and 16 seconds with distractions present. We found that the ADHD subjects made significantly larger reproduction errors than the controls during the 6- and 10-second trials as well as during the 10- and 16-second trials with distraction. As in the Cappella et al. (1977) studies, both groups made larger errors of reproduction as the duration to be reproduced increased in size. However, we did not find that the ADHD subjects showed greater increases in errors than the control group.

In the second study, 12 children with ADHD were compared to 26 normal children in their ability to reproduce durations of 12, 24, 36, 48, and 60 seconds. On half of the trials presented at each duration, a distraction was created. In Figure 10.1, results are shown for the measure of absolute discrepancies in the time reproductions (magnitude of the error above or below the sample duration expressed as an absolute number). They indicate that the ADHD subjects made greater errors of time reproductions than did the control subjects across these time

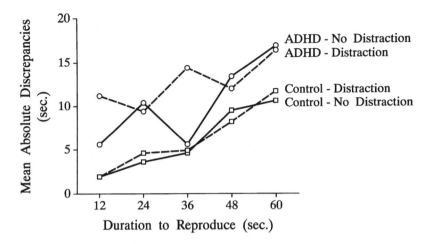

FIGURE 10.1. The mean absolute magnitude of errors in the time productions of ADHD and control children at five different durations with and without distraction. From Barkley, Koplowicz, Anderson, and McMurray (in press). Copyright 1997 by Cambridge University Press. Reprinted by permission.

intervals. Both groups made increasingly larger errors as the durations to be reproduced increased. The distractions affected the ADHD subjects rather than the control subjects, particularly at the 12- and 36-second durations.

These results can be recast as coefficients of accuracy to determine whether the errors made by the subjects tended to be in one direction more than another. That is, did the ADHD subjects tend to overreproduce or underreproduce the sample intervals? The score is created by dividing the subject's raw score for the duration of the reproduction by the actual duration of the sample interval. A score greater than 1.00 reflects a tendency to overreproduce the interval, while a score less than 1.00 indicates the opposite. These results are shown in Figure 10.2. As this figure illustrates, control subjects tended to slightly underreproduce the intervals. They also tended to increase the magnitude of their underreproductions as the sample intervals increased in duration. The presence of the distractor had no impact on their reproductions. In contrast, the ADHD subjects significantly overreproduced the shorter time durations (12 and 24 seconds). But, like the normal subjects, they moved toward a progressively greater likelihood of underreproducing the intervals as the sample durations increased in size. The effect of distraction was to increase the likelihood of overreproducing the interval, primarily at the 12- and 36-second intervals.

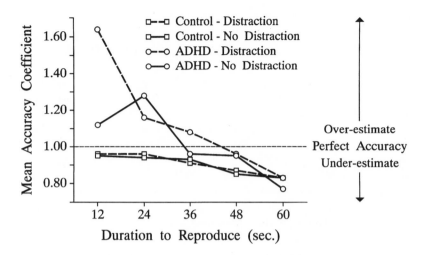

FIGURE 10.2. The mean coefficient of accuracy scores for the time productions of ADHD and control children at five different durations with and without distraction. From Barkley, Koplowicz, Anderson, and McMurray (in press). Copyright 1997 by Cambridge University Press. Reprinted by permission.

Overall, the results indicate that children with ADHD are less accurate in their sense of time than control subjects, as measured by this time reproduction method. The small sample sizes that may have limited the power of this study to detect other group differences were problematic, but would not be likely to have affected those numerous differences that were found to be significant.

It has been suggested that time reproductions can be interpreted as reflecting the individual's subjective sense of time (Zakay, 1992). If so, then this study suggests that subjects with ADHD tend to feel time is progressing more slowly than do normal subjects—durations feel longer than they actually are, especially at intervals below 36 seconds. At durations longer than this, their sense of time is becoming increasingly inaccurate but fluctuates more equally between feeling the interval as moving more slowly or more quickly than it does by clock time.

In another study in our laboratory using adults with ADHD, we investigated the use of both time estimation and time production methods (Barkley et al., 1996b). A small sample of young adults with ADHD (n = 23) were compared with 23 young adults without ADHD comprising a community control group. In the time estimation task, a research assistant signaled the beginning and end of a temporal interval. Subjects were tested at six different time intervals (2, 4, 12, 15, 45, and 60 seconds) and were then required to state the duration of the interval in seconds. In the production task, subjects were told the precise time interval in seconds and asked to reproduce that interval by signaling to the research assistant when it should begin and end. The results revealed a marginally significant difference ($p < .09$) between the groups, with the young adults with ADHD being less accurate in their time estimations than the control adults. The ADHD subjects tended to overestimate the intervals relative to the control subjects. This tendency to overestimate time is consistent with the time reproduction study, implying that ADHD subjects tend to experience time as moving more slowly than do their non-ADHD peers. Both groups became significantly less accurate as the sample duration increased. The fact that this difference was not statistically significant is likely the result of very low statistical power in this study.

The groups did not differ on the time production task, although both groups again became significantly less accurate as the sample duration increased. The failure to find a group difference on the time production task may reflect a problem with low power as well as the fact that time productions are considered the easiest of tasks in assessing sense of time. The precise interval to be produced is given to the subject, who can then use it as the basis for producing the duration.

Three other studies have evaluated sense of time in those with ADHD or hyperactivity, or rated as simply being impulsive. White, Barratt, and Adams (1979) reported that adolescents with hyperactivity made substantially larger errors than control subjects when asked to estimate the length of an interval presented to them (2 minutes). Senior, Towne, and Huessy (1979) observed that students with ADHD and emotional disturbance responded with significantly shorter time productions than did a control group when asked to produce a 30-second interval. Finally, Walker (1982) found that students identified as impulsive produced a significantly shorter time interval than those who were identified as reflective when asked to indicate when a 12-second interval had elapsed. The more impulsive children were on the Matching Familiar Figures Test, the shorter were their time reproductions ($r = .46, p < .05$). No group differences were found in the time production procedure, where subjects were given the precise interval they were to produce. The results of the Senior et al. (1979) and Walker (1982) studies are consistent with the conclusion that impulsive individuals or those with ADHD experience time as progressing more slowly than it does in reality. When asked to verbally report an estimate of how long an interval was, they will tend toward overestimation. However, when asked to physically reproduce an interval described to them, they will underreproduce it.

All of these studies on sense of time and ADHD or hyperactivity had a number of significant methodological flaws, making attempts at replication imperative. Their general consistency, however, tentatively suggests some support for the hypothesis that sense of time is probably impaired in those with ADHD.

Uninvestigated to date is the possibility that children with ADHD are less mature in their development of the strategies developed by normal children to estimate temporal durations. Individuals often rely on a variety of strategies when requested to estimate time durations (Michon & Jackson, 1984), the most common of which is counting to the self. This strategy is not typically used by young children when they are faced with estimating temporal durations but becomes a rule commonly used by children 13 years of age and older (Levin, Wilkening, & Dembo, 1984). It would be interesting to investigate whether those with ADHD are delayed in their reliance on this strategy for temporal estimations relative to normal children, as might be expected from the hybrid model.

The hybrid model of executive functions also predicts that the insertion of temporal delays into behavioral contingencies or tasks should more adversely affect the performance of those with ADHD than control groups, with longer durations associated with a correspondingly greater likelihood that such group differences will emerge. Numerous studies of ADHD have found that delays interposed in tasks as well as temporal uncertainties result in poorer performances on the tasks (Chee, Logan, Schachar, Lindsay, & Wachsmuth, 1989; Gordon, 1979; Sonuga-Barke, Taylor, & Hepinstall, 1992; Sonuga-Barke, Taylor, Sembi, & Smith, 1992; van der Meere, Shalev, Borger, & Gross-Tsur, 1995; van der Meere et al., 1992; Zahn, Krusei, & Rapoport, 1991). These results are supportive of a deficit in time, timing, and the cross-temporal organization of behavior in those with ADHD. Alternatively, delays may simply create boredom and so may increase off-task behavior in ADHD children that proves detrimental to their performance, as suggested in Zentall's (1985) optimal stimulation theory.

No research on ADHD has examined verbal references to time, plans for the future, the future more generally, and other aspects of hindsight and forethought as they might be evident in the discourse of ADHD individuals with others. In addition, just how well those with ADHD are able to temporally tag or organize their recall and internal representation of sequential events has not been studied. That such deficits are common in patients with prefrontal lobe injuries

(Gershberg & Shimamura, 1995; Godbout & Doyan, 1995) argues for their likely impairment in those with ADHD as well. The recent research on the verbal discourse of ADHD children (Tannock, 1996) found deficits that might imply such a difficulty in the children's organization of sequential material in the retelling of stories. Prior studies of narrative ability (Tannock, Purvis, & Schachar, 1992) and elicited language (Zentall, 1988) have also noted organizational deficits in ADHD children. While organizational deficits in discourse are suggested by these results, they may instead reflect the presence of comorbid language problems known to exist in a substantial minority of children with ADHD (Cantwell & Baker, 1992). Countering such an interpretation is the fact that Tannock (1996) used a control group of children with reading disorders who also were known to have language problems and still found greater organizational deficits in the ADHD group.

The model suggests that those with ADHD are less well controlled by internally represented information than are others. Like patients with prefrontal lobe injuries (Stuss & Benson, 1986), those with ADHD may be more controlled by external stimuli and display more utilization behavior (see Chapter 9). The model predicts that such behavior should be more evident in children with ADHD, yet no research has specifically studied the issue. Such research might profit from borrowing the methodologies used to study this issue in brain-injured patients (see Goldberg & Podell, 1995).

To summarize, some evidence presented here is consistent with the prediction that children with ADHD have difficulties with nonverbal working memory, planning, and sense of time. However, these results are not always consistent across studies, nor has there been a sufficient amount of research on this issue to support this hypothesis unequivocally. Few of these studies, with the exception of Barkley et al. (in press) on sense of time, specifically set out to test this hypothesis using tasks designed expressly for this purpose. Even then, sample sizes have been sufficiently small to pose serious limitations on the statistical power of the study to detect the hypothesized impairments. There is, nevertheless, sufficient promise within the present set of findings to encourage future research to specifically evaluate the predictions made by the hybrid model about nonverbal working memory and ADHD.

Verbal Working Memory

Verbal working memory tasks typically involve the retention and oral repetition of digit spans (especially in reverse order), mental computation or arithmetic, such as serial addition, and memory tasks that require the retention of verbal material across delay intervals. Often the latter tasks impose a demand for organizing the material in some way so as to more easily restate the material when called upon to do so. The hybrid model predicts that verbal working memory deficits should be associated with ADHD. Consistent with those predictions, children with ADHD have been found to be significantly less proficient in speed of mental computation (Ackerman, Anhalt, & Dykman, 1986; Barkley, DuPaul, & McMurray, 1990; Mariani & Barkley, 1997; Zentall & Smith, 1993; Zentall, Smith, Lee, & Wieczorek, 1994). More recently, adolescents with ADHD have been shown to have a similar deficiency (MacLeod & Prior, 1996). Both children and adults with ADHD have also shown more difficulties with digit span (particularly backwards) (Barkley et al., 1996b; Mariani & Barkley, 1997). The Freedom from Distractibility factor of the Wechsler Intelligence Scale for Children— Revised, or the WISC-III, comprises tests of Digit Span, Arithmetic, and Coding (Digit Symbol) and thus has been interpreted as reflecting executive processes, such as verbal working memory and resistance to distraction (Ownby & Matthews, 1985). ADHD children have been found to perform more poorly on this factor than do normal children (Anastopoulos, Spisto, & Maher, 1994; Golden, 1996; Lufi, Cohen, & Parish-Plass, 1990; Milich & Loney, 1979; van der Meere et al., 1996). A recent study of adults with ADHD documented similar deficiencies in the performance of these same tests on the Wechsler Adult Intelligence Scale (Matochik, Rumsey, Zametkin, Hamburger, & Cohen, 1996). By themselves, such findings might suggest a variety of problems besides working memory (i.e., deficient arithmetic knowledge, slow motor speed, etc.). However, Zentall and Smith (1993) were able to rule out some of these potential confounding factors in their study of mental computation in ADHD children, thus giving greater weight to the association of deficient verbal working memory with ADHD. The high comorbidity of learning disorders with ADHD, nevertheless, argues for some caution in interpreting these findings until further studies are able to distinguish to what extent those disorders may have contributed to such findings of group differences between ADHD and control subjects.

One study, by Siegel and Ryan (1989), at first blush seems to contradict the predictions of the hybrid model for ADHD; it focuses on the development of verbal working memory in four groups of children. These groups consisted of ADHD, reading-disabled, math-disabled, and normal control children. Three age groups were formed from the subjects within each group, ages 7–8, 9–10, and 11–13. Subjects were given tasks assessing their counting ability and memory for words in sentences as measures of verbal working memory. The sample sizes within each group were rather small (*n*'s of 8 and 7 for the ADHD 7–8- and 9–10-year-old groups, respectively), and some of the cells of the design were empty of subjects, including the 11–13-year-old ADHD group. Results of this study indicated that on the working memory task involving words in sentences, the 9–10-year-olds in both the normal and ADHD groups were significantly more proficient than the 7–8-year-olds. The 11–12-year-olds were not analyzed because of the lack of ADHD subjects at this age. The ADHD group performed significantly better than the reading-disabled group but was not different from the control group on this measure. For the counting task, the same results were found. In other words, the children classified as ADHD in this study showed no significant deficits on either test of working memory relative to the control group. Older children in both groups performed better than younger ones, implying age-related improvements in these working memory tasks.

Several problems plague this study, however, as an appropriate test of the hybrid model with respect to verbal working memory deficits in ADHD. First, the sample sizes for the ADHD group were so small as to raise serious doubts about the study's statistical power, and hence the internal validity, to detect group differences on these measures. Second, the definition of ADHD (or "ADD," in the published report) used to select subjects was exceptionally vague. Subjects merely had to have scored two standard deviations above the mean on the Conners Parent Questionnaire (Goyette, Conners, & Ulrich, 1978) to qualify as ADD. This questionnaire actually comprises a number of different dimensions of psychopathology, including conduct problems, learning problems, psychosomatic symptoms, and anxiety, in addition to items reflecting inattention and hyperactive–impulsive behavior. The actual composition of this group as to their specific psychopathologies is unknown. Whether or not any of these subjects would meet clinical diagnostic criteria for ADHD is open to doubt. Finally, it is not clear that the tasks used were sufficiently difficult for children at these developmental ages to be sensitive to the mild to moderate delay that may exist in verbal working memory in ADHD. Thus, there is reason to view this study as an inadequate test of the predictions of the hybrid model for working memory deficits associated with ADHD, especially in view of the substantial literature cited above in favor of such deficits.

The storage and recall of simple information using verbal memory tests has not been found to be impaired in those with ADHD (Barkley, DuPaul, & McMurray, 1990; Cahn & Marcotte, 1995; Douglas, 1983, 1988). Instead, it seems that when larger, more complex amounts of verbal information must be held in mind, especially over a lengthy delay period, such deficits become evident (Douglas, 1983, 1988;

Seidman, Biederman, et al., 1995; Seidman et al., 1996). Also, where strategies are required that assist with organizing material so as to respond to it or remember it more effectively, those with ADHD are less proficient than control groups (Amin, Douglas, Mendelson, & Dufresne, 1993; August, 1987; Benezra & Douglas, 1988; Borcherding et al., 1988; Douglas, 1983; Douglas & Benezra, 1989; Felton, Wood, Brown, Campbell, & Harter, 1987; Frost, Moffitt, & McGee, 1989; Shapiro, Hughes, August, & Bloomquist, 1993). This is true not only of ADHD children, but has more recently been demonstrated in adults with ADHD (Holdnack, Moberg, Arnold, Gur, & Gur, 1995).

As noted earlier, those with ADHD have more trouble in doing what they know, rather than in knowing what to do. Such a problem was evident in the study by Greve, Williams, and Dickens (1996) in which ADHD children displayed deficiencies in sorting cards by a rule on a task similar to the WCST, even when they were given the rule needed to do so by the examiner. Children with ADHD have been shown to have more difficulty not only in spontaneously developing a strategy to organize material to be memorized (August, 1987), but also in following that rule over time (August, 1987). Conte and Regehr (1991) also found that hyperactive children were less likely to transfer the rules they had acquired on a prior task to a new task, consistent with this hypothesis.

Other evidence, albeit less direct, is suggestive of this problem of extant knowledge poorly governing behavioral performance in those with ADHD. Past studies have found that hyperactive–impulsive children are more prone to accidents than normal children (Bijur, Golding, Haslum, & Kurzon, 1988; Methany & Fisher, 1984; Taylor et al., 1991), yet they are not deficient in their knowledge of safety or accident prevention (Mori & Peterson, 1995). Barkley, Murphy, and Kwasnik (1996a) also found that teens and young adults with ADHD have significantly more motor vehicle accidents and other driving risks (speeding), but demonstrated no deficiencies in their knowledge of driving, safety, and accident prevention.

Delayed Internalization of Speech in ADHD

I suggested in Chapters 5 and 7 that verbal working memory may actually represent the internalization of speech. Therefore, the literature on cognitive deficits in ADHD should demonstrate evidence not only of deficiencies in verbal working memory, but also of delays in the development of internalized speech and the rule-governed behavior it affords. The association of disinhibited behavior with less mature self-directed speech, rule governance of behavior, and moral reasoning, as stipulated in Chapter 7, has been suggested in studies of normal school children (Kochanska et al., 1994; Weithorn & Kagen, 1984; Zelazo, Reznick, et al., 1995). The few studies using hyperactive children or those with ADHD have also found such an immaturity (Berk & Potts, 1991; Copeland, 1979; Gordon, 1979; Rosenbaum & Baker, 1984).

The most informative and most rigorous of these studies on the development of internalized speech has been the research of Berk and her colleagues (Berk & Landau, 1993; Berk & Potts, 1991; Landau, Berk, & Mangione, 1996). In the initial study of ADHD children by Berk and Potts (1991), ADHD and normal children were observed in their natural classroom settings and the occurrences of private (self-directed but publicly observable) speech were recorded while the children were engaged in math work at their desks. Observations were collected on 19 boys with ADHD and 19 matched control boys without ADHD. The observations were classified into one of three levels of private speech believed to reflect the maturational progression of such private speech as originally proposed by Vygotsky (1978). Level 1 speech consisted of task-irrelevant utterances. Level 2 consisted of task-relevant externalized private speech, such as describing one's own actions and giving self-guiding comments; task-relevant, self-answered questions; reading aloud and sounding out words; and task-relevant affect expression. Level 3 was considered task-relevant external manifestations of inner speech. The latter included inaudible muttering, mouthing of clear words related to the task, and lip and tongue movements associated with the task.

The results indicated that the overall amount of private speech was not significantly different between groups, but differences were observed in the levels of private speech employed by each group. ADHD children were found to use significantly more Level 2 and significantly less Level 3 speech than their matched control counterparts. In contrast to the findings of Copeland (1979), the two groups did not differ in their use of Level 1 (task-irrelevant) speech. Berk and Potts (1991) analyzed their results as a function of age of the children in these groups and found significant differences in the developmental patterns. These are shown in Figure 10.3. No significant effects related to age were evident in Level 1 speech or total private speech, so these levels are not shown in the figure. ADHD children at all ages engaged in more Level 2 speech than control children. Both groups declined significantly in their use of this level of private speech with age. ADHD children were found to increase markedly in Level 3 speech between ages 6 to 7 years and 8 to 9 years, leveling off at the 10- to 11-year age group. Control subjects, in contrast, remained high in their use of this form of speech across the two youngest ages (6–7 and 8–9 years) and then declined in

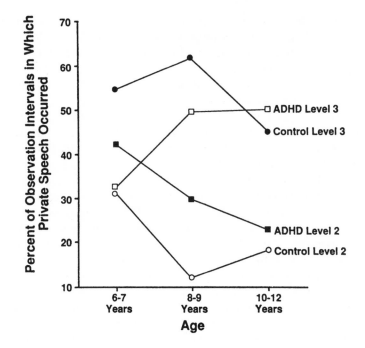

FIGURE 10.3. Developmental trends in Levels 2 and 3 private speech for ADHD and control children. From Berk and Potts (1991, p. 367). Copyright 1991 by Plenum Publishing Corp. Reprinted by permission.

their use of this level of speech by the oldest age group (10–11 years). This decline in Level 3 speech was interpreted by the authors as being consistent with Vygotsky's (1978) theoretical position that speech by this age is moving to being fully internalized (covert) and therefore less observable. The conclusion of this study was that ADHD and normal children show a similar pattern of development of private speech but that those with ADHD are considerably delayed in this process relative to control children.

It is important to demonstrate in such a study that the private speech of children is coming to serve a controlling or governing function over behavior. Berk and Potts (1991) correlated the private speech categories of these children with observations of the motor behavior associated with the task as well as with their attention to the task. Children in both groups who were more likely to have difficulty sustaining attention were found to display more Level 2 forms of private speech. Both Level 1 and Level 2 speech were also negatively correlated with focused attention and were positively correlated with diversions from seatwork. Level 2 speech was significantly and positively associated with the amount of task-facilitating behavior shown by the child. Greater degrees of Level 3 speech, thought to reflect greater maturity, were significantly correlated with degree of focused attention and were negatively associated with amount of task diversion (off-task behavior). Interestingly, only the ADHD boys showed a significant positive association between Level 3 speech and self-stimulating forms of behavior. The authors interpret such findings as indicative of a delay in the controlling effects of speech over behavior as the former proceeds to internalization.

Two additional studies provide further support to the conclusion that children with ADHD are delayed in the internalization of speech. Berk and Landau (1993) observed 56 LD children and 56 normal children in grades 3–6 while they performed their daily math and language assignments at their desks in their natural classroom settings. The LD children were further subdivided into those without ADHD ($n = 47$) and those with ADHD ($n = 9$) on the basis of teacher ratings on a behavior rating scale of ADHD symptoms. Note that the sample size for the LD/ADHD group was exceptionally small and thus severely limited the statistical power of this study to detect effects due to ADHD beyond those resulting from the presence of LD. Consistent with the earlier study, rates of private speech (self-directed yet public speech) during work were exceptionally high, and level of cognitive development (IQ) was significantly and negatively related to amounts of Level 2 speech ($r = -.25$). Again this suggests that the greater the mental maturity of children, the faster their rate of progression through the stages of internalization of speech. Both the LD and normal children showed a developmental (age-related) pattern similar to that found by Berk and Potts (1991): Level 2 speech declined linearly with increasing grade level while Level 3 speech demonstrated a quadratic effect. That is, Level 3 speech was found to increase from grades 3 to 4 and then decline from grades 4 to 5, after which it stabilized from grades 5 to 6. LD children engaged in more than twice as much private, task-relevant (Level 2) speech as normal children. However, there were no significant differences between LD and control children in Level 3 speech, nor did the LD children show more task-irrelevant (Level 1) speech. When the LD/ADHD children were separated and contrasted with the other two groups (pure LD and control), the results showed that the ADHD group displayed more than 3 times as much task-relevant, externalized (Level 2) speech as did the pure LD group and about 4 times as much as the control children. The ADHD children also demonstrated significantly less Level 3 speech, the most mature stage of internalization measured in this study, than did the pure LD or control children. Such significant group differences despite low statistical power in the ADHD subgroup suggest that this finding of delayed speech is rather robust. These findings also suggest that ADHD more than LD contributes to a delay in the internalization of speech, which is quite consistent with the findings of Berk and Potts (1991).

In a more recent and smaller study, Landau et al. (1996) compared the self-speech of impulsive and nonimpulsive children during their performance of math problems. These children were not clinically diagnosed as ADHD, but were 55 regular school students in first through third grade who were rated as either most or least impulsive by their teachers. Impulsive children were found to be significantly more dependent on externalized private speech for problem solving at their instructional level in math than were the nonimpulsive children. However, as the level of difficulty of the problems rose to becoming very challenging, the private speech of nonimpulsive children increased, as predicted by Vygotsky (1978) and shown in other research (Berk, 1992), while it decreased for impulsive children. In general, impulsive children used more task-irrelevant and less mature speech as the math problems became more challenging, while the nonimpulsive children did not use task-irrelevant speech at any level of difficulty and increased their task-relevant speech as problem difficulty increased. The results were interpreted as reflecting a more adaptive use of private speech by the nonimpulsive children. All of these studies provide considerable support for the prediction of the hybrid model that impulsiveness is associated with a greater delay in the internalization of speech as well as for the prediction that such internalization would be delayed in children with ADHD.

Delays in Rule-Governed Behavior in ADHD

The internalization of speech assists with the child's capacity to follow through on rules, instructions, and commands. Its delay in those with ADHD should therefore be manifest in a delay in the ability to comply with or complete such verbal instructions. ADHD children have been observed to be less compliant with directions and commands given by their mothers than are normal children (see Danforth, Barkley, & Stokes, 1991, for a review). ADHD children also appear to be less able to restrict their behavior in accordance with experimenter instructions during laboratory playroom observations where rewarding activities are available, although this finding is not consistently observed, however (see Luk, 1985, for a review). Some studies (noted in Chapter 4) have found ADHD children to be much less able to resist forbidden temptations than same-age normal peers. Such rule-following seems to be particularly difficult for ADHD children when the rules compete with rewards available for committing rule violations (Hinshaw, Heller, & McHale, 1992; Hinshaw, Simmel, & Heller, 1995). These results might indicate problems with the manner in which rules and instructions control behavior in children with ADHD.

Further evidence consistent with a developmental delay in rule-governed behavior comes from studies showing that ADHD children are less adequate than normal children at problem solving (Douglas, 1983; Hamlett et al., 1987; Tant & Douglas, 1982), and are also less likely to use organizational rules and strategies in their performance of memory tasks (August, 1987; Butterbaugh et al., 1989; Douglas & Benezra, 1990; Voelker et al., 1989). Problem solving and the discovery of strategies may be a direct function of rule-governed behavior and the self-questioning associated with it (Cerutti, 1989).

Hayes (1989) set forth a number of features that would characterize rule-governed behavior, as noted in Chapter 7. These features underlie my predictions about the types of deficiencies that might be evident in children with ADHD (Chapter 9). Some evidence does exist for these predicted deficiencies, in that ADHD children (1) demonstrate significantly greater variability in patterns of responding to laboratory tasks, such as those involving reaction time or CPTs (see Corkum & Siegel, 1993; Douglas, 1983; and Douglas & Peters, 1978, for reviews; van der Meere & Sergeant, 1988b, 1988c; Zahn et al., 1991); (2) perform better under conditions of immediate versus delayed rewards; (3) have significantly greater problems with task performance when delays are imposed within the task and as these delays increase in duration; (4) display a greater and more rapid decline in task performance as contingencies of reinforcement move from being continuous to intermittent; (5) show a greater disruption in task performance when noncontingent consequences occur during the task (see Barkley, 1989; Douglas, 1983; Haenlein & Caul, 1987; and Sagvolden, Wultz, Moser, Moser, & Morkrid, 1989, for reviews; also Douglas & Parry, 1994; Freibergs & Douglas, 1969; Parry & Douglas, 1983; Schweitzer & Sulzer-Azaroff, 1995; Sonuga-Barke, Taylor, & Heppinstall, 1992; Sonuga-Barke, Taylor, Sembi, & Smith, 1992; Zahn et al., 1991); and (6) are less able to work for delayed rewards in delay-of-gratification tasks (Rapport, Donnelly, Zametkin, & Carrougher, 1986).

However, as discussed later (in the section on self-regulation of affect/motivation/arousal), other researchers have not found evidence for item 4, that partial reinforcement schedules are necessarily detrimental to the task performances of ADHD children relative to their performance under continuous reinforcement. Instead, the schedule of reinforcement appears to interact with task difficulty in determining the effect of reinforcement on performance by ADHD children (Barber & Milich, 1989). It is also possible that differences in the delay periods between reinforcement contribute to these inconsistent findings; if delay intervals are sufficiently brief, no differences between ADHD and normal children under partial reinforcement should be noted. Thus, studies of reinforcement schedules and children with ADHD cannot be interpreted in a straightforward fashion as supportive of the view that poor rule-governed behavior underlies any problem ADHD children may have with partial reinforcement schedules. Barber, Milich, and Welsh (1996) have recently suggested that an inability to sustain effort over time may better explain these findings. Poor self-regulation of motivation may play a large role in these results.

The combination of deficits predicted to exist in both working memory and internalized speech also led to the prediction in Chapter 9 that children with ADHD would have difficulties with commands or instructions that included a reference to a delayed performance of a behavior. The prolongation of reference into the future afforded individuals by their working memory permits them to obey instructions in which the performance is delayed until a later time. This led me to predict in Chapter 9 that children with ADHD would have more difficulty complying with instructions involving such prolonged references to future behavioral performances; the further into the future the performance is delayed or prolonged, the more difficult it would prove to be for them relative to those not having ADHD. I could locate no research on ADHD that has investigated this issue, but the studies reviewed earlier regarding deficits in both working memory and rule-governed behavior would imply that such research on delayed behavioral performance would be fruitful.

Several prior investigators (Hayes et al., 1996; Kopp, 1982) have made the case that rule-governed behavior (internalized speech) along with working memory give rise to moral reasoning and the moral regulation of behavior. If this is so, then those with ADHD should be more likely to have delays in moral development and in the moral regulation of their behavior, given the impairments hypothesized to exist in both of these executive functions. Consistent with this prediction, moral reasoning has been shown to be less well developed in hyperactive–impulsive children or those with ADHD (Hinshaw et al., 1993; Nucci & Herman, 1982). Delays in moral development, especially if characterized by hedonistic moral reasoning, also have been found to be significantly predictive of disruptive and aggressive classroom behavior, diminished social competencies, and, consequently, diminished social status (Bear & Rys, 1994). That these findings stem from deficient internalization of speech cannot be determined from these studies.

Deficits in Reading Comprehension

I suggested in Chapter 7 that internalized speech, probably in concert with the retrospective and prospective functions of nonverbal working memory, contributes to reading comprehension. Therefore, those with ADHD were predicted to be less effective in reading comprehension. I could locate only two studies of ADHD children specifically focusing on reading comprehension. Cherkes-Julkowski and Stolzenberg (1991) found ADHD children to be significantly poorer in reading comprehension than other control groups of children, including those with learning disabilities. This problem with comprehension increased as passage length increased, as would be expected if working memory deficits were contributing to it. In a more recent study, Brock and Knapp (1996) compared 21 children with ADHD to 21 carefully matched control children on measures of reading comprehension. Care was taken to control for the effects of other reading abilities that might contribute to poor reading comprehension yet that were not executive in nature, as I have defined the term. These other abilities were word identification, word attack skills, reading speed, vocabulary, and background knowledge. Results indicated that the ADHD children were significantly poorer in their reading comprehension than were the control children. Both of these studies are consistent with the predictions from the hybrid model and suggest that the comprehension deficit is not the result of learning disabilities or differences in other, nonexecutive abilities that are important for reading. Even so, the link between the comprehension deficit and working memory deficits predicted by the model to exist would be more convincing had these studies also used measures of verbal and nonverbal working memory. Nevertheless, other researchers have shown a link between comprehension and working memory (Hulme & Roodenrys, 1995; Swanson & Berninger, 1995; Wadsworth et al., 1995).

EVIDENCE FOR DEFICITS IN SELF-REGULATION OF AFFECT/MOTIVATION/AROUSAL

The hybrid model makes the following predictions about those who have deficiencies in inhibition. They should show (1) greater emotional reactivity to emotionally charged immediate events; (2) less anticipatory emotional reactions to future emotionally charged events (in view of the decreased capacity for forethought); (3) decreased ability to act with the impact of their emotions on others in mind; (4) less capacity to induce and regulate emotional, drive or motivational, and arousal states in the service of goal-directed behavior (the further away in time the goal, the greater the incapacity to sustain the arousal and motivation toward the goal), with the corollary characteristic of (5) a greater dependence within the immediate context upon external sources affecting motivation and arousal in determining the degree of persistence of effort in goal-directed actions. In other words, those with ADHD should be found to apply less effort in circumstances that require self-regulation and goal-directed behavior, particularly in the absence of external rewards for doing so. Their effort should be found to be more erratic or variable given that their motivation is more contingency-shaped than internally guided or rule-governed.

Affect

Only a few of these predictions have been examined in research. The development of inhibition has been shown to be important for developing self-regulation of emotion and motivation (see Garber & Dodge, 1991; Kopp, 1989; Mischel et al., 1989, for reviews). Preschool children's emotional responses to disappointment also have been shown to be related to self-regulation and disruptive behavior patterns (Cole et al., 1994). Similarly, children's emotional intensity and negative emotion have been related to teacher ratings of resistance to distraction, or interference control (Eisenberg et al., 1993). Shoda et al. (1990) found significant associations between inhibition in a resistance-to-temptation task in children's preschool years and parent ratings of the same children's emotional control and frustration tolerance at adolescence.

The foregoing research implies some linkage between behavioral inhibition and emotional/motivational self-regulation. Therefore, the delay in behavioral inhibition in those with ADHD should be associated with less affective and motivational self-control. Irritability, hostility, excitability, and a general emotional hyperresponsiveness toward others have been frequently described in the clinical literature on ADHD (see Barkley, 1990; Still, 1902). Douglas (1983, 1988) anecdotally observed and later objectively documented the tendency of ADHD children to become overaroused and excitable in response to rewards and to be more visibly frustrated when past rates of reinforcement declined (Douglas & Parry, 1994; Wigal et al., 1993). Rosenbaum and Baker (1984) also reported finding greater negative affect expressed by ADHD children during a concept learning task involving noncontingent negative feedback. Cole et al. (1994) found that levels of negative affect were significantly and positively correlated with symptoms of and risk for ADHD, but only in boys. The opposite proved true for girls.

These studies intimate that emotional self-control may be problematic for children with ADHD. However, ADHD children may experience a greater number of failures on such tasks because of their other cognitive deficits (working memory) or comorbid learning disabilities, which could lead to greater frustration and other negative emotional reactions. Future studies must, therefore, take care to equate the levels of success between ADHD and normal children before concluding that ADHD children are more emotional during their performance on learning tasks.

Greater emotional reactivity has been reported as well in the social interactions of ADHD children. Mash (personal communication, February 1993) found that children with ADHD displayed greater emotional intonation in their verbal interactions with their mothers. Studies of peer interactions have also found ADHD children to be more negative and emotional in their social communications with peers (Hinshaw & Melnick, 1995). This greater level of expressed negative emotion in children with ADHD is most salient in that subgroup that has high levels of comorbid aggression (Hinshaw & Melnick, 1995). Consistent with such findings, Keltner, Moffitt, and Stouthamer-Loeber (1995) recorded the facial expressions of adolescent boys during a structured social interaction. Four groups of boys were created: one was rated as having high levels of externalizing symptoms (hyperactive–impulsive–inattentive–aggressive behavior); a second comprised boys rated as having more internalizing symptoms (anxiety, depression, etc.); a third group consisted of boys having elevations on ratings of both types of symptoms; and the fourth group comprised nondisordered adolescent boys. Boys showing high levels of externalizing symptoms were found to demonstrate significantly more facial expressions of anger than the other groups, who were low in externalizing symptoms. These results suggest the possibility that the commonly noted association of ADHD with defiant and hostile behavior (see Barkley, 1990, and Hinshaw, 1987, for reviews) may, at least in part, stem from a deficiency in emotional self-regulation in those with ADHD. Again, however, these findings are merely suggestive rather than confirmatory of a link between ADHD and emotional self-regulation and tend to imply that the poorest emotion modulation may be within the aggressive subgroup of ADHD children.

The hybrid model of executive functions extended to ADHD also would predict that the perception or recognition of others' emotions would not be affected by ADHD, as such recognition is typically nonexecutive in nature. The only study of this issue of which I am aware supports this view (Shapiro et al., 1993); children with ADHD were not observed to be significantly different in their processing of emotional information compared to normal children, except on two auditory tests that appeared to make demands on auditory–verbal working memory. However, caution must be exercised in interpreting these results, given that many possible explanations exist for a failure to reject a null hypothesis.

Motivation

As for ADHD being associated with less drive, motivation, or effort in the performance of goal-directed behaviors, researchers have frequently commented on such difficulties in tasks requiring repetitive responding that involve little or no reinforcement (Barber et al., 1996; Barkley, 1990; Douglas, 1972, 1983, 1989). Written productivity in arithmetic tasks, in particular, may be taken as a measure of persistence; those with ADHD have been found to be less productive on such tasks than control children (Barkley, DuPaul, & McMurray, 1990). Multiple studies also have documented an impairment in persistence of effort in laboratory tasks with ADHD children (August, 1987; Barber et al., 1996; Borcherding et al., 1988; Douglas & Benezra, 1990; Milich, in press; Ott & Lyman, 1993; van der Meere et al., 1995; Wilkison, Kircher, McMahon, & Sloane, 1995). Thus, the evidence for difficulties in the self-regulation of motivation (particularly persistence of effort) in ADHD is fairly impressive.

It is possible that this component of the model (self-regulation of motivation) provides an explanation for the apparent insensitivity to reinforcement reported in some studies of children with ADHD (see Barkley, 1989; Haenlein & Caul, 1987; and Sagvolden et al., 1989, for reviews). Studies using varying schedules of reinforcement typically find that ADHD and normal children do not differ in their task performances under immediate and continuous reward (Barber et al., 1996; Cunningham & Knights, 1978; Douglas & Parry, 1983, 1994; Parry & Douglas, 1983), as discussed earlier. In contrast, when partial reinforcement is introduced, the performance of ADHD children may decline relative to that of normal children (Parry & Douglas, 1983; Freibergs & Douglas, 1969). Just as many studies, however, have not found this decline (Barber et al., 1996; Pelham, Milich, & Walker, 1986) or have found that the difficulty of the task moderates the effect (Barber & Milich, 1989). In a similar vein, the performance of ADHD children during relatively tedious tasks involving little or no reward is often enhanced by the addition of reinforcement, yet so is the performance of normal children (Carlson & Alexander, 1993; Iaboni, Douglas, & Baker, 1995; Kupietz, Camp, & Weissman, 1976; Pelham, Milich, & Walker, 1986; Solanto, 1990; van der Meere, Hughes, Borger, & Sallee, 1995). These findings have been interpreted as suggesting that ADHD children have a reduced sensitivity to reinforcement (Haenlein & Caul, 1987) or are dominated by immediate reinforcement (Douglas, 1983; Sagvolden et al., 1989). But the similar enhancement of the performance of normal children by reward in the studies noted has challenged this interpretation (Pelham et al., 1986; Solanto, 1990). Douglas and her colleagues (Iaboni et al., 1995) also did not find the reward dominance effect that she earlier had hypothesized might be associated with ADHD (Douglas, 1983).

The hybrid model of executive functions suggests a more plausible explanation for these results. It focuses upon the observations that the performance of normal children is superior to that of ADHD children under conditions of little or no reward and may be less affected by reductions in schedules of reinforcement, depending upon the task duration and its difficulty level. Normal children may develop the capacity to bridge temporal delays between the elements of behavioral contingencies via the executive functions in the model. Combined with working memory as well as self-directed speech and the rule-governed behavior it permits, self-regulation of motivation may allow normal children not only to retain the goal of their performance in mind and subvocally encourage themselves in their persistence, but also, in so doing, to create the drive necessary for such persistence (Berkowitz, 1982; Mischel et al., 1988). This line of reasoning would suggest that, across development, the behavior of those with ADHD remains more contingency-shaped, that is, under the control of the immediate and external sources of reward, than the behavior of normal children. Therefore, it is not that ADHD children are either less sensitive to reinforcement or, conversely, are dominated by a tendency to seek immediate rewards. They instead have a diminished capacity to bridge delays in reinforcement and permit the persistence of goal-directed acts.

Arousal

Concerning the self-regulation of arousal, there is some evidence suggesting possible problems in the regulation of central and autonomic nervous system arousal to meet task demands in those with ADHD. Multiple reviews of the psychophysiological (Brand & van der Vlugt, 1989; Hastings & Barkley, 1978; Klorman, Salzman, & Borgstedt, 1988; Rosenthal & Allen, 1978; Rothenberger, 1995) and cognitive literatures (Douglas, 1983, 1988) have concluded that

ADHD children show greater variability in central and autonomic arousal patterns, and seem underreactive to stimulation in evoked response paradigms, particularly in the later P300 features of the evoked response, which have been shown to be associated with frontal lobe activation (Klorman, 1992; Klorman, Salzman, & Borgstedt, 1988; Knight et al., 1995). ADHD children have also been shown to display less anticipatory activation on electroencephalogram (EEG), known as the contingent negative variation, or "expectancy" wave (Hastings & Barkley, 1978), in response to impending events within tasks, and to have less recruiting of psychophysiological activity over the frontal regions when necessary for appropriate task performance relative to control groups (Brand & van der Vlugt, 1989; Rothenberger, 1995).

More recently, studies using PET scan as a means of measuring brain activity have also found diminished brain activation in adults as well as in adolescent females with ADHD (Ernst et al., 1995; Zametkin et al., 1990). Results have not been as reliably obtained with adolescent males (Zametkin et al., 1993). Similarly, studies using cerebral blood flow as a means of measuring brain activity have found decreased perfusion of the frontal regions and striatum in those with ADHD (Lou et al., 1984, 1989; Sieg et al., 1995).

Hypothesized deficits in nonverbal working memory (hindsight and forethought) in conjunction with those in self-regulated affect and motivation were predicted to create less anticipatory affect and motivation ahead of the arrival of future events in those with ADHD. The farther in the future the event, the less it would result in such anticipatory affect/motivation relative to the decrement expected in normal children. I could locate no research that has examined this prediction of the model.

To summarize, it seems that the evidence available to date is certainly suggestive of problems in the regulation of arousal or activation in those with ADHD. Much of this evidence implicates frontal lobe underactivity, particularly underreactivity to events.

EVIDENCE FOR DEFICITS IN RECONSTITUTION

Within the domain of verbal behavior, tests of verbal fluency, confrontational story narratives or writing, joint peer communication tasks, or other situations and tasks that demand the accurate and efficient communication of information should reflect the process of reconstitution. It should also be evident in similar nonverbal tasks, such as design fluency, and in problem-solving tasks requiring the generation of complex and novel motor sequences. Goal-directed behavioral flexibility and creativity are believed to reflect the executive function of reconstitution, and might be measured by tasks like the WCST.

The application of the hybrid model to ADHD in Chapter 9 predicts that those with ADHD should manifest greater difficulties with tasks and settings, in which reconstitution is essential. There is evidence suggestive of just such deficiencies within the domain of verbal behavior and discourse. Children with ADHD have been noted to perform more poorly on tests of simple verbal fluency (Carte et al., 1996; Grodzinsky & Diamond, 1992; Reader et al., 1994), although others have not documented such differences (Fischer et al., 1990; Loge, Staton, & Beatty, 1990; McGee et al., 1989; Weyandt & Willis, 1994). The discrepancy in findings may pertain, in part, to the type of fluency test used. Tests in which subjects generate words within semantic categories (Weyandt & Willis, 1994), such as names for animals or fruits, are easier and therefore not as likely to discriminate ADHD and control children as those using more subtle organizing cues, such as letters (Grodzinsky & Diamond, 1992; Reader et al., 1994). Age may also be a factor, given that older ADHD children may have far fewer difficulties on such simple fluency tests than younger ADHD children (Fischer et al., 1990; Grodzinsky & Diamond, 1992). Low statistical power and the use of nonclinical samples (Loge et al., 1990; McGee et al., 1989) could also contribute to failures to find differences between ADHD and control groups in these studies. It appears, then, that simple word fluency, particularly on tasks using letters as the generative rule, may be diminished in young children with ADHD, although the finding is not always evident in research. This deficit may dissipate with age, but this does not necessarily mean that a problem with reconstitution or behavioral diversity is dissipating. Recall my point at the beginning of this chapter that ADHD constitutes a relative delay in terms of the design of assessment measures. At some point in development even ADHD children will eventually master this simple fluency task, while more complex forms of fluency or reconstitution may now become deficient, as normal children move on to master such higher-order fluency tasks.

Illustrating this point are studies of more complex language fluency and discourse organization, which have been much more likely than other measures to reveal problems in this domain in children with ADHD. ADHD children appear to produce less speech in response to confrontational questioning than do normal children (Tannock, 1996; Ludlow, Rapoport, Brown, & Mikkelson, 1979), are less competent in verbal problem-solving tasks (Douglas, 1983; Hamlett et al., 1987), and are less capable of communicating task-essential information to peers in cooperative tasks (Whalen, Henker, Collins, McAuliffe, & Vaux, 1979). They also produce less information and less organized information in their story narratives (Tannock, 1996; Tannock, Purvis, & Schachar, 1992; Zentall, 1988) or in describing the strategies they used during task performance (Hamlett et al., 1987). Where no goal or task is specified, the verbal discourse of ADHD children does not appear to differ from that of normal children (Barkley, Cunningham, & Karlsson, 1983; Zentall, 1988). Studies of nonverbal motor or gestural fluency and behavioral simulation in children with ADHD, however, could not be located, so the predictions of the model for this domain of reconstitution remain untested.

The behavioral flexibility thought to arise from reconstitution may be reflected in certain scores from the WCST. A large number of studies have used the WCST with samples of ADHD children; these were mentioned in Chapter 4 as possibly indicating problems with aspects of response inhibition (cessation of ongoing responses) in ADHD. However, the WCST requires several of the executive functions contained in the model, as the factor analytic and neuroimaging studies reviewed in Chapter 6 indicate. Both working memory and response flexibility (reconstitution) were requirements of this task. Therefore, the WCST will be reviewed here for evidence of deficits in response flexibility in those with ADHD.

In Chapter 4, I discussed a total of 21 studies that used the WCST with subjects having ADHD. Using studies based on children and adolescents, a tally finds that 13 of them showed ADHD subjects to be deficient in their performance of the WCST. The score most often found to be deficient was perseverative errors, while the score for number of categories achieved correctly was also occasionally found to be deficient. Three more studies of adults with ADHD exist that used the WCST; they did not find group differences on this measure.

Perseverative responding on the WCST may reflect the capacity to use rules to govern behavior and to inhibit automatic forms of behavior when new rules become operative. The score of number of categories correctly achieved, however, may be more reflective of concept formation or the capacity to derive rules from relatively ambiguous information about performance. This distinction among the processes assessed by these scores was evident in some of the factor-analytic studies reviewed in Chapter 6. If this distinction is correct, the weight of the evidence from the WCST supports a problem primarily with rule following and inhibition of automatic responding (perseverative responding) in ADHD. Less consistent though still evident in some studies is difficulty with rule formulation or concept formation given feedback about errors. Consequently, these findings seem to support the predictions of the hybrid model that problems with verbal working memory (poor rule governance) and the inhibition of prepotent responses are most associated with ADHD. There is weaker evidence of problems with reconstitution (rule formulation and flexibility).

A recent study by Greve et al. (1996) attempted to disentangle this issue by using a test similar to the WCST, known as the California Card Sorting Test (CCST) with ADHD and control children. Although subjects must sort cards based upon rules, the test involves three different forms of administration. One includes telling the subject the rule to be used for sorting (Cued Sort), another includes the examiner sorting the cards but the child stating the rule from the sorting pattern (Structured Sort), and the third involves the subject both sorting the cards and stating the rule he or she is using (Free Sort). It was hypothesized that if ADHD children have problems with concept formation, they will have difficulties with Free Sort and Structured Sort, both of which require the child to identify or formulate the rule that is in effect. They will have no difficulty on Cued Sort because they have been explicitly told the rule to use for sorting. Conversely, if ADHD children have difficulty with rule-governed behavior (the control of the rule over motor responding), then deficits will be apparent in Cued Sort as well as the other sorting routines. In the other two sort procedures, however, they will be able to accurately describe the rule in use when they are correctly sorting. Their errors, then, in the latter two sorts are evidence of poor rule execution, not rule formulation.

The results of the CCST indicated that ADHD children differed on scores that implied a problem with rule execution. Applied to the WCST, this might indicate that the poor scores of ADHD children in the number of correct categories achieved do not occur because they cannot formulate the new sorting rule so much as that they cannot adhere to it in response execution. However, because of the relatively small sample sizes (24 ADHD and 39 control subjects), the statistical power of this study may be limited. The failure to find group differences may not necessarily be interpreted as a failure to find evidence of poor concept formation in children with ADHD. Still, the results are intriguing and are worthy of replication with larger sample sizes.

The evidence for a deficit in behavioral or verbal creativity (flexibility and originality), as opposed to simple fluency (total number of responses generated), in ADHD is considerably weaker, primarily because there are so few studies examining the issue, as well as problems in the very definition of creativity itself (Boden, 1994; R. T.

Brown, 1989; Sternberg & Lubart, 1996). Creativity during free play (Alessandri, 1992) and performance of nonverbal, figural creativity tasks (Funk, Chessare, Weaver, & Exley, 1993) have been noted to be significantly below normal in children with ADHD. However, Shaw and Brown (1990) did not find a deficit in creativity in a small sample of high-IQ ADHD children. However, these children gathered and used more diverse, nonverbal, and poorly focused information and displayed higher figural creativity. Using so small a sample and only bright ADHD children, however, hardly poses a reasonable test of the prediction. More research on creativity in ADHD is clearly needed.

EVIDENCE FOR DEFICITS IN MOTOR CONTROL/FLUENCY/SYNTAX

Inhibition and the executive functions described in the hybrid model contribute greater control, timing, persistence, flexibility, novelty, complexity, and syntax to goal-directed motor actions (Fuster, 1989, 1995). These effects may assist with the development of ever finer, more varied and complex, and hierarchically organized patterns of motor responses directed toward goals. Some evidence exists for a linkage of behavioral inhibition to this type of motor control. Within samples of normal children, deficiencies in inhibition have been associated with delays in both motor control and gestural fluency (Schonfeld, Shaffer, & Barmack, 1989). In the research literature on ADHD, motor problems also have been noted (Barkley, DuPaul, & McMurray, 1990; Douglas, 1972; Hartsough & Lambert, 1985; Stewart, Pitts, Craig, & Dieruf, 1966; Szatmari, Offord, & Boyle, 1989); but rarely discussed for their theoretical implications, except, perhaps by Denckla (1985). Neurological examinations for "soft" signs related to motor coordination and motor overflow movements find ADHD children to demonstrate more such signs and movements than control children, including those with purely learning disabilities (Carte et al., 1996; Denckla & Rudel, 1978; Denckla, Rudel, Chapman, & Krieger, 1985; McMahon & Greenberg, 1977; Shaywitz & Shaywitz, 1984; Werry et al., 1972). These overflow movements have been interpreted as indicators of delayed development of motor inhibition (Denckla et al., 1985).

Studies using tests of fine motor coordination, such as balance, fine motor gestures, electronic or paper-and-pencil mazes, and pursuit tracking often find children with ADHD to be less coordinated in these actions (Hoy, Weiss, Minde, & Cohen, 1978; Mariani & Barkley, 1997; McMahon & Greenberg, 1977; Moffitt, 1990; Shaywitz & Shaywitz, 1984; Ullman et al., 1978). Simple motor speed, as measured by finger-tapping rate or grooved pegboard tests, does not seem to be as affected in ADHD as is the execution of complex, coordinated sequences of motor movements (Barkley, Murphy, & Kwasnik, 1996b; Breen, 1989; Grodzinsky & Diamond, 1992; Mariani & Barkley, 1997; Seidman, Biederman, et al., 1995; Seidman et al., 1996). The bulk of the available evidence, therefore, supports the existence of deficits in motor control, particularly when motor sequences must be performed, in those with ADHD.

But the most rigorous and compelling body of evidence for a motor control deficit in ADHD comes from the substantial programmatic research of Sergeant, van der Meere, and colleagues in Holland (Sergeant & van der Meere, 1990). Employing an information-processing paradigm, these studies have isolated the cognitive deficit in those with ADHD to the motor control stage rather than to an attentional or information-processing stage. More specifically, their research suggests that the deficit is not at the response choice stage but at the motor presetting stage involved in motor preparedness to act (Oosterlaan & Sergeant, 1995; van der Meere et al., 1996). There appears to be both a greater sluggishness and greater variability in motor preparation. Fuster (1989) identified this type of motor preparedness, or anticipatory set, as one of the major effects that the executive functions would have on motor control. But he also identified a sensitivity to errors or response feedback as a second influence of the executive functions on the motor control system. Deficits in behavioral inhibition should lead to an insensitivity to errors and to a loss of behavioral flexibility as a consequence (Fuster, 1995; Knight et al., 1995; Milner, 1995), and, indeed, research has identified such an insensitivity in children with ADHD (Oosterlaan & Sergeant, 1995; Sergeant & van der Meere, 1988).

Complex motor sequencing and generating complex, novel motor responses as well as their syntax have not received much attention in research on ADHD. Handwriting, however, is just such a complex sequencing of simpler motor movements built into complex, novel patterns of new arrangements of letters, words, and sentences requiring great flexibility and fluency of fine motor movement. Handwriting has often been noted in the clinical literature to be less mature in those with ADHD (Sleator & Pelham, 1986). Difficulties with drawing have likewise been found in children with ADHD (Hoy et al., 1978; McGee et al., 1992). Speech certainly represents the ability to assemble complex fine motor sequences so as to articulate language. Those with ADHD have been found to be more likely to have speech problems relative to control groups (Barkley, DuPaul, & McMurray, 1990; Hartsough & Lambert, 1985; Munir, Biederman, & Knee, 1987;

Szatmari et al., 1989; Taylor et al., 1991). All of this might imply problems with the programming and rapid execution of complex, fine motor sequences in those with ADHD.

One test that seems to capture a simpler form of motor sequencing is the Hand Movements Test from the Kaufman Assessment Battery for Children (Kaufman & Kaufman, 1983). Patients with frontal lobe injuries have difficulties with such tasks (Kesner, Hopkins, & Fineman, 1994). Three studies have used this task with ADHD subjects, and all found the ADHD group to be significantly less proficient (Breen, 1989; Grodzinsky & Diamond, 1992; Mariani & Barkley, 1997), suggesting a problem with temporal ordering of motor sequences (Kesner et al., 1994). The developers of the test battery also commented that hyperactive children performed poorly on this task during the clinical validation trials of the battery (Kaufman & Kaufman, 1983). This could reflect simply a problem with the working memory demands of the task, as discussed earlier. However, some of the preceding research involved motor tasks with little or no working memory demands and still found motor control deficits in ADHD, implying that deficient performance on this task may involve both working memory and motor sequences problems in those with ADHD.

ADHD AND INTELLIGENCE (IQ)

At the end of Chapter 6, I presented evidence that the executive functions are not simply masquerading as general cognitive ability, or IQ, under another name. There I showed that the executive functions are dissociable from IQ. But this does not mean that the former have no relationship to or effects upon the latter. The inhibitory processes and the executive functions linked to them in the hybrid model could be expected to result in a small but significant relationship between ADHD and IQ, particularly for measures of more crystallized intelligence. The relationship may be more evident with verbal IQ, given the loading of verbal working memory tests such as Digit Span and Arithmetic on this component of IQ tests. The association of ADHD with IQ would likely be even stronger were IQ to be assessed more by measures thought to reflect fluid rather than crystallized forms of intelligence, given that the former are thought to make heavier demands on executive functioning (Duncan et al., 1995).

Studies using both normal samples (Halverson & Waldrop, 1976; Hinshaw, Morrison, Carte, & Cornsweet, 1987; McGee, Williams, & Silva, 1984) and behavior problem samples (Sonuga-Barke, Lamparelli, et al., 1994) have found significant negative associations between degree both of rated and observed hyperactive–impulsive behavior and of measures of intelligence. Likewise, the degree of difficulty in inhibiting motor responses has been observed to be significantly associated with IQ (Maccoby, Dowley, Hagen, & Degerman, 1965; Olson, Bates, & Bayles, 1990; Welsh & Pennington, 1988). Measures of omission and commission errors on CPTs, often found to distinguish ADHD and control children, are also significantly associated with IQ tests (Aylward, Verhulst, Bell, & Gordon, 1996a, 1996b; Krener et al., 1993), particularly those subtests presumed to reflect verbal working memory (Aylward et al., 1996a, 1996b; Rasile, Burg, Burright, & Donovik, 1995). The scores from the WCST most often found to distinguish ADHD and control groups (number of correct categories and perseverative responding and errors) have moderate and significant correlations (.35 to .48) with measures of intelligence (Riccio, Hall, Morgan, Hynd, & Gonzalez, 1994). All of this suggests that degree of ADHD symptoms, impairment in behavioral inhibition, and other executive functions hypothesized to be dependent on inhibition have small-to-moderate yet significant relationships to IQ.

In contrast, associations between ratings of conduct problems and intelligence in children are often much smaller or even nonsignificant, particularly when hyperactive–impulsive behavior is partialed out of the relationship (Hinshaw et al., 1987; Lynam, Moffitt, & Stouthamer-Loeber, 1993; Sonuga-Barke, Lamparelli, et al., 1994). This implies that the relationship between IQ and disruptive behavior in children is relatively specific to the hyperactive–impulsive element of the disruptive behavior disorders (see Hinshaw, 1992, for a review).

In keeping with the findings that ADHD and IQ have a low but significant association, studies have found that when samples of hyperactive or ADHD children are selected for study without specifically equating groups for IQ, the hyperactive or ADHD children are often found to differ significantly from control groups in their intelligence, particularly verbal intelligence (Barkley, Karlsson, & Pollard, 1985; Mariani & Barkley, 1997; McGee et al., 1992; Moffitt, 1990; Stewart et al., 1966; Werry et al., 1987). Differences in IQ have also been found between hyperactive boys and their normal siblings (Halperin & Gittelman, 1982; Tarver-Behring, Barkley, & Karlsson, 1985; Welner et al., 1977). All of this suggests that hyperactive–impulsive behavior generally, and ADHD specifically, has an inherent association with diminished IQ, particularly verbal IQ (Halperin & Gittelman, 1982; Hinshaw, 1992; McGee et al., 1992; Sonuga-Barke, Lamparelli, et al., 1994; Werry et al., 1987). This small but significant relationship implies that up to 10% or more of the variance in measures of crystallized IQ may be explained by symptoms of ADHD (hyperactive–impulsive behavior). The amount of variance accounted for by ADHD in tests of fluid IQ is probably even higher.

This relationship raises serious questions about the wisdom of statistically controlling out IQ as a covariate in studies of children with ADHD. Typically when this has been done, differences between children with hyperactive–impulsive behavior or with ADHD and control groups on various cognitive tests are often reduced or are no longer statistically significant. For example, Mariani and I (1997) observed significant differences between preschool ADHD and normal children on measures of verbal memory and some academic readiness skills in a factor-analytic study. When we then controlled for group differences in verbal IQ, these particular differences were no longer significant, although other group differences on motor and nonverbal tasks remained so. Werry et al. (1987) observed a similar loss of their initially significant group differences when doing much the same in their study contrasting ADHD children with other control groups on laboratory measures. They suggested that perhaps the cognitive deficits found in ADHD children simply reflect low intellectual ability. Grskovic et al. (1995) also lost their originally significant group differences on a time estimation task after controlling for IQ. Castellanos et al. (1994) found that an initially significant correlation between size of the caudate and behavior ratings of hyperactive–impulsive behavior in children with ADHD was no longer significant when controlling for IQ.

The repeated findings that ADHD symptoms are significantly related to IQ, in both normal and ADHD samples, challenges the wisdom of controlling for IQ. Such study design probably eliminates some of the differences between groups that are the result of the independent variable of interest, ADHD. It also removes some of differences that are a secondary consequence of the effects of ADHD on the executive functions. In the future, researchers on cognitive deficits associated with ADHD at the very least should report their findings with and without controlling for IQ so that other investigators can decide for themselves how any group differences should be interpreted in light of the association of ADHD with IQ deficits. Certainly, it should no longer be assumed that controlling for IQ automatically enhances the internal validity and rigor of the research, or that investigators who fail to do so are somehow less than rigorous, their findings about ADHD therefore open to doubt. Nor should it be assumed that initially significant group differences that become nonsignificant in the process of controlling for IQ therefore do not really reflect the effects of ADHD on those measures.

STIMULANT MEDICATION EFFECTS ON ADHD AND EXECUTIVE FUNCTIONS

The hybrid model of executive functions placed behavioral inhibition at a pivotal position, essentially arguing that the effectiveness of the other executive functions was conditional upon the functioning of that unit. By involving a deficit in behavioral inhibition, ADHD creates secondary deficits in those executive functions dependent upon it, in turn leading to significant problems with the control of motor behavior by the internally represented information they generate. If this set of conditional relations among components of the model as well as its extension to ADHD is correct, then it would also be predicted that any treatment that could be shown to improve or even ameliorate, if only temporarily, the inhibitory deficits related to this disorder should also result in an improvement or even temporary normalization of the deficiencies in the executive functions as well. There is only one form of treatment of which I am aware that is capable of such an improvement or temporary normalization of the inhibitory deficit in this neuropsychological model, and that is stimulant medication.

It is not necessary to engage in a detailed review of the vast literature on the effects of stimulant medications, such as methylphenidate (Ritalin), *d*-amphetamine (Dexedrine), or pemoline (Cylert), on those having ADHD. This has been done repeatedly by others, and the interested reader should consult those sources (Barkley, 1977; DuPaul & Barkley, 1993; Rapport & Kelly, 1993; Swanson, McBurnett, Christian, & Wigal, 1995). It is sufficient to show here that evidence exists in support of these predictions. Regrettably, despite its vastness, little of the literature on stimulant medication effects on ADHD has employed measures of the executive functions of interest here. However, some evidence is available for medication effects on some of the executive functions.

First, it must be shown that stimulant medications result in improvements in behavioral inhibition in those with ADHD. That requirement is handily met. One of the most common findings in this literature is an improvement in inhibition or impulse control in those with ADHD. The findings of significant improvements as evaluated in parent and teacher ratings of hyperactive–impulsive behavior as well as by direct observations of such behavior are ubiquitous and constitute another "fact in the bag" in the literature on ADHD (Barkley, 1977; Barkley, DuPaul, & McMurray, 1991; Swanson et al., 1995). Likewise, significant improvements as a function of stimulant medication have been found on many of the laboratory tests of inhibition discussed in Chapter 4, including the stop-signal paradigm, go/no-go test, commission errors on CPTs, the MFF Test, and resistance-to-temptation tasks (see Rapport & Kelly, 1993, and Solanto, 1991, for reviews; Hinshaw et al., 1992; Tannock, Schachar, Carr, Chajczyk, & Logan, 1989; Trommer, Hoeppner, & Zecker, 1991).

Given this clear demonstration of stimulant drug effects on response inhibition, are improvements found in the other executive functions as well? As with the ADHD literature generally, that dealing with stimulant medications and ADHD has not tended to employ measures of nonverbal working memory, so this domain of predicted effects remains underinvestigated. Some studies do exist that required children to learn visual stimuli and associate them with classes of such stimuli, which may have placed some demands on visual–spatial working memory. These studies have found positive effects of stimulant medications on such learning tasks (Rapport & Kelly, 1993). However, such tasks do not reflect relatively pure nonverbal working memory tasks, so the prediction of medication effects on this component of working memory remains to be more conclusively supported. Nor have measures of planning such as the TOL, thought to reflect in part nonverbal working memory, been employed in such research.

Only one study seems to have examined the effects of stimulants on time reproductions of those with ADHD (Barkley, Koplowicz, et al., 1997), and it found no significant effects, contrary to this model. However, the sample size was quite small (n = 12), and the subjects were typically evaluated in mid- to late afternoon, giving rise to the possibility that medication effects were well past their peak at the time of testing. Thus, medication effects on the various aspects of nonverbal working memory described in the model require much more research before the predicted improvement in this domain from stimulant medication can be said to have been fairly evaluated.

Some studies have employed measures of verbal working memory, such as mental arithmetic, digit span, and short-term memory for verbal material and have found them to improve with stimulant medication (Barkley et al., 1991; Rapport & Kelly, 1993; Tannock, Ickowitz, & Schachar, 1995). Berk and Potts (1991) also demonstrated a significant improvement in direct observations of self-directed speech (internalization of speech) in children with ADHD after placement on stimulant medication. If compliance with parental requests can be taken as evidence of rule-governed behavior, then studies have repeatedly found such compliance to improve in response to stimulant medication (see Danforth et al., 1991, for a review). Internalized speech and rule-governed behavior were suggested in the model as contributing to moral reasoning and conduct. Stealing, property destruction, and cheating can certainly be considered behavioral indicators of a child's moral conduct. Hinshaw et al. (1992) documented that ADHD children were more likely to engage in stealing and cheating than control subjects, but also found that stimulant medication reduced stealing and destruction of property by children with ADHD. This would imply an improvement from medication in the moral conduct of ADHD children. However, this study also found an increase in cheating by the ADHD children while taking medication, which the authors interpreted as being secondary to a medication-induced increase in investment in the academic tasks the children were required to perform.

The effects of stimulant medications on emotional self-control and motivation have not been well studied. Stimulant medications have been shown to reduce aggressive behavior in ADHD children (Hinshaw, Henker, Whalen, Erhardt, & Dunnington, 1989; Murphy, Pelham, & Lang, 1992). Research examining the capacity of children to persist in applying effort over extended periods of time frequently documents improvements in this aspect of sustained attention or goal-directed persistence (Barkley, 1977; Barkley et al., 1991; Douglas et al., 1995; Humphries, Swanson, Kinsbourne, & Yiu, 1979; Milich, Carlson, Pelham, & Licht, 1991; Wilkison et al., 1995). Such findings imply improvements in the self-regulation of motivation that is necessary for goal-directed persistence, although this cannot be considered conclusive evidence of a shift to internally guided motivation.

Little research exists on the effect of stimulant medication on aspects of reconstitution. However, at least one study examining the issue of rule learning and response flexibility using measures such as the WCST has documented improvements in response to medication treatment in ADHD children (Douglas et al., 1995). To my knowledge, measures of verbal and design fluency have not been employed in stimulant medication studies with ADHD children, so these aspects of reconstitution have not been evaluated. One study examining creativity, however, did not find any significant improvements due to medication (Funk, Chessare, Weaver, & Exley, 1993). The study, however, employed the Torrance Tests of Creativity, which have been criticized as primarily reflecting intelligence (R. T. Brown, 1989). Perhaps a better measure of creativity is one assessing ideational fluency, or the diversity of alternate uses that one can generate for a given object (R. T. Brown, 1989). Using such a test, Solanto and Wender (1989) found an increase in the total number of functional responses generated by their ADHD subjects as a result of stimulant medication. Others have also documented increases in word creativity in children with ADHD when placed on medication (Douglas, Barr, Amin, O'Neill, & Britton, 1986).

Stimulant effects on motor speed and performance are not routinely observed (Barkley, 1977; Rapport & Kelly, 1993). However, effects on more complex motor actions have been documented, including motor sequencing and fine motor coordination (Lerer & Lerer, 1976) and handwriting (Lerer, Lerer, & Artner, 1977). The interaction of inhibition with working memory was argued by Fuster (1989; see Chapter 5, this volume) to result in a sensitivity to errors that would be evident in motor performance. ADHD children, as noted earlier, do demonstrate a greater insensitivity to feedback than normal children. Several studies suggest that this sensitivity to feedback is significantly improved by stimulant medication (Klorman, Brumaghim, Fitzpatrick, & Borgstedt, 1991; Sonneville, Njiokiktjien, & Bos, 1994).

This cursory discussion of the possible effects of stimulant medication on executive functions cannot do justice to the complexities of such research or to the measurement and other methodological issues involved in such investigations. Virtually all of these studies did not intend to investigate this model, so the measures that they employed cannot be interpreted as an unequivocal test of this prediction of the model. Moreover, even if medication effects are found on executive functions, this does not necessarily mean that those effects are secondary to improvements in behavioral inhibition. They could just as easily be direct effects of the medication on those brain substrates that subserve these executive functions, apart from any effects the medications may have on inhibition. What concerns me here is not whether this evidence can provide unequivocal proof for the predictions of the model, for it cannot. My concern is whether the findings of this literature are at all inconsistent with the predictions of this model. To date, among what minimal research has explored stimulant medication effects on executive functions, the existing evidence does not contradict the predictions of the model.

ADHD, REPRODUCTIVE FITNESS, AND LIFE EXPECTANCY

The ultimate utility of the executive functions and the self-regulation they permit is the maximization of net long-term outcomes for the individual—in essence, net long-term self-interest. However, this could be considered "ultimate" only from the standpoint of a psychological analysis. If we step back further to encompass this analysis within the broader domain of biological evolution generally, and human evolution specifically, the ultimate utility function of self-regulation is enhanced survival and, particularly, enhanced reproductive fitness for the individual. Organisms that can hold or represent information in mind, or "on-line," and then act upon and manipulate that information to generate hypothetical futures are, in essence, engaging in a form of covert behavioral simulation of those futures (Bronowski, 1967/1977; Dennett, 1991, 1995; Popper & Eccles, 1977). The power to simulate those futures and the behaviors necessary to attain them permits plans or courses of actions to be tested out hypothetically for their likely outcomes before one is finally chosen to perform. This ability would convey a remarkable evolutionary advantage to an individual or its species, as it would greatly reduce the likelihood of the individual making errors that were harmful or even fatal. Individuals may confront problems they encounter in their environment by trial and error, generating a diversity of responses and testing each one out as they go until one is found that succeeds. This, as Dennett (1995) well described it, is a form of behavioral or conditioning plasticity that is represented by operant conditioning and is analogous to a process of natural selection acting at the level of behavior (Skinner, 1953). As Dennett (1995) further notes:

> Skinnerian conditioning is a fine capacity to have, so long as you are not killed by one of your early errors. A better system involves preselection among all of the possible behaviors or actions, weeding out the truly stupid options before risking them in the harsh world. We human beings are creatures capable of this third refinement, but we are not alone. We may call the beneficiaries of this . . . *Popperian creatures*, since, as Sir Karl Popper once elegantly put it, this design enhancement "permits our hypotheses to die in our stead." Unlike the merely Skinnerian creatures, many of whom survive only because they make lucky first moves, Popperian creatures survive because they're smart enough to make better-than-chance first moves . . . But how is this preselection in Popperian agents to be done? Where is the feedback to come from? It must come from a sort of *inner environment*. . . . (pp. 374–375)

The inner environment, I believe, is achieved by working or representational memory—the power to sense and resense to oneself. Dennett (1995, p. 377) discusses how Popperian creatures may have evolved into *Gregorian creatures* by a further step in the development of this inner environment, the acquisition of inner tools from outer tools, as psychologist Richard Gregory (1987) has described it. Tools are not just the result of intelligence but also endow intelligence, bringing with their use an enhancement in "Potential Intelligence," as Dennett (1995) describes it:

The better designed the tool (the more information embedded in its fabrication), the more Potential Intelligence it confers on its user. And among the pre-eminent tools, Gregory reminds us, are what he calls "mind-tools": *words* [emphasis added]. Words and other mind-tools give a Gregorian creature an inner environment that permits it to construct ever more subtle move-generators and move-testers. Skinnerian creatures ask themselves, "What do I do next?" and haven't a clue how to answer until they have taken some hard knocks. Popperian creatures make a big advance by asking themselves, "What should I think about next?" before they ask themselves, "What should I do next?" Gregorian creatures take a further big step by learning how to think better about what they should think about next—and so forth, a tower of further internal reflections with no fixed or discernible limit. (p. 378)

The development of self-speech and its progressive internalization to covert form provides the preeminent "mind-tools," greatly enhancing the Potential or Kinetic Intelligence of the individual, as Gregory and Dennett have discussed it. This same point was made even earlier by Bronowski (1967/1977), who recognized that internalized speech coupled with working memory and the hindsight and forethought it provides grants the individual tremendous powers not only to simulate environments, but to reconstitute them into new ones and, along with them, to reconstitute new behaviors that will respond to them—behaviors of increasing hierarchical complexity aimed at outcomes ever more distant on the temporal horizon.

Thus, to summarize, the evolution of the power to internally simulate environments and their associated behaviors and outcomes via representational memory and the mind-tools of internal speech affords the individual the power to test out responses before performing one, a significant survival advantage. Further, the greater the power to simulate and preselect, the greater the survival advantage. This line of reasoning, then, would suggest that the executive functions in the hybrid model and the self-regulation toward the future they permit have the ultimate utility function of conveying an enhanced survival and reproductive advantage to individuals and to the species at large. In contrast, *ADHD should be found to reduce the survival and reproductive advantage conveyed by the executive functions and self-regulation when observed to operate over substantial time periods of an evolutionary scale.*

The point is not merely idle, nor is it alarmist chatter. There is increasing evidence, though it is far from definitive, that ADHD may result in a reduced life expectancy (Barkley, 1996), as I will discuss further. There is also an intimation from the results of my ongoing follow-up study that ADHD children who are now adults suffer a

having this set of characteristics lived an average of 8 years less than those who did not (73 vs. 81 years). Given that subjects in this study were defined as impulsive by virtue of falling within the lowest 25% of the sample in impulse control, and that subjects defined as ADHD typically fall in the lowest 5–7% in this regard, the risk for reduced longevity in those with ADHD would seem to be even greater than was found among Terman's subjects. That conclusion would seem to be further supported by the fact that Terman's subjects were intellectually gifted and came from families of above average or higher economic backgrounds. Both of these factors probably would have conveyed a greater advantage toward longer life expectancy than would be the case for intellectually normal ADHD children who tend to come from middle or lower economic backgrounds. Thus, there is some reason to suspect that the implications of this model for reduced reproductive advantage and life expectancy as a function of ADHD are not without some merit, at least as issues deserving of future research.

UNRESOLVED ISSUES

An important issue deserving of research and critical to the model is the extent to which the deficits in inhibition and its associated executive functions are specific to ADHD or result from disorders often coexisting with it, such as aggression (oppositional defiant disorder) and CD or, less often, the learning disabilities. Few of the studies on ADHD cited in this volume attempted to disentangle these effects. Some of the more recent studies did so, however, and their findings suggest that these cognitive disturbances are more closely associated with ADHD than with these other disorders (see Pennington & Ozonoff, 1996, for a review).

Research suggests that impairment in behavioral inhibition is more characteristic of children with ADHD than those with academic underachievement, emotional disturbance CD, or autism (Milich et al., 1994; Pennington & Ozonoff, 1996; Schachar & Logan, 1990; Werry et al., 1987). Likewise, the disturbance in the motor inhibition, presetting, effort, and control stages of information-processing paradigms are specific to children with ADHD and are not seen in normal, anxious, or purely aggressive children (Oosterlaan & Sergeant, 1995). Direct observations of playroom behavior have also shown that problems with impulsive, undercontrolled behavior and adherence to rules to restrict behavior are more characteristic of ADHD than aggressive children (Milich, Loney, & Landau, 1982). These and other studies (Werry et al., 1987) suggest that children with mixed ADHD and conduct problems are likely to have as much or more cognitive impairment than those with ADHD alone. The difficulties with motor control, response perseveration, rule following, and verbal fluency have likewise been shown to associate more with ADHD than purely aggressive behavior (Carte et al., 1996; McBurnett et al., 1993; Seidman, Biederman, et al., 1995; Seidman et al., 1996; Werry et al., 1987). As other reviews have concluded (Hinshaw, 1987; Pennington & Ozonoff, 1996; Taylor et al., 1991; Werry, 1988), ADHD is most closely associated with cognitive impairments, while CD is more aligned with adverse child-rearing variables and social disadvantage.

Similarly, studies employing control groups of reading disabled or more generally learning disabled children have not found such children to demonstrate the inhibitory or executive function deficits characteristic of those with ADHD (Barkley, Grodzinsky, & DuPaul, 1990; Dykman & Ackerman, 1992; Epstein, Shaywitz, Shaywitz, & Woolston, 1992; Pennington & Ozonoff, 1996). Thus, while hardly definitive, what research does exist places the inhibitory, neuropsychological, and motor deficits described here in the domain of ADHD rather than in aggression/conduct problems or learning disabilities. Still unresolved, however, is whether the group having mixed ADHD and conduct problems represents a qualitatively different disorder, as some have suggested (Biederman et al., 1992; Schachar & Logan, 1990), or just a more severe form of the same disorder relative to those having ADHD alone.

There are numerous other unresolved issues related to this hybrid model of executive functions and ADHD that speak to its present limitations and the need for future research on it. These issues include determining (1) the precise strength of the relationship between behavioral inhibition and each of the executive functions; (2) the precise degrees to which each executive function contributes to the motor control module in the model; (3) the extent to which the subfunctions within each component of the model are best placed where they are now; (4) whether there is some hierarchical organization to these four executive functions; (5) whether the number of components of the model can be further reduced (i.e., is self-directed speech the source of verbal working memory, as current research implies? see Becker, 1994); (6) whether all four executive functions represent a larger process of the internalization and self-direction of all human behavior generally, rather than just that of speech (i.e., self-directed seeing, hearing, manipulation, etc.); (7) the neurological and neuropsychological mechanisms that cause behavior to be turned on the self and then slowly privatized; (8) the proper sequence of these executive functions in development; (9) to what degree each executive function and its subfunctions are impaired by the behavioral inhibition deficit in ADHD; (10) the degree to which stimulant medications differentially affect each of these domains of executive functions and motor control in ADHD; (11) whether the predominantly inattentive type of ADHD can be dissociated from the remaining hyperactive–impulsive types on measures of these executive functions; (12) the extent to which socialization affects the development and organization of these executive functions and the means by which it might do so; (13) the potential gender differences that may exist in the development of these executive functions and in their deficiencies in those with ADHD; and (14) whether and to what extent cultural factors influence the universal structure hypothesized here to exist for the executive functions and, if so, the mechanisms by which they do so.

The basic composition of the construct of behavioral inhibition as I have rendered it here is also uncertain. As I noted in Chapters 3 and 5, there is plenty of reason to suspect that the process of interference control is separable from that of inhibiting initial prepotent responses. Interference control, in fact, may be an inherent part of working or representational memory, as Goldman-Rakic (1995a, 1995b) has suggested from her research with primates. Activation of sensory representations during delays appears to simultaneously activate inhibition of competing sources of sensory–motor behavior as an inherent part of the working memory process. Roberts and Pennington (1996) have made a similar argument. If this view is correct, then interference control should be reassigned to the two working memory components of the model (nonverbal and verbal) and probably share top billing with them as critical to these executive functions.

In a similar manner, the process of behavioral inhibition associated with the cessation of ongoing responses, particularly if that cessation is a function of a sensitivity to errors (as may occur on the WCST or other laboratory tasks), may arise as a result of an interaction between the working memory and behavioral inhibition systems, as Fuster (1980, 1989) has suggested. Immediately past patterns of outcomes for responding are temporarily held in working memory and analyzed for information that would then feed forward to affect the presetting of immediately future responses. In so doing, such information may signal an increase in behavioral inhibition if the current pattern of responding is resulting in errors and is projected to be disadvantageous to the individual. If this is so, then the cessation of ongoing responding, like planning, goal-directed persistence, and moral reasoning, is the result of several executive functions acting in concert, not a subfunction of only one.

There is also evidence, reviewed in Chapters 5 and 6, that the function of reconstitution may not be a separate executive function. Instead, it may be a more advanced developmental stage of both nonverbal and verbal working memory. It would seem to be impossible to take apart and recombine information about behavioral contingencies and the responses within them if that information cannot be temporarily held in mind. This would suggest that the satisfactory development of representational memory is a precursor to the development of reconstitution. The latter may even be housed within the former function. The question of the dissociation of reconstitution from the two working memory systems is difficult to answer at the moment, given the contradictory evidence that seems to exist on the matter (Chapter 6). Studies using factor analysis appear to reliably identify a factor related to response fluency and flexibility, which seems to reflect reconstitution as I have rendered it, that is separate from a dimension of behavior reflecting working memory. However, the initial and fairly limited neuroimaging research using neuropsychological measures of these functions have, to date, shown that they occur largely within the same prefrontal regions, chiefly the dorsolateral prefrontal cortex. Within this cortex, reconstitution may well occur in a region separate but adjacent to that of working memory, it may be separable but heavily dependent upon working memory. More research is in order on this issue of the place of reconstitution, as a separate executive function or as an advanced stage of working memory.

CONCLUSION

This chapter has reviewed evidence for executive function deficits in children and adults with ADHD to determine if such deficits are consistent with the hybrid model of executive functions (Chapter 7) and my prediction that it applies to ADHD (Chapter 9). In general, the evidence seems consistent with the predictions of the model about ADHD, although this assertion must be qualified by the limited amount of research on each of the executive functions in those with ADHD. Nor are the findings uniformly consistent within or across the executive functions predicted to be impaired in those with ADHD. Considerable evidence shows ADHD to be associated with impairments in behavioral inhibition (see Chapter 4), the first component of the model. There is also supportive evidence presented here for deficits in working memory, mainly for impairments in verbal working memory and delays in the internalization of speech thought to underlie such working memory. The evidence available pertaining to the predicted deficits in nonverbal working memory is less impressive, primarily because there are very few studies of this area of cognitive functioning in children and adults with ADHD. Within that domain, however, more substantial evidence exists for delays in sense of time and in planning ability, both of which were hypothesized to be dependent on nonverbal working memory. There is some evidence for difficulties with emotional self-control in those with ADHD, particularly as regards persistence of effort or motivation. As with nonverbal working memory, research on reconstitution is quite limited. The extant research does suggest some difficulties with verbal fluency and response flexibility in those with ADHD, although age was clearly a factor in whether or not such findings were significant. Finally, the evidence is reasonably consistent that ADHD is associated with difficulties with motor control and fine motor sequencing abilities.

Regardless of its consistency with the hybrid model, the evidence reviewed here clearly indicates that ADHD is associated with deficits on many measures previously interpreted by others as reflecting executive functioning. Such research seriously undermines the current clinical consensus view that ADHD is primarily a disorder of attention. The next chapter will discuss the implications of the model for the clinical understanding, diagnosis, assessment and treatment of those with ADHD.

CHAPTER 11

———

Understanding ADHD and Self-Control: Social and Clinical Implications

MOST OF THIS BOOK HAS dealt with empirical research, its theoretical implications, and the building of a theory of executive functions and self-regulation that is intended to provide a better understanding not only of self-regulation but of ADHD as well. But this theory holds more than just a different way of scientifically conceptualizing self-control and ADHD, a different means for explaining research findings, or a different perspective that generates myriad testable hypotheses about ADHD for future research. The theory also contains a number of clinical implications as well. Some are rather obvious, such as ADHD being a disorder of inhibition rather than attention; others are not so readily apparent, such as ADHD resulting in a delay in the development of internally governed behavior that is aimed at the future. In this chapter, I discuss what I believe to be the clinical implications of what may be a rather radical shift in the conceptualization of ADHD engendered by the extrapolation of the hybrid model of executive functions to this disorder. I discuss these clinical implications under the domains in which I believe they fall: understanding, diagnosis, assessment, and treatment.

By their very nature, implications are speculations, conjectures from what seems to be known to what the consequences might be. They reduce theory to pragmatics, hypotheses to their likely outcomes for individuals or groups, and empirical findings to their practical cash value for us and society. The material that follows may include some inferential stretches; the radical shift in the viewpoint of ADHD associated with this theory compels me to attempt them. I wish to go beyond the flintiness of dustbowl empiricism, its love of cynicism, and its anathema for inference beyond the first order that are necessities of the scientific enterprise in which I spend most of my professional activities. Here I go to orders of inference that are of the second and third magnitude in many cases. If my flair for the dramatic, with which my friends, colleagues, and editors are well acquainted, has crept in here, then I trust I will be excused its presence, if only for the 25 years of scientific service I have rendered to ADHD to date. Here, in sum, I ask the question, "What does this all mean for understanding and caring for those with ADHD?"

SOCIAL IMPLICATIONS OF UNDERSTANDING ADHD

I began this book by presenting the modern clinical consensus view of ADHD as described in DSM-IV and as traced back through its predecessors. For nearly 30 years, this perspective has held that ADHD (or its earlier aliases) consists of impairments in the areas of excessive motor movement (hyperactivity), poor motor inhibition (impulsivity), and inattention (distractibility with poor sustained attention). For at least the past 18 of these 30 years, pride of place among these three symptoms has gone to inattention as the chief characteristic of this disorder. As I hope this volume has demonstrated by now, this view of ADHD is no longer scientifically defensible. Whether or not one accepts the model of self-regulation and its executive functions developed here as a useful heuristic tool for understanding ADHD, the conclusion is unavoidable that *ADHD is far more a deficit of behavioral inhibition than of attention.* At the very least, then, a term such as Behavioral Inhibition Disorder would better capture the current status of the scientific knowledge about ADHD than does its current name and acronym. Nowhere in this label is an inhibitory deficit emphasized except perchance by one of its earliest developmental manifestations— hyperactivity.

ADHD as a Developmental Delay
in Internalization and Self-Regulation

Beyond the rather mundane conclusion that ADHD is just a deficit in behavioral inhibition are the far-reaching implications for self-regulation. *The disinhibition that so characterizes those with ADHD results in a disruption of the four executive functions that comprise self-regulation.*

Those with ADHD must come to be seen as being less regulated and governed by internally represented information and aspects of time. They also must be seen as more controlled by the moment, its three-dimensional features, and its tantalizing offers of immediate reinforcement. Their behavior will be less directed at maximizing the future and more directed at maximizing the moment. Being less internally guided and rule-governed, their behavior will seem to others as more chaotic, reactive, ill considered, and emotional, and as less organized, purposive, reflective, and objective.

The totality of the deficits associated with ADHD serve to cleave thought from action, knowledge from performance, past and future from the moment, and the dimension of time from the rest of the three-dimensional world more generally. This, as I have said before, means that ADHD is not a disorder of knowing what to do, but of doing what one knows. It produces a disorder of applied intelligence by partially dissociating the crystallized intelligence of prior knowledge, declarative or procedural, from its application in the day-to-day stream of adaptive functioning. ADHD, then, is a disorder of performance more than a disorder of skill; a disability in the "when" and "where" and less in the "how" or "what" of behavior. Those with ADHD often know what they should do or should have done before, but this provides little consolation to them, little influence over their behavior, and often much irritation to others. Such knowledge seems to matter little when they are actually behaving at particular moments. This is more than just that knowledge is out of sight, out of mind; instead, knowledge out of sight, out of mind, and does not matter.

Events predicted to lie in the distant future will elicit planning and anticipatory behaviors in others at a far greater future time horizon than is likely to be seen in those with ADHD, who may not begin to make preparations, if they make any, until the event is far closer in time, is imminent, or even immediately upon them. This is a recipe for a life of chaos and crisis. If those with ADHD are like the first or second of the three little pigs in the children's fable of that name and the rest of us are like the third, their fate is clear even to a kindergart- ner—they deserve the wolf that comes for them. After all, anyone could have foreseen the consequences and could thereby have avoided them. Do those with ADHD actually "deserve what they get" when they fail to attend to the future? Many in society believe so. The caning of the ADHD teenager, Michael Fey, by the Singapore government in 1994 is testament to that point of view, as was the attitude of more than half of all Americans at the time who thought that he deserved what he got and that it would teach him a lesson. Would it? Did it? Apparently not. Fey has returned to the United States and his troubles have continued, owing to impulsive conduct. I will return to this general point later with regard to the issue of holding those with ADHD accountable for the consequences of their actions. For now, it is sufficient to conclude that ADHD greatly constricts the temporal window or time horizon over which those with the disorder consider the consequences of their actions, and it is through no fault of their own that they find themselves in this predicament.

ADHD and the Sources of Behavioral Control

It is not quite correct to say that ADHD represents a loss of control or an undercontrol of behavior. It would be more accurate to say that the nature of the sources of control have shifted as a consequence of having this disorder. The executive functions and the self-control they permit do not free behavior from control by the environment, but merely shift the sources of such control from external to internally represented information, or from outer to self (inner) control. However, this shift is but a means to another end, a move from control by the moment to control by time—the past and the future. Behavior is internalized during child development to anticipate change (time) and to prepare for it, so as to maximize long-term outcomes. This shift from external to internal control, then, represents a change in the control of behavior from that of a three-dimensional world of space within the temporal now to control by a four-dimensional world of space wedded to time, or space–time. The development of self-control, it seems to me, is but the means to this end of shifting the source of behavioral control from space to space–time.

That being the case, ADHD represents a delay in the development of this shift in sources of control. Behavior is more regulated by the immediate context and less by covert executive functions, time, and the future. From this vantage point, the behavior of those with ADHD makes perfect sense once time, or the lack of it, is taken into account in the analysis of their behavior.

ADHD and Human Will

Given the information presented in this volume, I would go so far as to say that *ADHD impairs the human will and one's volition,* as earlier philosophical psychologists (James, 1890/1992) and neurologists (Bastian, 1892) conceived of those terms. I am not the first to reach this conclusion. George Still (1902), the first clinician to describe the disorder, was also the first to make this point when he concluded that these children had a defect in volitional inhibition and in the moral control of behavior. An organism that is less internally guided in its actions is less free in its choice of actions and is less free of momentary influences. It is, consequently, less willful or volitional in its conduct. ADHD greatly narrows the range of options/outcomes available for consideration by those with the disorder and the time frame in which those choices are to be considered. This makes the will less free, one's actions less voluntary, one's choices more limited, and one's time frame or horizon more narrowed as a consequence of having ADHD.

ADHD and Personal Responsibility

I fully appreciate the conundrum such conclusions about ADHD pose for the notion of personal accountability and responsibility within society. The argument here could be used by some to seek a finding of "diminished capacity" in the mental status of those with ADHD, as that capacity was originally conceived to be in common law—the power to consider one's actions in light of past experience and future consequences, to deliberate the outcomes of one's acts relative to time. In a way, those who might seek to make such a case would be correct in this analysis: ADHD does create a diminished capacity to deliberate upon the outcomes of one's actions.

It is clear that ADHD is disrupting the cross-temporal organization of behavior, loosening the binding of past and future consequences to the deliberations on current behavior, and lessening the capacity to bridge delays among the elements of a behavioral contingency. Given this circumstance, I submit that *the required response of others to the poor self-control shown by those with ADHD, then, is not to eliminate the outcomes of their actions and to excuse them from personal accountability. It is to temporally tighten up those consequences, emphasizing more immediate accountability.* Consequences must be made more immediate, increased in their frequency, made more "external" and salient, and provided more consistently than is likely to be the case for the natural consequences associated with one's conduct. More feedback, more often is the resulting conclusion; more accountability and holding to responsibility, not less, are the watchwords in helping those with ADHD. Their problem is not so much in being held accountable for the outcomes of their actions but *the delays in that accountability* that are often inherent in those natural outcomes. The most salient natural outcomes of our behavior are often those that are delayed in time, such as eventually being retained in grade after several years of poor school performance, of being suspended from school after years of repeated misconduct in that environment, and being arrested and jailed for years of impulsive criminal conduct. The provision of more proximal outcomes more often should preclude or minimize the likelihood of these more harmful, socially damaging, yet temporally distal natural outcomes of the conduct of those with ADHD.

ADHD is, therefore, not an excuse but an explanation, not a reason to dismiss outright the ultimate consequences of one's actions but a reason to increase accountability by making it more temporally contiguous with those actions. Time, not consequences, is the problem in life's behavioral contingencies for those with ADHD, so removing time, not removing outcomes, is the solution to their problem of "diminished capacity." It is time and the future that are the nemeses of those with ADHD, not outcomes and personal responsibility. It is through no fault of their own that they find themselves in this temporal dilemma. Thus, society should not absolve those with ADHD of accountability or responsibility for their actions, but it should absolve them of the moral indignation of others that often accompanies this issue.

ADHD, Self-Control, and Society

Leaping farther out into inferential space, let me ponder the meaning of all of this for the rest of us. *ADHD appears to represent the lower end of a continuum of a normal trait or set of traits. That trait certainly comprises behavioral inhibition and the self-regulation associated with it.* In a very real sense, then, ADHD comprises the lower tail of a distribution of self-control in the population. This is much like most forms of mental retardation, which represent the lower end of the continuum of general cognitive ability or intelligence. It is also like most forms of dyslexia, which comprise the lower end of the continuum of reading ability (phonological awareness). Granted, there are cases of more severe ADHD that arise out of pathological processes, just as more severe cases of mental retardation (IQ < 50) or the most severe cases of dyslexia are more likely to be the result of various brain injuries before or after birth. But the point here is that most cases of ADHD reflect the lower end of a dimension of inhibition and self-control. As I discussed in Chapter 2, the dimension of behavior believed to comprise ADHD (e.g., inhibition/self-regulation), along with the disorder of ADHD that rests upon it has a large genetic contribution to it.

So far I do not believe that most behavioral scientists would argue the points that I have just made. The evidence that ADHD reflects the extreme of a dimension has been around for some time. The evidence that this dimension represents behavioral inhibition is very compelling, and the link of inhibition to self-control is rather obvious. Finally, the substantial heritability of the dimension along which ADHD falls is increasingly accepted among behavioral scientists in this field. This

makes the behavioral dimension comprising ADHD (behavioral inhibition) very much a trait, like human height, for instance. But the next
step in this sequence of events may be of substantial social import.
Before discussing the social ramifications, I will propose and examine
the evidence for the next step.

The first part of the next step is the assertion that human
self-regulation is a trait, or at least a set of traits. As I stated in Chapter
8, self-control may be a trait that is as natural and instinctive to
humans as is the instinct for language (Pinker, 1995). The second part
of the step is that individual differences in the trait of behavioral
inhibition, and the set of traits comprising the executive functions
based upon it, appear to be largely due to genetic factors. This may
seem quite an inferential leap, and many of my colleagues would
consider it highly speculative at this stage of scientific discovery, but
I believe this is the direction in which the data are taking us if current
trends in research on ADHD and self-control continue their present
course.

I admit that the evidence for the heritability of some of the
executive functions is lacking at the moment, primarily because, as I
said in Chapter 6, they have not been studied for the contributions
genetics makes to them. But behavioral inhibition (hyperactive–impulsive–inattentive behavior) and working memory (particularly verbal)
have been so studied, and the ratio of genetic to environmental
influences for both is rather lop-sided, favoring heredity at least 3:1.
Moreover, the rationale I gave earlier (Chapter 8) for viewing the
executive functions as largely instinctive would suffice just as well in
support of the idea of viewing differences in them among individuals
as largely genetically determined: They are founded on forms of human
behavior that are just as instinctive, namely, sensing, speech, affect/mo-
tivation/arousal, and play/experimentation.

If one accepts that *human inhibition and self-control are traits and that
individual differences along those traits are largely, though not solely, genetically determined,* the implications for how society views not only ADHD
but also variations in self-control in the normal population are quite
extraordinary, given that this can hardly be considered the view now
held by most people. That view could generally be characterized as the
belief that our capacity for self-control is pretty much self-determined
(no circularity of reasoning intended), that with the exception of the
truly insane we are all pretty much granted an equal amount of this
capacity at birth, and that just how well we may put it to use in
day-to-day functioning reflects in part the proficiency with which our
parents imparted it to us. Self-control from this vantage point is equal
across most individuals in the population, and the extent of its use by

any individual is largely self and socially (parentally) determined. From this perspective, if you fail to use your powers of self-control, others have the right to legally and morally judge you (and, by inference, the quality of your parents' child rearing). I cannot help but point out here the very obvious conflict between the implications of research on ADHD, self-control, and executive functions as discussed in this volume and the general societal view of self-control.

Let us presume for the moment that the implications of this research as I have described them to this point are correct and the societal view is wrong. What would this mean? Well, first it would clearly mean that those who have ADHD largely cannot help behaving in the more impulsive and less self-regulated way that they do. It would mean that differences among individuals in the extent of having symptoms of ADHD are largely the result of genetic factors. Their lack of self-control would have little to do with how proficient at child rearing their parents may have been or how free of sugar and other dietary evils the ADHD child and their family's nutrition had been as well, as I discussed in Chapter 2. As I stated there, the genetic contribution to individual differences in ADHD symptoms is similar to that for human height (about .80, or 80%). Knowing this, we realize that it is absurd to make moral judgments about the worth or character or parents of those who may be somewhat shorter in height than us. But it should also, then, be just as absurd to make moral judgments about the worth, character, or parents of those having more symptoms of ADHD, or less self-control, than us.

This leads to an equally interesting and provocative corollary. If we are not to blame those with ADHD, or those with less self-control, for their self-regulatory failings, then can we give so much credit to those who are extraordinarily well self-controlled and socially well-off as a result? And can we give their parents, by inference, so much credit for the accomplishments of their offspring that stem from such exceptional self-regulation? If the parents of those with ADHD are not to blame for their children's lack of self-control, then the parents of those with exceptional self-control are not so deserving of our adoration. Would not a little more humility about one's successes in life or the successes of one's offspring that are the result of exceptional self-control be a consequence of this perspective?

This state of affairs, reflecting as it may a conflict between the emerging scientific view of ADHD and society's view of self-control, explains much to me. It helps me to understand why the widespread social acceptance of ADHD as a disability has been so difficult to attain and remains the minority view. The public simply finds it hard to accept the fact that such undercontrolled, poorly regulated, and impulsive patterns of behavior are anything but willful misconduct. They find it equally as difficult to accept that it does not arise from a lousy family upbringing and poor diet. This conflict also helps me to appreciate one source for the periodic media firestorms that erupt around the use of stimulant medications for those with ADHD. If the misbehavior of these children is largely self and familially determined, as society seems to believe, then giving a brain-altering medication to these children is not just scandalous, but ethically reprehensible, and any evidence of an increase in such medication use would be equally as scandalous and reprehensible. Yet if the speculations in which I have engaged here about ADHD and self-control are at all accurate, then it is perfectly understandable why medication can and should be used to assist them with their self-regulation and why a historically and relatively transient rise in medication use would be rational, ethical, and humane care.

The conflict between scientific and social views of ADHD and self-control may even help to explain why there is little sympathy or compassion for the families seeking to gain services and accommodations for their ADHD children, and also why compassion is equally lacking for the adults with ADHD who now seek recognition for the disorder in this age group as well. After all, why should accommodations be made for children or adults who are willfully misbehaving, choosing not to regulate their own behavior, and repeatedly making the wrong decisions in life? They deserve what they get out of life, do they not? All of this would suggest that *before society will accept ADHD as a developmental disorder of self-control and admit it into the realm of the other developmental disorders, societal views about self-control will need to change.*

IMPLICATIONS FOR CLINICAL DIAGNOSIS

The new model of ADHD which I have proposed brings with it several implications for the development and utilization of diagnostic criteria for ADHD. One of the most important of these is the clarification that the model provides of the nature of the inattention that exists in the disorder. Because internally represented information and its associated motivational states are not regulating behavior as well as is normal, the power of the ADHD individual to persist toward goals and assigned activities that require such endurance will be deficient. Those with ADHD are not so much inattentive, as the current clinical view has emphasized, but are *impersistent* toward activities that require self-motivation and self-regulation. Their proneness to distraction is now seen to be somewhat limited in scope and more erratic in its likelihood of appearance, owing as it does to their more limited capacity for interference control. The distractibility associated with ADHD should only be evident in situations where protection of the executive functions from interference is critical—situations requiring planning, self-control, and persistence. Where the executive functions and self-control are unnecessary or of limited assistance, distractibility should be less evident and less detrimental. The hyperactivity and inattentiveness demonstrated by those with ADHD can now be seen to be but the most obvious and perhaps more superficial by-products of their disinhibition and delayed self-regulation, by-products better conceptualized as excessive task-irrelevant and contextually reactive activity as well as poor persistence and interference control.

This may explain the rather puzzling nature of the development of symptoms of ADHD, as noted in Chapter 1—the apparently earlier onset of symptoms of hyperactivity and their earlier decline observed across childhood relative to the symptoms of inattention, which appear to arise somewhat later and to persist longer into development. The symptoms of hyperactive–impulsive behavior often found in parent and teacher rating scales (and the DSM-IV) that are used in studies of ADHD are heavily weighted toward hyperactivity. Only a few symptoms of poor inhibition are contained in these instruments. We should not be surprised to find then that this hyperactivity is but an initial manifestation of poor inhibition and self-control, as those would be expressed at young developmental periods. Hyperactivity may decline, but the difficulties with behavioral inhibition will remain and give rise now to deficits in self-regulation as the executive functions that subserve it begin to start their maturational courses by late preschool to early elementary ages.

The delay in these executive functions will no longer appear as exaggerated activity levels but will be manifest as deficiencies in working memory, private speech, rule-governed behavior, and emotional/motivational self-regulation, and even later as deficiencies in problem solving, behavioral flexibility and creativity, sense of time, and the management of one's behavior relative to it. I believe it is those early deficiencies in the executive functions of working memory, rule-governed behavior, and self-motivation, along with the poor interference control ADHD comprises, that now give rise to poor goal-directed persistence, rather than poor sustained attention.

Problems in Diagnosing ADHD across the Life Span

The theoretical model of ADHD developed here suggests that several problems are likely to arise in using the DSM-IV items to diagnose

ADHD across the life span. First, much of the content of the inattention items actually refers to the persistence of goal-directed responding and resistance to distraction (interference control). The items relating to forgetfulness, poor organization, and appearing not to listen to others may well be reflecting the deficits predicted to exist in working memory. Certainly, the capacity for initiating and sustaining motivation and effort toward goal-directed tasks is evident in some of these items as well. Still others reflect rule-governed behavior (follows through on directions) that must await the development of self-directed speech in normal children sufficient to make comparisons with those having ADHD useful. The term inattention, then, is in many ways misleading, as distraction and impersistence have nothing to do with perception of information processing, which are usually associated with attention.

A second problem is that items reflecting poor behavioral inhibition are grossly underrepresented relative to their importance to identifying the disorder. Out of 18 items, only 3 are formally acknowledged to represent impulsivity, as that might be seen beyond the preschool years. Even these are going to prove limited in the age span over which they will be developmentally sensitive to the disorder, given their wording. The substantial scientific evidence on the inhibitory deficits associated with ADHD discussed in Chapter 4, alone, would justify a heavier weighting of the symptom list with items reflecting behavioral inhibition as it is manifest across the life span. That course of action is even further supported by the model of ADHD developed here, wherein behavioral inhibition is proposed to play a central role in the disorder and the poor self-regulation seen in conjunction with it. All of this argues for a greater inclusion of items reflecting poor self-regulation as it may be evident and as it may change across development, rather than weighting the item sets so heavily to inattention and excessive movement.

A third problem is that the hybrid model would predict an increasing insensitivity of the current DSM-IV cutoff scores for the disorder with increasing age of the population to which they are being applied. In Chapter 1, the case was made for viewing ADHD as a developmental disorder and therefore one in need of developmentally referenced criteria. Like mental retardation, ADHD represents a delay in the development of certain cognitive abilities. While the delay may remain relatively constant across development, the manifestations of that delay will change with each new stage of development. Old skills, talents, and demands will eventually be mastered, even by the person suffering such a developmental delay, although often at an age that is later than the age at which most normal individuals have mastered those abilities and the tasks that initially challenged them. But as the normal individual is developing new or more advanced abilities, the individual with the delay will not do so at the same developmental pace or at the same age level as the normal individual. Therefore, the symptom list and cutoff scores on those lists that are useful for one age group will be much less likely to be so for other age groups if those groups fall markedly outside of the "window of developmental delay" formed by the difference between normal individuals and those delayed by the disorder. Select items that are very difficult or requiring a high degree of advanced development, and both normal and ADHD individuals who are quite young will not succeed at them; both will appear to be deficient.

For example, consider the items reflecting inattention in the DSM-IV (see Table 1.1). Scanning these items, we can see that they are unlikely to prove very sensitive to disorder with preschool age children because most of these items reflect the goal-directed persistence, rule-governed behavior, and temporal organization abilities that arise with maturation of the executive functions. These abilities are present to a minimal degree, if at all, even in normal preschool children, who are quite impersistent and distractible, forgetful and poorly organized, and have trouble following directions, especially below 3–4 years of age. Items pertaining to inattention therefore will become useful only after sufficient executive functioning has developed in normal children to permit worthwhile comparisons with those thought to have ADHD.

This phenomenon could easily explain why the predominantly hyperactive–impulsive subtype of ADHD had to be invented from the results of DSM-IV field trials. Those symptoms would prove to be the only ones characterizing the disorder that DSM-IV was sufficiently sensitive to this preschool-age level, because they directly reflect the inhibitory deficiency as it may be evident in this age group.

Now consider the hyperactive–impulsive items in Table 1.1. These items likely reflect the early difficulties with behavioral inhibition as they would be seen in a poorly regulated motor control system. In the preschool years, the failure to develop adequate inhibition results in a near-renegade motor control system that is quite context- or environmentally driven and controlled, eliciting multiple and excessive forms of action in response to ongoing environmental events. This means that the inverse of the developmental sensitivity problem for the inattention items is likely to prove true for the symptoms of hyperactivity. As inhibition develops and behavior moves toward becoming internalized, even ADHD children will eventually come to a point where they can inhibit task-irrelevant activity, climbing on furniture, acting as if driven by a motor, and talking excessively. Thus, these symptoms, which proved so useful to detecting ADHD in young children, are increasingly less likely to do so by late childhood and adolescence.

Note that even though the symptoms of inattention become useful discriminators of ADHD in school-age children, they may become increasingly less useful by adulthood, though clearly on a different and more protracted schedule of diminishing sensitivity to disorder than the symptoms of hyperactivity. By adulthood, even those with ADHD will have developed some ability to sustain attention, hold items in working memory, persist toward goals, and resist distraction. Only the more serious cases of ADHD would be likely to be detected by these inattention items, and even then not particularly well. Conversely, the selection of symptoms or items that are relatively elementary, requiring little by way of advanced development, means that both groups will have little or no difficulty with them; both will appear normal or unimpaired.

Thus, at each age level or limited age range that we examine individuals for the presence of ADHD, symptoms that reflect developmental talents only recently mastered by normal individuals will have to be used as criteria. Then the delay in those with ADHD should be evident. Also notice, however, that this same set of items will not be as useful in its sensitivity to the disorder for much older or much younger children. The same difficulties will apply to any numerical cutoff score that might be chosen using a list of symptoms for ADHD. A fixed cutoff score will prove optimally sensitive to the disorder only within a relatively narrow range of ages, being much less sensitive for individuals much younger or considerably older than this optimum age range.

The foregoing problems with the DSM item set suggest that follow-up studies of hyperactive or ADHD children that have used these sets to determine persistence of disorder over time have a significant methodological problem. Such studies are likely to provide underestimates of the true extent of persistence of disorder within their subject groups. The item sets are likely to be proving significantly less sensitive to the disorder with age. This gives the illusion that the subjects in the studies have outgrown their disorder, whereas, in actuality, the diagnostic criteria used in the studies are being outgrown. The extent of the underestimation of persistence of disorder is likely to increase with advancing age of the subjects, making it appear as if ADHD undergoes a developmental extinction, as some have claimed (Hill & Schoener, 1996).

To circumvent this problem of increasing developmental insensitivity of assessment instruments to the disorder, we must do what has already been done in the diagnosis of mental retardation or learning disabilities such as reading disorders. A wide range of items must be used that represent the broad developmental span for the cognitive impairment of interest. A flexible cutoff score also must be chosen that is developmentally referenced so as to continue to reflect the same degree of deviance at all ages. Consider again the analogy of mental retardation. Whether using IQ tests or adaptive inventories to assess individuals for mental retardation, we recognize that they must contain a large number of items that are developmentally speeded. That is, the item sets demonstrate an increasing level of difficulty and thus require an increasingly advanced stage of cognitive development to demonstrate the ability needed to master that level of difficulty. Examine the items on the Vocabulary, Similarities, Arithmetic, Block Designs, or other subtests of the Wechsler IQ tests; the developmental speededness, or increasing difficulty, of the item sets is readily apparent. The absolute score for the number of items that will not itself define the person as having mental retardation based on the IQ test; instead, the comparison of this score to the average number of items answered correctly by the normal individual of identical chronological age makes the determination. This norm-referenced comparison is a critical element in the diagnostic process for mental retardation.

The hybrid model of ADHD makes the same case for that disorder. If we wish to have a set of symptom lists that are part of our diagnostic criteria for ADHD and that remain sensitive to the disorder across a broad age span, then this item set must not only be lengthier than it currently is, but more importantly, it must be developmentally speeded. It must demonstrate a hierarchy of increasing developmental complexity or advancement. Items chosen to represent impaired behavioral inhibition at the preschool age level are unlikely to represent it at adulthood.

To select items that are going to be useful for detecting the delay in behavioral inhibition that comprises ADHD, we will need to learn more from the developmental psychology literature about the developmental progression of this cognitive ability and its likely manifestations at each stage of advancement. Likewise, if we continue to insist that symptoms of inattention, or what I have shown here to be impersistence and distractibility, are to be diagnostic features of the disorder, then these items will also have to be chosen to represent the developmental advancement of these abilities across their maturation. Cutoff scores based on these item lists cannot be fixed, but must move with development, always reflecting a comparison between what is normal for that age and the degree of delay thought to be characteristic of ADHD.

This last point about flexible, developmentally moving cutoff scores may require some clarification. Let us say for the moment that ADHD represents a 30% delay in the development of inhibition, resistance to interference (distractibility), and goal-directed persistence. Then it is this degree of difference between normal and ADHD individuals that defines ADHD at each age level one wishes to consider. The absolute number of items that an individual does or does not demonstrate is not as critical as its comparison to what is normal for that age. That comparison must reveal the individual to be 30% or more discrepant from normal as one of the diagnostic criteria. Just as maintaining an IQ of 70 as the demarcation for mental retardation requires an ever-changing (increasing) number of items on an IQ test that a person must meet as a function of advancing age, so, too, will the absolute number of symptoms required to diagnose ADHD need to change with age in order to maintain the same degree of relative developmental delay to demarcate the disorder. Holding the cutoff score on the item list fixed at the same number across development results in a threshold for the disorder that will prove increasingly difficult for individuals to achieve, thus making it appear as if they are outgrowing the disorder. This is a statistical illusion, however, achieved by continually moving the developmentally relative threshold for the disorder in the direction of increasing deviance. The same problem would arise with mental retardation by using a fixed set of items on an IQ test. This absolute number could wind up representing an IQ of 70 in childhood, then an IQ of 50 in adolescence, and finally an IQ of 25 in adulthood. The net effect is that increasingly fewer people would be diagnosed as mentally retarded as a function of their increasing age. In summary, when fixed cutoff scores are applied to a developmental disorder, they give the appearance of individuals outgrowing their disorder with age when they are simply outgrowing the criteria for the disorder. To diagnose ADHD properly, then, the cutoff score on the symptom lists will need to change with the age group of the individual being evaluated in order to reflect the relative delay in inhibition, distractibility, and persistence that ADHD seems to represent.

The Problem of Too Few Diagnostic Items
Reflecting Executive Functions and Self-Regulation

The model of executive functions that was extrapolated to ADHD also implies that items reflecting the four executive functions might prove useful in detecting the disorder across development, particularly in older age groups. Once these executive functions have emerged and advanced in their development, those with ADHD are likely to be delayed in the proficient utilization of these functions compared to normal individuals of that age. For instance, once working memory has become sufficiently advanced to permit normal children to readily hold information in mind and manipulate it, as in mental arithmetic, then items reflecting working memory might become useful for the diagnosis of ADHD, whereas they would not be so in the early preschool years. That is because working memory, though emerging, is not particularly advanced enough to begin discriminating children who are significantly delayed in its development. Or, for example, consider the use of items reflecting sense of time, hindsight, and forethought. They may not be especially sensitive to the disorder in preschool children but might become so by late childhood or adolescence, and certainly by adulthood, when individuals are expected to be regulating their behavior via these capacities. Examples of other items could be drawn from the executive functions related to self-control, such as internalized speech, the self-regulation of affect and motivation, and reconstitution. Recall, for instance, from Chapter 7, the numerous features listed that are believed to characterize rule-governed behavior. Such features might prove useful as guidelines for item construction that would make the DSM symptom list more sensitive to the disorder at later ages, such as adulthood. It is not my intention here to formally develop such items for a new symptom list for ADHD, only to point out the possible implications the model of ADHD developed in this volume may have for doing so.

The Problem of Separating a Continuum of Self-Control into a Diagnostic Category

A further implication of the model of ADHD I have tried to develop is that it would make the demarcation of a diagnostic threshold for ADHD a vexing issue. I have tried to show that ADHD, in most cases, probably represents the relatively extreme end of a normal dimension of a trait, namely, behavioral inhibition and self-regulation. If ADHD is but a zone along this continuum, establishing where the boundary of that "clinically significant" zone should begin will be a thorny issue indeed. Attempting to distinguish, using a continuum, a qualitatively distinct category of individuals with normality of self-control is doomed to fail, as no such clear-cut demarcation is going to exist. It is as if one tried to say exactly when day ends and night begins, or when a person is truly mentally retarded rather than just intellectually "slow." Setting the line of demarcation along the dimension is going to be a bit arbitrary and more often the result of a consensus of opinion rather than some true demarcation in reality. This demarcation will then determine the prevalence of the "disorder" within the population.

All of this is not to say that establishing such a cutoff or boundary for the disorder is unhelpful or unnecessary—far from it. Many decisions that are made about clinical cases are categorical in nature (i.e., to medicate or not), so demarcating a category of ADHD is necessary to determine when treatment should be instituted. Nor does stipulating that exactly where the line is to be drawn for diagnosis is somewhat arbitrary make the exercise of doing so meaningless. Research demonstrates that the further out on this dimension of inhibition an individual places, the greater the impairments he or she is likely to experience. Consequently, drawing a line at the 93rd or 95th percentile for disinhibition is not meaningless, as individuals exceeding this cutoff are more likely to be impaired, to be more impaired, and to suffer from more impairments than are those who do not exceed it. It is just that the precision of the specific demarcation must of necessity remain relatively vague. That demarcation will more likely be decided by social ("Who should be called mentally ill?"), political ("What proportion of the population must become so ill before action should be taken to give them government assistance?"), legal ("How severe must ADHD be to result in diminished capacity?"), or financial considerations ("How many children can a school district afford to label as ADHD for whom accommodations and special education must be provided?") than by purely scientific ones.

This problem is not specific to ADHD alone but plagues the definition and delineation of all developmental and mental disorders that represent simply extreme ends along a continuum of normality (e.g., mental retardation, the learning disabilities, major depression, generalized anxiety disorder, Tourette syndrome, obsessive–compulsive disorder, etc.). DSM has chosen to escape this dilemma by stipulating that evidence of significant impairment in some domain of adaptive functioning must be present for an individual to qualify as having a mental disorder. A disorder is not present just because someone is statistically deviant along some dimension of a normal trait. But this is a quasi-political solution that should not obscure the underlying conundrum that will always plague identifying as disorders such problems as ADHD that represent relative positions along continuums. Some slop and unreliability of diagnosis is inevitable unless all clinicians dogmatically adhere to the exact same threshold for establishing presence of disorder. Even if they should do so, that threshold still remains one that was arbitrarily chosen.

The Problem of Age of Onset

The model of ADHD advocated here likewise suggests a similar problem for establishing the age of onset for the disorder. Making the age of onset a precise one, as the successive editions of DSM have done in specifying age 7 years, is to suggest that symptoms developed before this age signify a qualitatively different condition and a valid disorder from those conditions/disorders associated with symptom onset after 7 years of age. As Joseph Biederman and I (Barkley & Biederman, in press), have recently concluded there simply is no evidence that would support so precise a delineation of age of onset of 7 years, or of any other specific age for that matter. If ADHD is itself a matter of degree, not one of kind, then its onset must also be a matter of degree. Severity of the inhibitory deficits associated with ADHD may well function to create an earlier age of onset of symptoms and impairment. Level of intelligence may well auger for the opposite effect, delaying the age of onset of impairment. But none of this can support any precision in stipulating to an age of onset.

To say that there is a precise age of onset for ADHD is, therefore, to say that their is a precise age of onset to behavioral inhibition, working memory, internalized speech, and the other executive functions. This would be folly, as one readily recognizes that there is a range of onsets for these executive functions across individuals. Further, those onsets are not really all-or-nothing events like turning on a light switch, they most likely reflect developmentally progressive events. The rates of those events, as they occur, may change, reflecting a steeper slope to their development at some ages more than others. Those changes in slope might be loosely interpreted as the onset of the development of those functions, yet rudiments of those functions are likely to be evident even before the stipulated age of onset, as is the case in the onset of language development, for instance. Here again, my point is not to attack DSM or other laudable efforts to develop a diagnostic taxonomy, as these are necessary endeavors in guiding clinical decision making. But having endeavored to create them, we should neither reify nor elevate the DSM playbook of diagnostic rules as near-religious dogma or view it as representing the true state of the disorder with any finality. To do so is to guarantee that some conceptual egg will be on our dogmatic faces as new scientific findings clarify the inevitable errors in our earlier thinking that such endeavors naturally incur. Efforts to develop more precise theories and descriptions of disorders, as I have attempted to do here for ADHD, can and should result in marked changes to diagnostic rules, as needed, so as to result in a more precise delineation of disorders like ADHD from normal and from among the other disorders.

The Problem of Symptom Pervasiveness

Finally, there seems to be an implication of this theoretical model for any attempts at making pervasiveness of the symptoms associated with ADHD a prerequisite for diagnosis of a valid disorder. This requirement was added only to the most recent DSM. Impairment from the symptoms of ADHD must now be present in at least two of three rather global contexts (at school, or work, or at home). For children, who do not have a job, this essentially requires impairment at both home and school settings, or a globally pervasive form of disorder before the diagnosis can be rendered.

The present model suggests that the nature of these particular contexts, the particular demands for self-regulation contained within them, the extent to which those demands are modified by the assistance provided by others, the consistency of those demands across time in that setting, as well as the severity of the individual's inhibitory and self-regulatory deficits, among other factors, are all likely to determine whether the impairment from the disorder is globally pervasive or not. As with the issues of specifying a precise cutoff score for demarcating the disorder or a precise age of onset for it, that of pervasiveness of impairment is likewise going to prove a matter of degree and is not likely to delineate valid from invalid cases of disorder. Like those other issues, we may have to settle for the fact that while specifying some pervasiveness of impairment is desirable, any precision in this specification may be difficult to achieve in such matters of degree.

In addressing this problem of pervasiveness of symptoms or impairment, it might be more helpful if more specific and more numerous settings were stipulated in the diagnostic criteria and if quantitative means of assessing them were employed, so as to permit developmentally relative comparisons. For example, I have previously created the Home and School Situations Questionnaires (HSQ/SSQ; see Barkley, 1981, 1990) to assess the pervasiveness of a child's behavior problems *within* each of these settings. Pervasiveness is reported by a single individual witnessing the child across numerous contexts within those settings. Parents rate 16 different contexts within and outside the home environment on the HSQ, while teachers make judgments on the SSQ about 12 different contexts within and outside the school environment with which they are likely to be familiar. Pervasiveness can then be determined by examining the number of settings rated as problematic as well as by their mean severity of problem behaviors across contexts. These scores can then be compared to norms available on these questionnaires (Barkley, 1990).

This has the advantage of not confounding the source of the information on pervasiveness (parent or teacher) with the contexts of interest (home or school), which will automatically inject a methodological artifact into a diagnostic criterion. It also permits the determination of the degree of pervasiveness relative to a normal population of similar-age individuals. I am not saying here that the HSQ and SSQ should be used for this purpose. The original set of these forms was developed to assess "behavior problems" generically, not ADHD. The subsequent revised forms did focus specifically on inattention, but as this volume has made plain, that may not have been the best symptom to choose for evaluating ADHD. Behavioral inhibition and self-control would have been better candidates to target in these ratings. What I am saying here is that similar instruments could be developed specifically for rating the behavioral inhibition, self-regulation, and persistence/distractibility problems characterizing ADHD across a number of contexts. This would also permit some normative data to be collected to assist with making developmentally referenced comparisons on the matter which would help objectify this diagnostic criterion, if it is to be retained in DSM in the future.

IMPLICATIONS FOR CLINICAL ASSESSMENT

Issues of Measurement

An obvious implication of the present model for the evaluation of ADHD is that measures of behavioral inhibition are likely to prove more discriminating of the disorder than are measures of attention or those of other psychological constructs. Specifically, measures that evaluate the capacity to inhibit responding, to cease ongoing responding quickly when demanded to do so or when confronted with errors of performance, and to protect periods of self-regulation from disruption by distracting events (interference control) should prove most useful. Measures of the executive functions that are dependent on behavioral inhibition in the model may also prove useful in evaluating individuals with ADHD. Unfortunately, satisfactory measures having good psychometric properties and norms supporting their clinical use are lacking at the moment for many of the executive functions shown in the model. Even where good clinical measures of some of the executive functions may exist, they are probably less useful than are those of behavioral inhibition in detecting ADHD, considering the point made earlier—that the degree of deficit in executive functions in ADHD will not be identical to the degree of deficit in inhibition, even though they are correlated with each other. The correlation is far from perfect, and thus the deficit in the executive function will be of a smaller magnitude than that in behavioral inhibition. But there is another caveat placed on these various measures that derives from the next implication of the model.

Settings and Durations

Measures that assess inhibition, self-regulation, the executive functions, or the capacity to organize behavior *across time* or over longer temporal durations will prove more useful than measures of relatively brief temporal durations. This means that measures taken in clinics or laboratory assessments over relatively brief temporal durations are going to prove less sensitive to the identification of the disorder and its associated cognitive deficits than will measures collected repeatedly over longer time periods or measures encompassing considerably longer durations as part of their procedures. For instance, a rating scale of behavioral inhibition on which parents or teachers rate the child on multiple items of this construct based on observations over the past 6–12 months will likely prove much more valuable in evaluating the presence and degree of this disorder than will a laboratory or clinical measure that assesses response inhibition over a period of just 6–12 minutes on a single occasion. The latter measure, then, would probably perform better if it involved a longer duration (say, 12–24 minutes) or if it were to be collected on multiple occasions, say, 3–5 times, each 1 week apart. Even then, it may not approach the same level of sensitivity to disorder as that measure of behavior ratings provided by caregivers whose observations of the individual being evaluated have been taken over a period of months to years.

This issue may seem obvious to many clinical researchers who study ADHD and who routinely use parent and teacher rating scales to identify their subjects or to diagnose patients. But it seems to have been lost on others with a predilection toward heavily weighting psychometric test batteries in their evaluations of patients, such as some school or clinical psychologists or some clinical neuropsychologists. The training of many of these professionals has greatly emphasized the employment of objective psychological tests and laboratory measures in evaluating various cognitive deficiencies in students or clinical patients. This is fine insofar as the limitations of such tests are kept in mind. But some of these professionals have gone so far as to then use these same measures in determining the presence or absence of a disorder based on the test score when very few, if any, of the tests they are employing have been validated for this purpose.

"Hit Rates," or Classification

I have come across a number of reports from clinical psychologists and neuropsychologists who evaluated children or adults for ADHD and used various neuropsychological tests of executive or frontal lobe functions in making their diagnosis. This practice may have arisen from the fact that differences between groups of ADHD individuals and normal individuals have been reported in the scientific literature on many, though by no means all, of these executive function tests (see Chapter 10). Apparently lost on these clinicians is the issue that tests on which such group differences may be statistically significant are not necessarily useful in clinical diagnosis. Research studies in which such group findings are reported are comparing the means between groups. This is not what clinicians are doing in the exercise of clinical diagnosis. They are classifying individuals. None of the vast number of studies reviewed in Chapter 4 that used measures of behavioral inhibition or those in Chapter 10 that employed some measures of executive functions reported such classification statistics, or hit rates. The three studies that attempted to examine this issue found these measures to be exceptionally disappointing in predicting the likely diagnosis of individuals as ADHD (Barkley & Grodzinsky, 1994; Grodzinsky & Barkley, 1996; Matier-Sharma, Perachio, Newcorn, Sharma, & Halperin, 1995). Abnormal scores are most likely to indicate the presence of disorder but not necessarily the disorder of ADHD, while normal scores on these measures predict the absence of ADHD at or below levels of chance.

This does not mean that such tests are not useful in evaluating deficits in executive functions in patients presenting to clinics. However, clinicians must bear in mind that such tests (1) have unacceptably high rates of false negative classifications (calling people normal who may have ADHD), (2) are much worse at discriminating among various disorders than at determining the presence or absence of disorder compared to normal, and (3) may only weakly predict, if at all, the adaptive performance of these individuals in more ecologically valid settings, such as school, occupational, or home activities (Barkley, 1991). Because they are taken over relatively brief durations and usually only on a single occasion, these tests are most likely to underestimate the degree of actual impairment in an executive function as it is applied in naturalistic settings across time. They are therefore likely to misclassify patients as normal when they actually do have ADHD or some other disorder that impairs executive functions.

Office Behavior

The problem of assessing ADHD, inhibition, or executive functions over short time periods may also explain why behavioral observations taken in the clinical setting on single occasions will not prove as useful in detecting the disorder as those collected on multiple occasions, especially in natural settings and over considerably longer durations. Again, the ratings and observations of natural caregivers that are collapsed over months or years are likely to prove far more instructive about the presence of ADHD in an individual than will clinical behavioral observations. The few studies that have examined this issue, like those studying the neuropsychological tests, found that the correlation of these observations with measures of behavior in natural settings (home or school) as well as the classification rates for determining a diagnosis of ADHD are quite disappointing (Barkley, 1991; Barkley, Grodzinsky, & DuPaul, 1992). Others have also found that behavior in the clinic is not predictive of the presence of hyperactivity in a child (Sleator & Ullmann, 1981).

In a recent study in our clinic which has not been prepared for publication as yet, we examined how well the misbehavior of young children in the clinic over a 3–4 hour period was likely to predict parent and teacher ratings of behavioral problems at home and school, respectively. As with the neuropsychological tests, normal scores on behavior ratings in the clinic were not predictive of normal behavior at home or school. However, abnormal behavior ratings in the clinic predicted abnormal teacher ratings in the classroom with an accuracy of about 70%. Even so, most children were well behaved in the clinic, again resulting in an inflated rate of false negatives if clinic behavior were to be used to predict school behavior. The foregoing discussion, then, suggests that the observations of caregivers made across long spans of time are far more useful to evaluating presence and degree of ADHD than tests or behavioral observations taken in clinic settings are likely to be.

Executive Functions as Topics in a Clinical Interview

In interviewing parents and teachers of children with ADHD, or family members of adults being evaluated for ADHD, clinicians may find that the hybrid model of executive functions applied to ADHD yields a rich vein of topics, the areas of potential deficits, about which these caregivers and family members can be interviewed. Instead of interviewing these people only about symptoms of inattention, hyperactivity, or even impulsivity, as DSM diagnostic criteria might suggest, clinicians should find it useful to go further. They should inquire about functioning of the patient with regard to working memory and sense of time, internalized speech and rule-governed behavior, the self-control of affect and motivation, and goal-directed creativity and persistence. These additional areas may yield useful information that may corroborate the diagnosis of ADHD or be helpful in treatment planning.

Since we have started doing so, our own patients (in the case of adults) or their caregivers (in the case of children) often report being pleasantly surprised that someone is asking them about these areas of functioning. Such areas as remembering to do things, their time-management abilities, the capacity to organize behavior across time toward distant goals, their ability to resist distractions in this process, the fluency of their thoughts, speech, and behavior, and the ability to sequence these activities properly, as well as their powers of persistence, may all be fruitful avenues of inquiry during the clinical interview. The surprise of patients or family members often results from the fact that we are the first clinicians to inquire into such areas and to provoke them to think about these domains of functioning. We have often found doing so to be richly rewarding, as many patients describe these deficits and the serious impact they have had on their day-to-day adaptive functioning at home, at work, in pursuing an education, in social relationships, and so forth.

Deficits in Performance Rather Than Knowledge

This leads to another implication of the model of ADHD for clinical assessment: Focusing on measures of deficits in behavioral performance will prove more useful in indicating the presence of the disorder than will measures of deficits in knowledge. Again, *ADHD is more a problem of doing what one knows rather than of knowing what to do.* Therefore, evaluating how the individual is performing in meeting daily demands, responsibilities, and other academic, social, occupational, or familial obligations will be far more sensitive indicators of ADHD than will evaluations of the individual's knowledge about how to do these things. For example, measures of adaptive functioning, such as the Vineland Adaptive Behavior Scales (Sparrow, Baila, & Cichetti, 1984) or the Normative Adaptive Behavior Checklist (Adams, 1984) may be more useful in evaluating ADHD, as they are more likely to reveal these performance deficits, compared to tests of knowledge, such as those assessing IQ or academic achievement. The latter areas may be deficient in those having ADHD, typically because of comorbid learning disabilities, but measures of them are not especially useful indicators of ADHD (Barkley, 1990). In contrast, measures of adaptive functioning, particularly when contrasted with levels of IQ to reveal discrepancies between them, appear to be more useful indicators of the disorder or of its impact on daily functioning (Green et al., 1996; Stein, Szumowski, Blondis, & Roizen, 1995).

Time and Impairment

Impairment in the ability to organize behavior relative to time in those with ADHD suggests that *the depth, scope, and seriousness of the impairments rendered by ADHD cannot be clinically appreciated immediately.* ADHD creates a diminution in the individual's ability to bind events with their responses and outcomes when time interposes among those elements. This will be difficult to detect upon meeting someone with ADHD or even after a short time with them. They may seem to be, in fact, no different from anyone else. The subtlety of their disability owes itself in large part to the subtlety of time as an aspect of daily life. Yet that subtlety becomes an increasingly important dimension relative to which one must regulate oneself in order to be successful in adult adaptive functioning. At most, what will be evident about someone with ADHD when observed over short periods of time, especially the younger they are, may be the more obvious by-products of their poor behavioral inhibition—excessive unnecessary movement or restlessness, excessive speech, interrupting others, an inability to wait, distractibility, and a certain impersistence at things boring. To appreciate the larger, more important handicap ensuing from this disorder would require observing the individual with ADHD over considerably longer time periods than anyone except parents, long-time friends, teachers, and employers are likely to have experienced. The more time that a clinician spends with someone with ADHD, the more months and years he or she comes to counsel them, the more the clinician will come to appreciate the magnitude of the impairment that ADHD creates in the lives of those having the disorder.

Summary of Assessment Issues

To summarize, the hybrid model as applied to ADHD suggests the following: (1) Measures of inhibition should be more useful than those of inattention; (2) measures of executive functions may be somewhat useful but not as much as those of inhibition, yet such measures are typically lacking for use in clinical settings; (3) information collected over longer time intervals and on repeated occasions will be more informative about ADHD than will brief clinic office observations or single-session testing; (4) the opinions of others who know the patient well are likely to be vastly more informative about the presence and degree of ADHD than are clinical observations or psychometric tests; (5) multiple observations taken in natural settings will prove more useful than brief observations in contrived or clinical settings; (6) measures of behavioral performance, such as daily adaptive functioning, will be far more useful than measures of knowledge; and (7) the magnitude of impairment and its scope becomes increasingly evident with time.

IMPLICATIONS FOR TREATMENT

There are numerous implications for the clinical treatment or management of ADHD that stem from the model of executive functions and self-regulation developed here and extrapolated to ADHD. Space permits a brief discussion of only the more important or obvious ones.

Time as the Ultimate Disability

This volume has taken as its premise that *time is the ultimate yet nearly invisible disability afflicting those with ADHD.* If one cannot see spatial distances very well, the solution is corrective lenses. If one neglects to respond to events at visual–spatial distances as a consequence of brain injury, the prescription is cognitive rehabilitation. But what are the solutions to those with a myopia or blindness to time and a neglect of distances that lie ahead in time? How can those individuals be expected to benefit from any corrective or rehabilitative treatments when the very cognitive mechanisms that subserve the use of these treatments— the self-regulatory or executive functions—are precisely where the damage caused by ADHD lies?

Teaching time awareness and management to a person who cannot *perform* time awareness or time management, no matter how much they may *know* about time and time management, is not going to prove especially fruitful. Given what you have learned from this text, one should not be surprised to find that the person with ADHD may not even show up for the appointments for such rehabilitation most of the time or may not show up on time, given their disability in performing within time. Understanding time and how one comes to organize behavior within it and toward it, then, is a major key to the mystery of understanding ADHD. To misunderstand this fundamental point is to misjudge those with the disorder, to misconduct their evaluation, and to misguide them in their management.

Point-of-Performance Treatment

It should be apparent that if ADHD results in a disability of behavioral performance rather than a deficit in knowledge or skill, then methods of effective management will prove to be those that assist individuals with *performing* what they know *when* it should be performed and not simply with giving them more knowledge or skills. Two predictions about treatment seem evident to me from this implication of the model of ADHD. First, treatments focusing on skill training, such as social skills, self-control, or cognitive-behavioral training, will not prove of much benefit to those with ADHD. This certainly seems to be the case given the treatment outcome studies conducted with these approaches to date, especially for self-control training (Abikoff, 1985, 1987; Barkley, 1990; Diaz & Berk, 1995). Such is likely to be the case with other skill training programs developed in the future for ADHD. This is not to say that some children with ADHD with relatively deprived upbringings or education may not need some skill training. But that has little to do with their ADHD, and such training would not likely influence those social performance problems that are directly related to the ADHD.

The second prediction from this implication is that *the most useful treatments will be those that are in place in natural settings at the point of performance where the desired behavior is to occur.* This "point of performance" would seem to be a key concept in the management of those with ADHD, as Ingersoll and Goldstein (1993) have stated. The farther away in space and time the location of the intervention from the point of performance, the less effective the former should prove to be for managing or treating ADHD. This immediately suggests that clinic-delivered treatments, such as play therapy, counseling of the child, neurofeedback, or other such therapies are not as likely to produce clinically significant improvement in ADHD, if any, in comparison to treatments undertaken by caregivers in natural settings at the places and times where the performance of the desired behavior is to occur. The latter treatments would be programs such as behavior modification that undertake to restructure the natural setting and its contingencies so as to achieve a change in the desired behavior *and so as to maintain that desired behavior over time.*

Symptomatic Treatment

This raises an additional implication of the model for treating those with ADHD—that any such treatment will be purely symptomatic. That is, treatments that serve to alter the natural environment so as to increase desired behavior at critical points of performance will result in changes in that behavior and its maintenance over time only insofar as the treatments are maintained in those places over time. Behavioral treatments or any other such method of management applied at the point of performance is not altering the underlying neuropsychological and largely genetic deficits in behavioral inhibition. It is only serving to provide immediate relief from them by reducing or restructuring those environmental factors that appear to handicap the performance of the individual with ADHD in that setting. Eliminate the behavioral treatments and environmental structure created to sustain the behavior and there should occur a reversal of the treatment effects to a large degree. This, in fact, appears to be the case with many studies of behavioral treatments for ADHD (Abikoff & Gittelman, 1984; Barkley, 1990; Barkley et al., 1980).

One should not expect to find that such treatments, even when in place, produce generalization of treatment effects to other settings where no such treatments are in place.

Thus, treatment of the individual with ADHD is not a "cure" that eliminates the underlying cause of the disorder. It is, instead, a means of providing temporary improvement in the symptoms of the disorder, and even then only in those settings in which such treatments are applied. While this may be done to reduce those future risks that are secondary consequences of having unmanaged ADHD, there is as yet little or no evidence that such long-term benefits accrue from these short-term treatments unless they are sustained over the long-term. Nevertheless, the management of behavior in the immediate environments in which it is problematic for those with ADHD is a laudable goal, in and of itself, even if it is not shown to produce additional benefits for the individual in later years. After all, the reduction of distress and improvement in success is a legitimate treatment outcome for improving the immediate quality of life for the individual.

Inhibition and Stimulant Medications

A more specific implication of this model for the management of ADHD is that only a treatment that can result in improvement or normalization of the underlying neuropsychological deficit in behavioral inhibition is likely to result in an improvement or normalization of the executive functions dependent on such inhibition. To date, the only existing treatment that has any hope of achieving this end is stimulant medication or other psychopharmacological agents that improve or normalize the neural substrates in the prefrontal regions that likely underlie this disorder. As discussed in Chapter 10, evidence to date suggests that this improvement or normalization in inhibition and some of the executive functions may occur as a temporary consequence of active treatment with stimulant medication, yet only during the time course the medication remains within the brain. Research shows that clinical improvement in behavior occurs in as many as 75–92% of those with the hyperactive–impulsive form of ADHD and results in normalization of behavior in approximately 50–60% of these cases, on average. The model of ADHD would imply that stimulant medication would be not only a useful treatment approach for the management of ADHD but the predominant treatment one, because it is the only treatment known to date to produce such improvement/normalization rates.

As I suggested in the last chapter, society may view medication treatment of ADHD children as anathema largely due to a misunderstanding of both the nature of ADHD specifically and the nature of self-control more generally. In both instances, many in society wrongly believe the causes of both ADHD and poor self-control to be chiefly social in nature, with faulty upbringing and child management by the parents of the poorly self-controlled child seen as the most likely culprit. The hybrid model states that not only is this view of ADHD incorrect, but so is this view of self-regulation. The model would also imply that using stimulant medication to temporarily improve or alleviate the underlying neuropsychological dysfunction is a commendable, ethically and professionally responsible, and humane way of proceeding with treatment for those with ADHD.

Discrepancy between Scientific and Societal Views of Medication Use

This discrepancy between scientific and societal views of ADHD means that any initiation of use of stimulant medication for ADHD in a country in which such has not previously been the case (such as in Great Britain, Australia [other than New South Wales], and, especially countries in Europe), should not be taken by that society or its media as immediate cause for alarm or scandal. Nor should any increase in prior rates of use of stimulants to treat ADHD (such as in the United States, Canada, Scandinavia, and New South Wales, Australia), be similarly interpreted. Such changes in prescribing practices should not be a reason for the smearing of professionals doing so with the tag of unethical drug-pusher, as has been the case with some of my professional colleagues in various countries. Such an attitude not only bespeaks a stunning scientific illiteracy of the nature, effects, and side effects of stimulant medications and their largely nonaddictive nature when used properly, but also reveals an unfamiliarity with the extant scientific literature on ADHD as well. As John Werry, MD, Professor Emeritus of Child Psychiatry, has so well stated, in any other medical or psychiatric condition where the evidence for drug efficacy is this substantial and for drug side effects is this benign, the failure of a physician to consider medication treatment for the disorder would be considered tantamount to malpractice.

Yet somehow many less-informed individuals have come to believe that it is the withholding of stimulant medication treatment for those with ADHD that is the more noble, ethical, and humane approach. Clearly, this can now be seen to be largely the result of naiveté or even a misunderstanding, unintentional or otherwise, of the extant scientific literature on ADHD and these medications. The model of ADHD developed here will simply not support that naive perspective any longer. It should be discarded on history's conceptual scrap heap of ideas that may have been well intentioned initially, yet which have proved increasingly ill-informed. If this model continues to prove correct, next on that scrap heap may be the idea that the capacity for human self-control is largely self-determined and largely instilled by one's parents during childhood. Until such time as more effective treatments having even fewer side effects have been scientifically identified, the use of stimulant medication as part of a larger treatment package for the management of ADHD should be a first-line and mainstay treatment, without apology.

Externalization of Information to Manage Behavior

Turning to more specific implications of this model of ADHD for treatment, it can be reasoned that if ADHD results in undercontrol of behavior by internally represented forms of information, then caregivers should get that information "externalized" as much as possible, whenever feasible. The internal forms of information, if they have been generated at all, appear to be extraordinarily weak in their ability to control and sustain behavior toward its future, beneficial purposes for the individual with ADHD. Self-directed visual imagery, audition, and the other covert resensing activities that form nonverbal working memory, as well as covert self-speech (verbal working memory), if they are functional at all, at certain times and contexts are not yielding up information of sufficient power to capture the control of behavior, which remains largely under the control of the salient aspects of the immediate three-dimensional context. The solution to this problem is not to carp at the ADHD individual simply to try harder or to remember what he or she is supposed to be working on or toward. It is, instead, to take charge of that immediate context and fill it with forms of stimuli that are comparable to the internal counterparts that are proving so ineffective. In a sense, clinicians treating those with ADHD must beat the environment at its own game. Sources of high-appealing distracters that may serve to subvert, pervert, or disrupt task-directed behavior should be minimized where possible. In their place should be forms of stimuli and information that are just as salient and appealing yet which are directly associated with or an inherent part of the task that is to be accomplished.

Moving to some specifics, parents or educators of children with ADHD may need to rely on external prompts, cues, reminders, or even physical props that serve to supplement the internal forms of information that are proving ineffective. If the rules that are understood to be operative during classroom individual desk work, for instance, do not seem to be controlling the ADHD child's behavior, then externalize them. This could be achieved by posting signs about the classroom that are related to these rules, creating a poster displayed at the front of the class, or typing in the rules on a card that will be taped to the child's desk. Having the child verbally self-state these rules out loud before and during these individual work performances may also be helpful. Tape recording these reminders onto a cassette tape which the child listens to through an earphone while working would be another means of externalizing the rules and putting them at the points of performance. It is not my intention to articulate the details of the many treatments that could be designed from this model. That is a textbook unto itself. All I wish to achieve here is to show that with the knowledge this model provides and a little ingenuity, many of these forms of internally represented information could be externalized for better management of the child or adult with ADHD.

Chief among these internally represented forms of information that either need to be externalized or removed entirely from the task would be those related to time. As I stated in the previous chapter, time and the future are the enemies of people with ADHD when it comes to task accomplishment or performance toward a goal. An obvious solution, then, is to reduce or eliminate these elements of a task when that is feasible. For instance, rather than assign a behavioral contingency that has large temporal gaps among its elements to someone with ADHD, reduce those temporal gaps where possible. Make the elements more contiguous, in other words.

Take the example of a book report assigned to an ADHD student. That report is assigned today but stipulates that the report is due in 2 weeks, after which it will be at least a week or more before the grade for it is returned to the student. There is a 2-week gap between the event (assignment) and response (report) in this contingency, as well as a 1-week gap between the response and its consequence (the grade). Moreover, the grade is a rather weak source of motivation for someone with ADHD as it is symbolic, secondary, and a formative type of augmental in rule-governed behavior (see Chapter 7). (This is another implication of this model that will be discussed, which deals with the requirement for more external sources of behavioral motivation to undergird task or goal-directed performances for those with ADHD.) The important point here is that large gaps in time exist within this temporal contingency that are detrimental to its successful performance by those with ADHD. This model suggests that the task, instead, should be structured more as follows for the child with ADHD: (1) read five pages right now from your book, then (2) write two to three sentences for me right now based on what you have read, after which (3) I will give you five tokens (or some other immediate privilege) that you have earned for following this rule. While the example may seem simplistic, the concepts underlying it are not; those concepts are critical to developing effective management programs for those with ADHD according to this model. Gaps in time within behavioral contingencies must be reduced or eliminated whenever possible.

When the gaps cannot be eliminated, then the sense of time itself, or its passage, needs to be externalized by some means. If the individual's internal, cognitive clock is not working well, then put an external clock in the immediate context that becomes part of the task's performance. For instance, instead of telling a child with ADHD that he or she has 30 minutes to get some classwork or school homework or a chore done, it would be much more helpful to do the following. Not only does the rule of the assignment need to be externalized, as in the use of printed rules on chore, homework, or classwork cards, but the time interval itself should be as well. This could be done by writing that number on the card to signify the time limit, but also by setting a spring-loaded kitchen cooking timer to 30 minutes and placing it before the child while he or she performs the task. Now there is little need for the child to fall back on an internal sense of this temporal duration, inaccurate as I have shown that is likely to be (Chapter 10). There are many ways in which time can be externalized within tasks or settings that simply require some cleverness to construct. Likewise, there may be other ways of "bridging" temporal delays that may help those with ADHD, limited only by the creativity of the clinician or caregiver. The point here I wish to emphasize, once again, is not the method, but the concept—externalize time and the bridges we use across it!

Externalization of Sources of Motivation and Drive

A major caveat to all of these suggestions for externalizing forms of internally represented information stems from the component of the model that deals with self-regulation of affect, motivation, and arousal: No matter how much you externalize the internalized forms of information you desire the person with ADHD to be guided by (stimuli, events, rules, images, sounds, etc.), this is likely to prove only partially successful, and even then only temporarily, if internal sources of motivation are not augmented with more powerful external forms as well. It is not simply the internally represented information that is weak in those with ADHD, but also the internally generated sources of motivation associated with it. These are critical to driving goal-directed behavior toward tasks, the future, and the intended outcome in the absence of external motivation to do so in the immediate context. Addressing one form of internalized information without addressing the other is a sure recipe for ineffectual treatment. Anyone wishing to treat or manage those with ADHD must come to understand that sources of motivation must also be externalized in those contexts in which tasks are to be performed, rules followed, and goals accomplished. Complaining to the ADHD individual about his or her lack of motivation (laziness), drive, willpower, or self-discipline will not suffice. Pulling back from assisting them so as to let the natural consequences occur as if this will teach them a lesson that will correct their behavior, is courting disaster. Instead, artificial means of creating external sources of motivation must be arranged in the context where the work or behavior is desired *at the point of performance* where it is to occur.

For example, token systems provide one of the best means for creating artificial reward programs for children 5 years of age and older that can subserve the weak internal sources of motivation in ADHD children. Plastic poker chips can be given throughout and at the end of the work performance, as suggested in the book report example. These chips can be exchanged for access to other more salient privileges, rewards, treats, and the like that the child with ADHD may desire. The point here is not so much the technique as the concepts. Rewards, in most cases artificial or socially arranged ones, must be instituted more immediately and more often throughout a performance context for those with ADHD and must be tied to more salient reinforcers that are available within relatively short periods of time if the behavior of those with ADHD is to be improved. This point applies as much to mild punishments for inappropriate behavior or poor work performance as it does to rewards. As I noted earlier, such artificial sources of motivation must be maintained over long periods of time or the gains in performance they initially induce will not be sustained.

The methods of behavior modification are particularly well-suited to achieving these ends, and many techniques exist within this form of treatment that can be applied to those with ADHD (see Barkley, 1990, 1996; DuPaul & Stoner, 1994; Parker, 1992, for such methods). What first needs to be recognized, as this model of ADHD stipulates, is that (1) internalized, self-generated forms of motivation are weak at initiating and sustaining goal-directed behavior; (2) externalized sources of motivation, often artificial, must be arranged within the context at the point of performance; and (3) these compensatory, prosthetic forms of motivation must be sustained for long periods of time.

Concerning the latter recommendation, it is certainly likely that with neurological maturation, those with ADHD will come to improve their ability to self-generate motivation, as is implied in the concept of a developmental delay. But, as a group at least, they never catch up with normal individuals. They merely lag behind their normal peers in this capacity at each age one wishes to examine them. Thus, like normal children, one can diminish their reliance on external sources of motivation and the intensity and frequency with which they are arranged as they mature and develop the capacity for self-motivation. Thus, behavior modification programs using artificial rewards can be "thinned," or reduced in their frequency and immediacy, over time, as the ADHD child's maturation results in an increase in ability to self-motivate. But this model also argues that at any age at which one is working with an individual with ADHD, such external sources of motivation must still be relied upon more than is normal for the child's age, even though with less rigor, immediacy, frequency, and consistency as may have been necessary at earlier ages.

Deficits in Reconstitution

So far, I have tried to address the treatment implications for deficits in the first three executive functions in the model: working memory, internalized speech, and self-regulated motivation. Just how one may deal with the predicted problem of deficient reconstitution in those with ADHD seems to me to be more difficult to address. If more were known about the process of analysis/synthesis and the behavioral creativity it gives rise to, ways of externalizing this process might be more evident and useful to those with ADHD. Perhaps taking the problem assigned to the ADHD child and placing its parts on some externally represented material would help, along with prompting and guidance as to how to take apart these forms of information and move them about so as to recombine them into more useful forms. Crick and Watson (1974) seem to have resorted to just such a neat trick when struggling to discover the structure of DNA; they reduced the amino acids to puzzle pieces and then simply began rearranging them into random combinations until they noticed the one that solved their dilemma. Adults likewise seem to do this when struggling with a difficult problem; they make their previous internal forms of problem-solving behavior external. For instance, we see this when people talk to themselves out loud while solving a difficult puzzle or learning a complex procedure, begin to doodle on a pad to play with certain designs, free associate publicly to the topic of the problem under discussion, or even reduce a number of words to slips of paper or pieces of magnets and then randomly reshuffle them to create new arrangements. (The recently marketed game Magnetic Poetry does this with words on small magnetic strips; Boggle, Scrabble, and anagrams achieve the same thing with letters.) In any case, the point is the same as for the other executive functions—by externalizing what should otherwise be internally represented information and even externalizing the process by which that information is being generated one may be able to assist those with ADHD to compensate for their weak executive functions. Again, such structuring of tasks and contexts would need to be sustained over long periods of time if the gains they initially achieve are to be sustained as well.

ADHD as a Chronic Disability

All of the foregoing leads to a much more general implication of this model of ADHD: The approach taken to the management of this disorder must be the same as is taken in the management of other chronic medical or psychiatric disabilities. I have frequently used the example of diabetes as a condition analogous to ADHD in trying to assist parents and other professionals in grasping this point. At the time of diagnosis, it is realized that there is no cure as yet for the condition, yet there are multiple means of providing symptomatic relief from its deleterious effects, some of which include taking daily doses of medication, while others involve changing settings, tasks, and lifestyles. A treatment package of these options is designed and brought to bear on the condition immediately following diagnosis. This package must be maintained over long periods of time so as to maintain the symptomatic relief initially achieved by the treatments. It is hoped that the treatment package, so maintained, will reduce or eliminate the secondary consequences of leaving the condition unmanaged. However, it is also realized that each patient is different, as is each instance of the chronic condition. As a result, symptom breakthroughs and crises are likely to periodically occur over the period of treatment and may necessitate reintervention or the design and implementation of entirely new packages of treatment. Throughout all of this, the goal of the clinician, family members, and patient is to try to achieve an improvement in the quality of life and in success for the individual, though his or her life may never be totally normal.

Alteration of Others' View of ADHD

This approach to conceptualizing treatment suggests the final implication I wish to discuss here, the attitude on the part of the patient, clinician, family members, and even society more generally that must be achieved if the lives of those chronically disabled with ADHD are to be improved in quality and outcome. That attitude is *compassion.* Individuals afflicted with ADHD will not be helped by ostracism, censure, criticism, or derogatory judgments of their moral worth. As this model clearly implies, the source of their disability is not of their own doing and largely not of their parents' doing either. The attitude of others that will prove most beneficial for them does not involve moral denigration of them or impugning their character or that of their families of origin. It is, instead, an attitude comprising compassion, accommodation, and acceptance. It is obvious that those who must live with, teach, and manage individuals with ADHD will need to adopt this posture if they are to be of much help, and so they can avoid the resentments, animosities, anger, guilt, and retribution that would otherwise accompany the daily interactions caregivers must have with one less self-controlled than others. Yet it is just as obvious from this model that this is precisely the same viewpoint that must be adopted by society at large if these individuals are to find any peace and success within society and for society to make peace with them—compassion, accommodation, and acceptance.

CONCLUSION

In this volume, I have attempted to show that ADHD is far more than just a disorder of attention. Indeed, while I have shown that the problem central to the disorder is one of inhibiting behavior, I have also tried to show that ADHD is far more than just a deficit in behavioral inhibition. For it appears from research in both neuropsychology and developmental psychology that behavioral inhibition is instrumental to the development and effective performance of the brain's executive functions and the self-regulation they permit. In surveying previous models of the executive functions, I have tried to cull from them those general functions that have been repeatedly identified by others as likely to qualify for the term "executive." These functions are executive in nature in that they assist us with the management of our own behavior.

The general executive functions appear to be the power to engage in covert sensing to the self, or nonverbal working memory, covert speaking to oneself, or verbal working memory, covert emoting and motivating to oneself, and covert experimenting with one's behavior to oneself, or reconstitution. I have tried to show that these functions share a common origin and a common purpose. They originate in public forms of behavior that come to be turned on the self and then become private or covert in form—that is, certain behavior becomes internalized across development, and functions to permit self-regulation relative to time so as to direct behavior toward the anticipated future.

These executive functions result in a shift in the control of behavior from external to internally represented information, from control by the immediate context and temporal now to control by contexts across time and the long-term consequences they may hold. This process of internally guided and motivated behavior serves to organize behavior across time and direct it toward the future to maximize the long-term outcomes for the individual. Therein rests its ultimate psychological utility.

I have argued in this volume that ADHD, through the delay in behavioral inhibition it represents, serves to delay and disrupt the overall developmental process of the internalization of behavior that creates self-regulation. Those with ADHD, therefore, are less able to covertly sense to themselves, speak to themselves, motivate and emote to themselves, and manipulate and reconstitute their own behavior to themselves as well as others of their age. The forms of thought these internalized behaviors give rise to will be diminished by ADHD, such that forms of thought will be more external than internal in form and behavior will be less internally simulated, selected, guided, and motivated across time than normal. The ADHD person is therefore more under the control of the immediate context, external information and sources of motivation, and the temporal now, and considerably less under the control of time, their past, the future, and the internally generated motivation that drives behavior away from the moment and toward that future. Those with ADHD have a form of temporal nearsightedness or time blindness that will produce substantial social, educational, and occupational devastation via its disruption of their day-to-day adaptive functioning relative to time and the future.

I have tried to show that a number of important implications arise from the proposed change in perspective concerning ADHD, not the least of which is the recognition that the inhibitory, self-regulatory, and temporal disabilities comprising ADHD are not of the person's own doing. The weight of the research points to hereditary and neurological factors as having the lion's share of influence over the expression of this disorder, not poor parenting, diet, or excessive television viewing. Genetic effects seem to account for as much as 80% of differences among individuals in these symptoms; the common environment accounts for very little, if any, of them. The yoke of moral indignation from others, character indictment, sinfulness, and willful neglect of social responsibilities can therefore finally be lifted from the shoulders of those with ADHD; they need bear it no longer, for it is clear now that to continue to hold such views will bespeak a stunning scientific ignorance about this disorder. If we are to effectively assist with the management of ADHD, it will not only be in casting aside such moral judgments. Nor will it just be in the recognition that environments must be restructured around those with the disorder and that medications may be needed for many and humanely applied to symptomatically improve their inhibitory deficiencies. It must also be done with the idea that such efforts at management are for the long-term and must be accompanied with compassion and acceptance of the disabled individuals.

Moving to the larger societal perspective, I have tried to demonstrate that those with ADHD represent a mirror on ourselves. For they have shown us the nature of our own self-control through their own disability in this area. They have shown us as well that there is probably a universal instinct for self-control enmeshed in our neuropsychological development and that the capacity for this instinct is not uniformly distributed across our species. If individual differences in degree of ADHD symptoms are largely genetically determined, then so must be individual differences in self-regulation and the power to direct behavior toward the future in the larger general population. This must be so, for ADHD merely represents the more extreme end of the distribution or continuum of a human trait, one that is unevenly distributed about the population. Those with the disorder differ from the rest of us, then, as a matter of degree alone. We must therefore take care, because to judge them harshly is to similarly judge all of us who fall even the slightest bit short in our own self-control. We have no more right to do so than we have to judge those who fall below the norm on traits having similar disproportionately genetic contributions to them, such as that of human height or even that of human intelligence.

It is my final hope for this book that it provide not only a richer scientific understanding of the nature of ADHD, but a more dignifying view of the disorder and those who may suffer from it. If lessons about our own self-control and society have been learned along the way, and if the veil of our ignorance about this universal human trait has been even slightly lifted, then so much the better for all of us.

References

Abikoff, H. (1985). Efficacy of cognitive training intervention in hyperactive children: A critical review. *Clinical Psychology Review, 5,* 479–512.

Abikoff, H. (1987). An evaluation of cognitive behavior therapy for hyperactive children. In B. B. Lahey & A. E. Kazdin (Eds.), *Advances in clinical child psychology* (Vol. 10, pp. 171–216). New York: Plenum.

Abikoff, H., & Gittelman, R. (1984). Does behavior therapy normalize the classroom behavior of hyperactive children? *Archives of General Psychiatry, 41,* 449–454.

Achenbach, T. M. (1986). *Child Behavior Checklist—Direct Observation Form.* Burlington, VT: Author.

Achenbach, T. M. (1991). *Manual for the Child Behavior Checklist/4–18 and 1991 Profile.* Burlington, VT: University of Vermont, Department of Psychiatry.

Achenbach, T. M., & Edelbrock, C. (1983). *Manual for the Child Behavior Checklist and Revised Child Behavior Profile.* Burlington, VT: Author.

Achenbach, T. M., & Edelbrock, C. (1986). *Manual for the Teacher Report Form and the Child Behavior Profile.* Burlington, VT: Author.

Achenbach, T. M., & Edelbrock, C. S. (1987). Empirically based assessment of the behavioral/emotional problems of 2- and 3-year-old children. *Journal of Abnormal Child Psychology, 15,* 629–650.

Ackerman, P. T., Anhalt, J. M., & Dykman, R. A. (1986). Arithmetic automatization failure in children with attention and reading disorders: Associations and sequela. *Journal of Learning Disabilities, 19,* 222–232.

Adams, G. L. (1984). *Normative Adaptive Behavior Checklist.* San Antonio, TX: Psychological Corporation.

Akshoomoff, N. A., & Courchesne, E. (1992). A new role for the cerebellum in cognitive operations. *Behavioral Neurosciences, 106,* 731–738.

Alessandri, S. M. (1992). Attention, play, and social behavior in ADHD preschoolers. *Journal of Abnormal Child Psychology, 20,* 289-302.

Altepeter, T. S., & Breen, M. J. (1992). Situational variation in problem behavior at home and school in attention deficit disorder with hyperactivity: A factor analytic study. *Journal of Child Psychology and Psychiatry, 33,* 741–748.

Aman, M. G., & Turbott, S. H. (1986). Incidental learning, distraction, and sustained attention in hyperactive and control subjects. *Journal of Abnormal Child Psychology, 14,* 441–455.

American Psychiatric Association. (1968). *Diagnostic and statistical manual of mental disorders* (2nd ed.). Washington, DC: Author.

American Psychiatric Association. (1980). *Diagnostic and statistical manual of mental disorders* (3rd ed.). Washington, DC: Author.

American Psychiatric Association. (1987). *Diagnostic and statistical manual of mental disorders* (3rd ed., rev.). Washington, DC: Author.

American Psychiatric Association. (1994). *Diagnostic and statistical manual of mental disorders* (4th ed.). Washington, DC: Author.

Amin, K., Douglas, V. I., Mendelson, M. J., & Dufresne, J. (1993). Separable/integral classification by hyperactive and normal children. *Development and Psychopathology, 5,* 415–431.

Anastopoulos, A. D., Spisto, M. A., & Maher, M. C. (1994). The WISC-III Freedom from Distractibility factor: Its utility in identifying children with attention deficit hyperactivity disorder. *Psychological Assessment, 6,* 368–371.

Anderson, C. A., Hinshaw, S. P., & Simmel, C. (1994). Mother–child interactions in ADHD and comparison boys: Relationships with overt and covert externalizing behavior. *Journal of Abnormal Child Psychology, 22,* 247–265.

Applegate, B., Lahey, B. B., Hart, E. L., Waldman, I., Biederman, J., Hynd, G. W., Barkley, R. A., Ollendick, T., Frick, P. J., Greenhill, L., McBurnett, K., Newcorn, J., Kerdyk, L., Garfinkel, B., & Shaffer, D. (in press). The age of onset for DSM-IV attention-deficit hyperactivity disorder: A report of the DSM-IV field trials. *Journal of the American Academy of Child and Adolescent Psychiatry.*

Arnsten, A. F. T., Steere, J. C., & Hunt, R. D. (1996). The contribution of alpha2 noradrenergic mechanism to prefrontal cortical cognitive function. *Archives of General Psychiatry, 53,* 448–455.

August, G. J. (1987). Production deficiencies in free recall: A comparison of hyperactive, learning-disabled, and normal children. *Journal of Abnormal Child Psychology, 15,* 429–440.

August, G. J., & Stewart, M. A. (1983). Family subtypes of childhood hyperactivity. *Journal of Nervous and Mental Disease, 171,* 362–368.

Aylward, G. P., Verhulst, S. J., Bell, S., & Gordon, M. (1996a, January). *The relationship between computerized CPT scores and measures of intelligence, achievement, memory, learning, and visual–motor functioning.* Paper presented at the annual meeting of the International Society for Research in Child and Adolescent Psychopathology, Santa Monica, CA.

Aylward, G. P., Verhulst, S. J., Bell, S., & Gordon, M. (1996b, January). *Relationships among ADHD dimensions and cognitive abilities using an optimality approach.* Paper presented at the annual meeting of the International Society for Research in Child and Adolescent Psychopathology, Santa Monica, CA.

Azmitia, M. (1992). Expertise, private speech, and the development of self-regulation. In M. Diaz & L. E. Berk (Eds.), *Private speech: From social interaction to self-regulation* (pp. 101–122). Mahwah, NJ: Erlbaum.

Baddeley, A. D. (1986). *Working memory.* Oxford, England: Oxford University Press.

Baddeley, A. D., & Hitch, G. J. (1994). Developments in the concept of working memory. *Neuropsychology, 8,* 485–493.

Baker, S. C., Rogers, R. D., Owen, A. M., Frith, C. D., Dolan, R. J., Frackowiak, R. S. J., & Robins, T. W. (1996). Neural systems engaged by planning: A PET study of the Tower of London task. *Neuropsychologia, 34,* 515–526.

Baloh, R., Sturm, R., Green, B., & Gleser, G. (1975). Neuropsychological effects of chronic asymptomatic increased lead absorption. *Archives of Neurology, 32,* 326–330.

Barber, M. A., & Milich, R. (1989, February). *The effects of reinforcement schedule and task characteristics on the behavior of attention-deficit hyperactivity disordered boys.* Paper presented at the annual meeting of the Society for Research in Child and Adolescent Psychopathology, Miami.

Barber, M. A., Milich, R., & Welsh, R. (1996). Effects of reinforcement schedule and task difficulty on the performance of attention deficit hyperactivity disordered and control boys. *Journal of Clinical Child Psychology, 25,* 66–76.

Barkley, R. A. (1977). A review of stimulant drug research with hyperactive children. *Journal of Child Psychology and Psychiatry, 18,* 137–165.

Barkley, R. A. (1981). *Hyperactive children: A handbook for diagnosis and treatment.* New York: Guilford Press.

Barkley, R. A. (1985). The social interactions of hyperactive children: Developmental changes, drug effects, and situational variation. In R. McMahon & R. Peters (Eds.), *Childhood disorders: Behavioral-developmental approaches* (pp. 218–243). New York: Brunner/Mazel.

Barkley, R. A. (1989). The problem of stimulus control and rule-governed behavior in children with attention deficit disorder with hyperactivity. In J. Swanson & L. Bloomingdale (Eds.), *Attention deficit disorders* (pp. 203–234). New York: Pergamon Press.

Barkley, R. A. (1990). *Attention-deficit hyperactivity disorder: A handbook for diagnosis and treatment.* New York: Guilford Press.

Barkley, R. A. (1991). The ecological validity of laboratory and analogue assessments of ADHD symptoms. *Journal of Abnormal Child Psychology, 19,* 149–178.

Barkley, R. A. (1994a). Impaired delayed responding: A unified theory of attention deficit hyperactivity disorder. In D. K. Routh (Ed.), *Disruptive behavior disorders: Essays in honor of Herbert Quay* (pp. 11–57). New York: Plenum Press.

Barkley, R. A. (1994b). *ADHD in adults* [Videotape]. New York: Guilford Press.

Barkley, R. A. (1995). Linkages between attention and executive functions. In G. R. Lyon & N. A. Krasnegor (Eds.), *Attention, memory, and executive function* (pp. 307–326). Baltimore: Paul H. Brookes.

Barkley, R. A. (1996). Attention-deficit/hyperactivity disorder. In E. J. Mash & R. A. Barkley (Eds.), *Child psychopathology* (pp. 63–112). New York: Guilford Press.

Barkley, R. A. (1997). Behavioral inhibition, sustained attention, and executive functions: Constructing a unifying theory of ADHD. *Psychological Bulletin, 121,* 65–94.

Barkley, R. A., Anastopoulos, A. D., Guevremont, D. G., & Fletcher, K. F. (1992). Adolescents with attention deficit hyperactivity disorder: Mother–adolescent interactions, family beliefs and conflicts, and maternal psychopathology. *Journal of Abnormal Child Psychology, 20,* 263–288.

Barkley, R. A., & Biederman, J. (in press). Towards a broader definition of the age of onset criterion for attention deficit hyperactivity disorder. *Journal of the American Academy of Child and Adolescent Psychiatry.*

Barkley, R., Copeland, A., & Sivage, C. (1980). A self-control classroom for hyperactive children. *Journal of Autism and Developmental Disorders, 10,* 75–89.

Barkley, R. A., & Cunningham, C. E. (1979a). The effects of methylphenidate on the mother–child interactions of hyperactive children. *Archives of General Psychiatry, 36,* 201–208.

Barkley, R. A., & Cunningham, C. E. (1979b). Stimulant drugs and activity level in hyperactive children. *American Journal of Orthopsychiatry, 49,* 491–499.

Barkley, R., Cunningham, C., & Karlsson, J. (1983). The speech of hyperactive children and their mothers: Comparisons with normal children and stimulant drug effects. *Journal of Learning Disabilities, 16,* 105–110.

Barkley, R. A., DuPaul, G. J., & McMurray, M. B. (1990). A comprehensive evaluation of attention deficit disorder with and without hyperactivity. *Journal of Consulting and Clinical Psychology, 58,* 775–789.

Barkley, R. A., DuPaul, G. J., & McMurray, M. B. (1991). Attention deficit disorder with and without hyperactivity: Clinical response to three doses of methylphenidate. *Pediatrics, 87,* 519–531.

Barkley, R. A., & Edelbrock, C. S. (1987). Assessing situational variation in children's behavior problems: The Home and School Situations Questionnaires. In R. Prinz (Ed.), *Advances in behavioral assessment of children and families* (Vol. 3, pp. 157–176). Greenwich, CT: JAI Press.

Barkley, R. A., Fischer, M., Edelbrock, C. S., & Smallish, L. (1990). The adolescent outcome of hyperactive children diagnosed by research criteria: I. An 8-year prospective follow-up study. *Journal of the American Academy of Child and Adolescent Psychiatry, 29,* 546–557.

Barkley, R. A., Fischer, M., Edelbrock, C. S., & Smallish, L. (1991). The adolescent outcome of hyperactive children diagnosed by research criteria: III. Mother–child interactions, family conflicts, and maternal psychopathology. *Journal of Child Psychology and Psychiatry, 32,* 233–256.

Barkley, R. A., Fischer, M., Fletcher, K., & Smallish, L. (1997). *Adult outcome of hyperactive children: I. Psychiatric status and psychological adjustment.* Manuscript in preparation.

Barkley, R. A., & Grodzinsky, G. (1994). Are neuropsychological tests of frontal lobe functions useful in the diagnosis of attention deficit disorders? *Clinical Neuropsychologist, 8,* 121–139.

Barkley, R. A., Grodzinsky, G., & DuPaul, G. (1992). Frontal lobe functions in attention deficit disorder with and without hyperactivity: A review and research report. *Journal of Abnormal Child Psychology, 20,* 163–188.

Barkley, R. A., Guevremont, D. C., Anastopoulos, A. D., DuPaul, G. J., & Shelton, T. L. (1993). Driving-related risks and outcomes of attention deficit hyperactivity disorder in adolescents and young adults: A 3–5 year follow-up survey. *Pediatrics, 92,* 212–218.

Barkley, R. A., Karlsson, J., & Pollard, S. (1985). Effects of age on the mother–child interactions of hyperactive children. *Journal of Abnormal Child Psychology, 13,* 631–638.

Barkley, R. A., Koplowicz, S., Anderson, T., & McMurray, M. B. (in press). Sense of time in children with ADHD: Effects of duration, distraction, and stimulant medication. *Journal of the International Neuropsychological Society.*

Barkley, R. A., Murphy, K. R., & Kwasnik, D. (1996a). Motor vehicle driving competencies and risks in teens and young adults with ADHD. *Pediatrics, 98,* 1089–1095.

Barkley, R. A., Murphy, K. R., & Kwasnik, D. (1996b). Psychological adjustment and adaptive impairments in young adults with ADHD. *Journal of Attention Disorders, 1,* 41–54.

Barkley, R. A., & Ullman, D. G. (1975). A comparison of objective measures of activity level and distractibility in hyperactive and nonhyperactive children. *Journal of Abnormal Child Psychology, 3,* 213–244.

Bastian, H. C. (1892). On the neural processes underlying attention and volition. *Brain, 15,* 1–34.

Baumgardner, T. L., Singer, H. S., Denckla, M. B., Rubin, M. A., Abrams, M. T., Colli, M. J., & Reiss, A. L. (1996). Corpus callosum morphology in children with Tourette syndrome and attention deficit hyperactivity disorder. *Neurology, 47,* 477–482.

Bear, G. G., & Rys, G. S. (1994). Moral reasoning, classroom behavior, and sociometric status among elementary school children. *Developmental Psychology, 30,* 633–638.

Becker, J. T. (1994). Special section: Working memory. *Neuropsychology, 8,* 483–562.

Benton, A. (1991). Prefrontal injury and behavior in children. *Developmental Neuropsychology, 7,* 275–282.

Bench, C. J., Frith, C. D., Grasby, P. M., Friston, K. J., Paulesu, E., Frackowiak, R. S. J., & Donal, R. J. (1993). Investigations of the functional anatomy of attention using the Stroop test. *Neuropsychologia, 31,* 907–922.

Benezra, E., & Douglas, V. I. (1988). Short-term serial recall in ADDH, normal, and reading-disabled boys. *Journal of Abnormal Child Psychology, 16,* 511–525.

Bennett, L. A., Wolin, S. J., & Reiss, D. (1988). Cognitive, behavioral, and emotional problems among school-age children of alcoholic parents. *American Journal of Psychiatry, 145,* 185–190.

Benton, A. (1991). Prefrontal injury and behavior in children. *Developmental Neuropsychology, 7,* 275–282.

Berk, L. E. (1992). Children's private speech: An overview of theory and the status of research. In R. M. Diaz & L. E. Berk (Eds.), *Private speech: From social interaction to self-regulation* (pp. 17–54). Mahwah, NJ: Erlbaum.

Berk, L. E. (1994, November). Why children talk to themselves. *Scientific American, 271,* 78–83.

Berk, L. E., & Garvin, R. A. (1984). Development of private speech among low-income Appalachian children. *Developmental Psychology, 20,* 271–286.

Berk, L. E., & Landau, S. (1993). Private speech of learning disabled and normally achieving children in classroom academic and laboratory contexts. *Child Development, 64,* 556–571.

Berk, L. E., & Potts, M. K. (1991). Development and functional significance of private speech among attention-deficit hyperactivity disorder and normal boys. *Journal of Abnormal Child Psychology, 19,* 357–377.

Berkowitz, M. W. (1982). Self-control development and relation to prosocial behavior: A response to Peterson. *Merrill–Palmer Quarterly, 28,* 223–236.

Berman, K. F., Ostrem, J. L., Randolph, C., Gold, J., Goldberg, T. E., Coppola, R., Carson, R. E., Herscovitch, P., & Weinberger, D. R. (1995). Physiological activation of a cortical network during performance of the Wisconsin Card Sorting Test: A positron emission tomography study. *Neuropsychologia, 33,* 1027–1046.

Berman, K. F., Randolph, C., Gold, J., Holt, D., Jones, D. W., Goldberg, T. E., Carson, R. E., Herscovitch, P., & Weinberger, D. R. (1991). Physiological activation of frontal lobe studied with positron emission tomography and oxygen-15 water during working memory tasks. *Journal of Cerebral Blood Flow and Metabolism, 11,* S851.

Berman, K. F., Zec, R. F., & Weinberger, D. R. (1986). Physiological dysfunction of dorsolateral prefrontal cortex in schizophrenia: II. Role of neuroleptic treatment, attention, and mental effort. *Archives of General Psychiatry, 43,* 126–135.

Biederman, J., Faraone, S., Milberger, S., Curtis, S., Chen, L., Marrs, A., Ouellette, C., Moore, P., & Spencer, T. (1996). Predictors of persistence and remission of ADHD into adolescence: Results from a four-year prospective follow-up study. *Journal of the American Academy of Child and Adolescent Psychiatry, 35,* 343–351.

Biederman, J., Faraone, S. V., Keenan, K., Knee, D., & Tsuang, M. T. (1990). Family-genetic and psychosocial risk factors in DSM-III attention deficit disorder. *Journal of the American Academy of Child and Adolescent Psychiatry 29,* 526–533.

Biederman, J., Faraone, S. V., & Lapey, K. (1992). Comorbidity of diagnosis in attention-deficit hyperactivity disorder. In G. Weiss (Ed.), *Child and adolescent Psychiatry Clinics of North America: Attention deficit hyperactivity disorder* (pp. 335–360). Philadelphia: Saunders.

Biederman, J., Faraone, S. V., Mick, E., Spencer, T., Wilens, T., Kiely, K., Guite, J., Ablon, J. S., Reed, E., & Warburton, R. (1995). High risk for attention deficit hyperactivity disorder among children of parents with childhood onset of the disorder: A pilot study. *American Journal of Psychiatry, 152,* 431–435.

Biederman, J., Milberger, S., Faraone, S. V., Guite, J., & Warburton, R. (1994). Associations between childhood asthma and ADHD: Issues of psychiatric comorbidity and familiality. *Journal of the American Academy of Child and Adolescent Psychiatry, 33,* 842–848.

Biederman, J., Wilens, T., Mick, E., Faraone, S. V., Weber, W., Curtis, S., Thornell, A., Pfister, K., Jetton, J. G., & Soriano, J. (1996). Is ADHD a risk factor for psychoactive substance use disorders? Findings from a four-year prospective follow-up study. *Journal of the American Academy of Child and Adolescent Psychiatry, 36,* 21–29.

Bijur, P., Golding, J., Haslum, M., & Kurzon, M. (1988). Behavioral predictors of injury in school-age children. *American Journal of Diseases of Children, 142,* 1307–1312.

Bivens, J. A., & Berk, L. E. (1990). A longitudinal study of the development of elementary school children's private speech. *Merrill–Palmer Quarterly, 36,* 443–463.

Bjorklund, D. F., & Harnishfeger, K. K. (1990). The resources construct in cognitive development: Diverse sources of evidence and a theory of inefficient inhibition. *Intelligence, 10,* 48–71.

Blasi, A. (1980). Bridging moral cognition and moral action: A critical review of the literature. *Psychological Bulletin, 88,* 1–45.

Blum, K., Cull, J. G., Braverman, E. R., & Comings, D. E. (1996). Reward deficiency syndrome. *American Scientist, 84,* 132–145.

Boden, M. A. (1994). Précis of *The creative mind: Myths and mechanisms. Behavioral and Brain Sciences, 17,* 519–570.

Borcherding, B., Thompson, K., Krusei, M., Bartko, J., Rapoport, J. L., & Weingartner, H. (1988). Automatic and effortful processing in attention-deficit/hyperactivity disorder. *Journal of Abnormal Child Psychology, 16,* 333–345.

Brady, K. D., & Denckla, M. B. (1994). *Performance of children with attention deficit hyperactivity disorder on the Tower of Hanoi task.* Unpublished manuscript, Johns Hopkins University School of Medicine, Baltimore.

Brand, E., & van der Vlugt, H. (1989). Activation: Base-level and responsivity—A search for subtypes of ADDH children by means of electro-cardiac, dermal, and respiratory measures. In T. Sagvolden & T. Archer (Eds.), *Attention deficit disorder: Clinical and basic research* (pp. 137–150). Hillsdale, NJ: Erlbaum.

Breen, M. J. (1989). ADHD girls and boys: An analysis of attentional, emotional, cognitive, and family variables. *Journal of Child Psychology and Psychiatry, 30,* 711–716.

Bremer, D. A., & Stern, J. A. (1976). Attention and distractibility during reading in hyperactive boys. *Journal of Abnormal Child Psychology, 4,* 381–387.

Breslau, N., Brown, G. G., DelDotto, J. E., Kumar, S., Exhuthachan, S., Andreski, P., & Hufnagle, K. G. (1996). Psychiatric sequelae of low birth weight at 6 years of age. *Journal of Abnormal Child Psychology, 24,* 385–400.

Brock, S. W., & Knapp, P. K. (1996). Reading comprehension abilities of children with attention-deficit/hyperactivity disorder. *Journal of Attention Disorders, 1,* 173–186.

Bronowski, J. (1977). Human and animal languages. In *A sense of the future* (pp. 104–131). Cambridge, MA: MIT Press. (Reprinted from 1967, *To Honor Roman Jakobson,* Vol. 1. The Hague, Netherlands: Mouton)

Brown, J. W. (1990). Psychology of time awareness. *Brain and Cognition, 14,* 144–164.

Brown, R. T. (1989). Creativity: What are we to measure? In J. A. Glover, R. R. Ronning, & C. R. Reynolds (Eds.), *Handbook of creativity* (pp. 3–32). New York: Plenum Press.

Brown, S. W. (1985). Time perception and attention: The effects of prospective versus retrospective paradigms and task demands on perceived duration. *Perception and Psychophysics, 38,* 115–124.

Burks, H. (1960). The hyperkinetic child. *Exceptional Children, 27,* 18.

Buschke, H., & Fuld, P. A. (1974). Evaluating storage, retention, and retrieval in disordered memory and learning. *Neurology, 11,* 1019–1025.

Butterbaugh, G., Giordani, B., Dillon, J., Alessi, N., Breen, M., & Berent, S. (1989, October). *Effortful learning in children with hyperactivity and/or depressive disorders.* Paper presented at the annual meeting of the American Academy of Child and Adolescent Psychiatry, New York.

Butters, M. A., Kaszniak, A. W., Glisky, E. L., Eslinger, P. J., & Schachter, D. L. (1994). Recency discrimination deficits in frontal lobe patients. *Neuropsychology, 8,* 343–353.

Cadoret, R. J., & Stewart, M. A. (1991). An adoption study of attention deficit/hyperactivity/aggression and their relationship to adult antisocial personality. *Comprehensive Psychiatry, 32,* 73–82.

Cahn, D. A., & Marcotte, A. C. (1995). Rates of forgetting in attention deficit hyperactivity disorder. *Child Neuropsychology, 1,* 158–163.

Campbell, S. B., Breaux, A. M., Ewing, L. J., & Szumowski, E. K. (1984). A one-year follow-up of parent-identified "hyperactive" preschoolers. *Journal of the American Academy of Child Psychiatry, 23,* 243–249.

Campbell, S. B., Douglas, V. I., & Morganstern, G. (1971). Cognitive styles in hyperactive children and the effect of methylphenidate. *Journal of Child Psychology and Psychiatry, 12,* 55-67.

Campbell, S. B., Endman, M., & Bernfield, G. (1977). A three-year follow-up of hyperactive preschoolers into elementary school. *Journal of Child Psychology and Psychiatry, 18,* 239–250.

Campbell, S. B., Pierce, E. W., March, C. L., Ewing, L. J., & Szumowski, E. K. (1994). Hard-to-manage preschoolers: Symptomatic behavior across contexts and time. *Child Development, 65,* 836–851.

Campbell, S. B., Szumowski, E. K., Ewing, L. J., Gluck, D. S., & Breaux, A. M. (1982). A multidimensional assessment of parent-identified behavior problem toddlers. *Journal of Abnormal Child Psychology, 10,* 569–592.

Cantwell, D. (1975). *The hyperactive child.* New York: Spectrum.

Cantwell, D. P., & Baker, L. (1992). Association between attention deficit-hyperactivity disorder and learning disorders. In S. E. Shaywitz & B. A. Shaywitz (Eds.), *Attention deficit disorder comes of age: Toward the twenty-first century* (pp. 145–164). Austin, TX: Pro-ed.

Cappella, B., Gentile, J. R., & Juliano, D. B. (1977). Time estimation by hyperactive and normal children. *Perceptual and Motor Skills, 44,* 787–790.

Cardebat, D., Demonet, J. F., Viallard, G., Faure, S., Puel, M., & Celsis, P. (1996). Brain functional profiles in formal and semantic fluency tasks: A SPECT study in normals. *Brain and Language, 52,* 305–313.

Cardon, L. R., Fulker, D. W., DeFries, J. C., & Plomin, R. (1992). Multivariate genetic analysis of specific cognitive abilities in the Colorado Adoption Project at age 7 years. *Intelligence, 16,* 383–400.

Carlson, C. (1986). Attention deficit disorder without hyperactivity: A review of preliminary experimental evidence. In B. Lahey & A. Kazdin (Eds.), *Advances in clinical child psychology* (Vol. 9, pp. 153–176). New York: Plenum Press.

Carlson, C. L., & Alexander, D. K. (1993, February). *Effects of variations in reinforcement and feedback strategies on the performance and intrinsic motivation of ADHD children.* Paper presented at the annual meeting of the Society for Research in Child and Adolescent Psychopathology, Sante Fe, NM.

Carte, E. T., Nigg, J. T., & Hinshaw, S. P. (1996). Neuropsychological functioning, motor speed, and language processing in boys with and without ADHD. *Journal of Abnormal Child Psychology, 24,* 481–498.

Casey, B. J., Castellanos, F. X., Giedd, J. N., Marsh, W. L., Hamburger, S. D., Schubert, A. B., Vauss, Y. C., Vaituzis, A. C., Dickstein, D. P., Sarfatti, S. E., & Rapoport, J. L. (1997). Implication of right frontostriatal circuitry in response inhibition and attention-deficit/hyperactivity disorder. *Journal of the American Academy of Child and Adolescent Psychiatry, 36,* 374–383.

Caspi, A., Henry, B., McGee, R. O., Moffitt, T. E., & Silva, P. A. (1995). Temperamental origins of child and adolescent behavior problems: From age three to age fifteen. *Child Development, 66,* 55–68.

Caspi, A., Moffitt, T. E., Newman, D. L., & Silva, P. A. (1996). Behavioral observations at age 3 years predict adult psychiatric disorders: Longitudinal evidence from a birth cohort. *Archives of General Psychiatry, 53,* 1033–1039.

Caspi, A., & Silva, P. A. (1995). Temperamental qualities at age three predict personality traits in young adulthood: Longitudinal evidence from a birth cohort. *Child Development, 66,* 486–698.

Castellanos, F. X., Giedd, J. N., Eckburg, P., Marsh, W. L., Vaituzis, C., Kaysen, D., Hamburger, S. D., & Rapoport, J. L. (1994). Quantitative morphology of the caudate nucleus in attention deficit hyperactivity disorder. *American Journal of Psychiatry, 151,* 1791–1796.

Castellanos, F. X., Giedd, J. N., Marsh, W. L., Hamburger, S. D., Vaituzis, A. C., Dickstein, D. P., Sarfatti, S. E., Vauss, Y. C., Snell, J. W., Lange, N., Kaysen, D., Krain, A. L., Ritchhie, G. F., Rajapakse, J. C., & Rapoport, J. L. (1996). Quantitative brain magnetic resonance imaging in attention-deficit hyperactivity disorder. *Archives of General Psychiatry, 53,* 607–616.

Cataldo, M. F., Finney, J. W., Richman, G. S., Riley, A. W., Hook, R. J., Brophy, C. J., & Nau, P. A. (1992). Behavior of injured and uninjured children and their parents in a simulated hazardous setting. *Journal of Pediatric Psychology, 17,* 73–80.

Ceci, S. J., & Tishman, J. (1984). Hyperactivity and incidental memory: Evidence for attentional diffusion. *Child Development, 55,* 2192–2203.

Cerutti, D. T. (1989). Discrimination theory of rule-governed behavior. *Journal of the Experimental Analysis of Behavior, 51,* 259–276.

Chee, P., Logan, G., Schachar, R., Lindsay, P., & Wachsmuth, R. (1989). Effects of event rate and display time on sustained attention in hyperactive, normal, and control children. *Journal of Abnormal Child Psychology, 17,* 371–391.

Chess, S. (1960). Diagnosis and treatment of the hyperactive child. *New York State Journal of Medicine, 60,* 2379–2385.

Clore, G. L. (1994). Why emotions are felt. In P. Ekman & R. J. Davidson (Eds.), *The nature of emotion: Fundamental questions* (pp. 103–111). New York: Oxford University Press.

Coccaro, E. F., Bergeman, C. S., & McClearn, G. E. (1993). Heritability of irritable impulsiveness: A study of twins reared together and apart. *Psychiatry Research, 48,* 229–242.

Cohen, J. (1992). A power primer. *Psychological Bulletin, 112,* 155–159.

Cohen, N. J., Weiss, G., & Minde, K. (1972). Cognitive styles in adolescents previously diagnosed as hyperactive. *Journal of Child Psychology and Psychiatry, 13,* 203–209.

Cole, P. M., Zahn-Waxler, C., & Smith, D. (1994). Expressive control during a disappointment: Variations related to preschoolers behavior problems. *Developmental Psychology, 30,* 835–846.

Conners, C. K. (1995). *The Conners Continuous Performance Test.* North Tonawanda, NY: Multi-Health Systems.

Conte, R., & Regehr, S. M. (1991). Learning and transfer of inductive reasoning rules in overactive children. *Cognitive Therapy and Research, 15,* 129–139.

Cook, E. H., Stein, M. A., Krasowski, M. D., Cox, N. J., Olkon, D. M., Kieffer, J. E., & Leventhal, B. L. (1995). Association of attention deficit disorder and the dopamine transporter gene. *American Journal of Human Genetics, 56,* 993–998.

Cook, E. H., Stein, M. A., & Leventhal, D. L. (1997). Family-based association of attention-deficit/hyperactivity disorder and the dopamine transporter. In K. Blum (Ed.), *Handbook of psychiatric genetics* (pp. 297–310). New York: CRC Press.

Copeland, A. P. (1979). Types of private speech produced by hyperactive and nonhyperactive boys. *Journal of Abnormal Child Psychology, 7,* 169–177.

Corkum, P. V., & Siegel, L. S. (1993). Is the continuous performance task a valuable research tool for use with children with attention-deficit-hyperactivity disorder? *Journal of Child Psychology and Psychiatry, 34,* 1217–1239.

Courtney, S. M., Ungerleider, L. G., Keil, K., & Haxby, J. V. (1996). Object and spatial visual working memory activate separate neural systems in human cortex. *Cerebral Cortex, 6,* 39–49.

Crick, F. (1994). *The astonishing hypothesis.* New York: Touchstone.

Crowe, S. F. (1992). Dissociation of two frontal lobe syndromes by a test of verbal fluency. *Journal of Clinical and Experimental Neuropsychology, 14,* 327–339.

Cummings, J. L. (1995). Anatomic and behavioral aspects of frontal-subcortical circuits. In J. Grafman, K. J. Holyoak, & F. Boller (Eds.), *Structure and functions of the human prefrontal cortex: Vol. 769. Annals of the New York Academy of Sciences* (pp. 1–13). New York: New York Academy of Sciences.

Cunningham, C. E., Benness, B. B., & Siegel, L. S. (1988). Family functioning, time allocation, and parental depression in the families of normal and ADDH children. *Journal of Clinical Child Psychology, 17,* 169–177.

Cunningham, S. J., & Knights, R. M. (1978). The performance of hyperactive and normal boys under differing reward and punishment schedules. *Journal of Pediatric Psychology, 3,* 195–201.

Daehler, M. W., Bukato, D., Benson, K., & Myers, N. (1976). The effects of size and color cues on the delayed response of very young children. *Bulletin of the Psychonomic Society, 7,* 65–68.

Daigneault, S., Braun, C. M. J., & Whitaker, H. A. (1992). An empirical test of two opposing theoretical models of prefrontal function. *Brain and Cognition, 19,* 48–71.

Damasio, A. R. (1994). *Descartes' error: Emotion, reason, and the human brain.* New York: Putnam.

Damasio, A. R. (1995). On some functions of the human prefrontal cortex. In J. Grafma, K. J. Holyoak, & F. Boller (Eds.), *Structure and functions of the human prefrontal cortex: Vol. 769. Annals of the New York Academy of Sciences* (pp. 241–251). New York: New York Academy of Sciences.

Danforth, J. S., Barkley, R. A., & Stokes, T. F. (1991). Observations of parent–child interactions with hyperactive children: Research and clinical implications. *Clinical Psychology Review, 11,* 703–727.

Daniel, D. G., Winberger, D. R., Jones, D. W., Zigun, J. R., Copploa, R., Handel, S., Bigelow, L. B., Goldberg, T. E., Berman, K. F., & Kleinman, J. E. (1991). The effect of amphetamine on regional cerebral blood flow during cognitive activation in schizophrenia. *Journal of Neuroscience, 11,* 1907–1917.

Dawkins, R. (1974). *The selfish gene.* Cambridge, England: Cambridge University Press.

Darwin, C. (1992). *The descent of man and selection in relation to sex.* Chicago: Enclyclopedia Britannica. (Original work published 1871)

David, O. J. (1974). Association between lower level lead concentrations and hyperactivity. *Environmental Health Perspective, 7,* 17–25.

Davidson, L. L., Hughes, S. J., & O'Connor, P. A. (1988). Preschool behavior problems and subsequent risk of injury. *Pediatrics, 82,* 644–651.

Davidson, L. L., Taylor, E. A., Sandberg, S. T., & Thorley, G. (1992). Hyperactivity in school-age boys and subsequent risk of injury. *Pediatrics, 90,* 697–702.

Davies, P. (1995). *About time: Einstein's unfinished revolution.* New York: Simon & Schuster.

Dawkins, R. (1982). *The extended phenotype.* New York: Oxford University Press.

Dehaene, S., & Changeux, J. P. (1995). Neuronal models of prefrontal cortical functions. In J. Grafman, K. J. Holyoak, & F. Boller (Eds.), *Structure and functions of the human prefrontal cortex: Vol. 769. Annals of the New York Academy of Sciences* (pp. 305–319). New York: New York Academy of Sciences.

de la Burde, B., & Choate, M. (1972). Does asymptomatic lead exposure in children have latent sequelae? *Journal of Pediatrics, 81,* 1088–1091.

de la Burde, B., & Choate, M. (1974). Early asymptomatic lead exposure and development at school age. *Journal of Pediatrics, 87,* 638–642.

Dellis, D. C., Squire, L. R., Bihrle, A., & Massman, P. (1992). Componential analysis of problem-solving ability: Performance of patients with frontal lobe damage and amnesic patients on a new sorting test. *Neuropsychologia, 30,* 683–697.

Dempster, F. N. (1991). Inhibitory processes: A neglected dimension of intelligence. *Intelligence, 15,* 157–173.

Dempster, F. N. (1992). The rise and fall of the inhibitory mechanism: Toward a unified theory of cognitive development and aging. *Developmental Review, 12,* 45–75.

Denckla, M. B. (1985). Motor coordination in dyslexic children: Theoretical and clinical implications. In F. H. Duffy & N. Geschwind (Eds.), *Dyslexia: A neuroscientific approach to clinical evaluation* (pp. 187–195). Boston: Little, Brown.

Denckla, M. B. (1994). Measurement of executive function. In G. R. Lyon (Ed.), *Frames of reference for the assessment of learning disabilities: New views on measurement issues* (pp. 117–142). Baltimore: Paul H. Brookes.

Denckla, M. B. (1996). A theory and model of executive function: A neuropsychological perspective. In G. R. Lyon & N. A. Krasnegor (Eds.), *Attention, memory, and executive function* (pp. 263–277). Baltimore: Paul H. Brookes.

Denckla, M. B., & Rudel, R. G. (1978). Anomalies of motor development in hyperactive boys. *Annals of Neurology, 3,* 231–233.

Denckla, M. B., Rudel, R. G., Chapman, C., & Krieger, J. (1985). Motor proficiency in dyslexic children with and without attentional disorders. *Archives of Neurology, 42,* 228–231.

Dennett, D. C. (1991). *Consciousness explained.* Boston: Little, Brown.

Dennett, D. C. (1995). *Darwin's dangerous idea: Evolution and the meaning of life.* New York: Simon & Schuster.

Denson, R., Nanson, J. L., & McWatters, M. A. (1975). Hyperkinesis and maternal smoking. *Canadian Psychiatric Association Journal, 20,* 183–187.

D'Esposito, M., Detre, J. A., Alsop, D. C., Shin, R. K., Atlas, S., & Grossman, M. (1995). The neural basis of the central executive system of working memory. *Nature, 378,* 279–281.

Dewey, D., & Kaplan, B. J. (1994). Subtyping of developmental motor deficits. *Developmental Neuropsychology, 10,* 265–284.

Diamond, A., Cruttenden, L., & Neiderman, D. (1994). AB with multiple wells: 1. Why are multiple wells sometimes easier than two wells? 2. Memory or memory + inhibition? *Developmental Psychology, 30,* 192–205.

Diaz, R. M. (1992). Methodological concerns in the study of private speech. In R. M. Diaz & L. E. Berk (Eds.), *Private speech: From social interaction to self-regulation* (pp. 55–84). Hillsdale, NJ: Erlbaum.

Diaz, R. M., & Berk, L. E. (1992). *Private speech: From social interaction to self-regulation.* Mahwah, NJ: Erlbaum.

Diaz, R. M., & Berk, L. E. (1995). A Vygotskian critique of self-instructional training. *Development and Psychopathology, 7,* 369–392.

Diaz, R. M., Neal, C. J., & Amaya-Williams, M. (1990). The social origins of self-regulation. In L. C. Moll (Ed.), *Vygotsky and education: Instructional implications and applications of sociohistorical psychology* (pp. 127–154). New York: Cambridge University Press.

Dickman, S. J. (1994). Impulsivity and information processing. In W. G. McCown, J. L. Johnson, & M. B. Shure (Eds.), *The impulsive client* (pp. 151–184). Washington, DC: American Psychological Association.

Dolphin, J. E., & Cruickshank, W. M. (1951). Pathology of concept formation in children with cerebral palsy. *American Journal of Mental Deficiency, 56,* 386–392.

Douglas, V. I. (1972). Stop, look, and listen: The problem of sustained attention and impulse control in hyperactive and normal children. *Canadian Journal of Behavioural Science, 4,* 259–282.

Douglas, V. I. (1980a). Higher mental processes in hyperactive children: Implications for training. In R. Knights & D. Bakker (Eds.), *Treatment of hyperactive and learning disordered children* (pp. 65–92). Baltimore: University Park Press.

Douglas, V. I. (1980b). Treatment and training approaches to hyperactivity: Establishing internal or external control. In C. Whalen & B. Henker (Eds.), *Hyperactive children: The social ecology of identification and treatment* (pp. 283–318). New York: Academic Press.

Douglas, V. I. (1983). Attention and cognitive problems. In M. Rutter (Ed.), *Developmental neuropsychiatry* (pp. 280–329). New York: Guilford Press.

Douglas, V. I. (1988). Cognitive deficits in children with attention deficit disorder with hyperactivity. In. L. M. Bloomingdale & J. A. Sergeant (Eds.), *Attention deficit disorder: Criteria, cognition, intervention* (pp. 65–82). London: Pergamon Press.

Douglas, V. I., Barr, R. G., Desilets, J., & Sherman, E. (1995). Do high doses of stimulants impair flexible thinking in attention-deficit hyperactivity disorder? *Journal of the American Academy of Child and Adolescent Psychiatry, 34,* 877–885.

Douglas, V. I., Barr, R. G., O'Neill, M. E., & Britton, B. G. (1986). Short term effects of methylphenidate on the cognitive, learning and academic performance of children with attention deficit disorder in the laboratory and the classroom. *Journal of Child Psychology and Psychiatry, 27,* 191–211.

Douglas, V. I., & Benezra, E. (1990). Supraspan verbal memory in attention deficit disorder with hyperactivity, normal, and reading disabled boys. *Journal of Abnormal Child Psychology, 18,* 617–638.

Douglas, V. I., & Parry, P. A. (1983). Effects of reward on delayed reaction time task performance of hyperactive children. *Journal of Abnormal Child Psychology, 11,* 313–326.

Douglas, V. I., & Parry, P. A. (1994). Effects of reward and non-reward on attention and frustration in attention deficit disorder. *Journal of Abnormal Child Psychology, 22,* 281–302.

Douglas, V. I., & Peters, K. G. (1978). Toward a clearer definition of the attentional deficit of hyperactive children. In G. A. Hale & M. Lewis (Eds.), *Attention and the development of cognitive skills* (pp. 173–248). New York: Plenum Press.

Draeger, S., Prior, M., & Sanson, A. (1986). Visual and auditory attention performance in hyperactive children: Competence or compliance. *Journal of Abnormal Child Psychology, 14,* 411–424.

Drew, E. A. (1974). The effect of type and area of brain lesion on Wisconsin Card Sorting Test performance. *Cortex, 10,* 159–170.

Dubois, B., Levy, R., Verin, M., Teixeira, C., Agid, Y., & Pillon, B. (1995). Experimental approaches to prefrontal functions in humans. In J. Grafman, K. J. Holyoak, & F. Boller (Eds.), *Structure and functions of the human prefrontal cortex: Vol. 796. Annals of the New York Academy of Sciences* (pp. 41–60). New York: New York Academy of Sciences.

Dunbar, K., & Sussman, D. (1995). Toward a cognitive account of frontal lobe function: Simulating frontal lobe deficits in normal subjects. In J. Grafman, K. J. Holyoak, & F. Boller (Eds.), *Structure and functions of the human prefrontal cortex: Vol. 769. Annals of the New York Academy of Sciences* (pp. 289–304). New York: New York Academy of Sciences.

Duncan, J., Burgess, P., & Emslie, H. (1995). Fluid intelligence after frontal lobe lesions. *Neuropsychologia, 33,* 261–268.

DuPaul, G. J., Anastopoulos, A. D., Power, T. J., Reid, R., Ikeda, M. J., & McGoey, K. E. (1996). *Parent ratings of attention-deficit/hyperactivity disorder symptoms: Factor structure, normative data, and psychometric properties.* Manuscript submitted for publication.

DuPaul, G. J., & Barkley, R. A. (1992). Situational variability of attention problems: Psychometric properties of the Revised Home and School Situations Questionnaires. *Journal of Clinical Child Psychology, 21,* 178–188.

DuPaul, G. J., & Barkley, R. A. (1993). Stimulants. In J. Werry & M. Aman (Eds.), *Practitioners guide to psychoactive drugs for children and adolescents* (pp. 206–238). New York: Plenum.

DuPaul, G. J., Power, T. J., Anastopoulos, A. D., Reid, R., McGoey, K. E., & Ikeda, M. J. (in press). Teacher ratings of attention-deficit/hyperactivity disorder symptoms: Factor structure, normative data, and psychometric properties. *Psychological Assessment.*

DuPaul, G. J., & Stoner, G. (1994). *ADHD in the schools: Assessment and intervention strategies.* New York: Guilford Press.

Ebaugh, F. G. (1923). Neuropsychiatric sequelae of acute epidemic 89-97.

Edelbrock, C. S., Rende, R., Plomin, R., & Thompson, L. (1995). A twin study of competence and problem behavior in childhood and early adolescence. *Journal of Child Psychology and Psychiatry, 36,* 775–786.

Ehri, L. C., & Wilce, L. S. (1985). Movement into reading: Is the first stage of printed word learning visual or phonetic? *Reading Research Quarterly, 20,* 163–179.

Eisenberg, N., Fabes, R. A., Bernzweig, J., Karbon, M., Poulin, R., & Hanish, L. (1993). The relations of emotionality and regulation to preschoolers' social skills and sociometric status. *Child Development, 64,* 1418–1438.

Ekman, P., & Davidson, R. J. (1994). *The nature of emotion: Fundamental questions.* New York: Oxford University Press.

Elkins, I. J., McGue, M., & Iacono, W. G. (1997). Genetic and environmental influences on parent–son relationships: Evidence for increasing genetic influence during adolescence. *Developmental Psychology, 33,* 351–363.

Embretson, S. E. (1995). The role of working memory capacity and general cognitive control processes in intelligence. *Intelligence, 20,* 169–189.

Engle, R. W., Conway, A. R. A., Tuholski, S. W., & Shisler, R. J. (1995). A resource account of inhibition. *Psychological Science, 6,* 122–125.

Epstein, M. A., Shaywitz, S. E., Shaywitz, B., A., & Woolston, J. L. (1992). The boundaries of attention deficit disorder. In S. Shaywitz & B. A. Shaywitz (Eds.), *Attention deficit disorder comes of age: Toward the twenty-first century* (pp. 197–219). Austin, TX: Pro-ed.

Ernst, M., Liebenauer, L. L., King, A. C., Fitzgerald, G. A., Cohen, R. M., & Zametkin, A. J. (1994). Reduced brain metabolism in hyperactive girls. *Journal of the American Academy of Child and Adolescent Psychiatry, 33,* 858–868.

Eslinger, P. J., & Grattan, L. M. (1993). Frontal lobe and frontal-striatal substrates for different forms of human cognitive flexibility. *Neuropsychologia, 31,* 17–28.

Faraone, S. V. (1996). Discussion of: "Genetic influence on parent-reported attention-related problems in a Norwegian general population twin sample." *Journal of the American Academy of Child and Adolescent Psychiatry, 35,* 596–598.

Faraone, S. V., Biederman, J., Chen, W. J., Krifcher, B., Keenan, K., Moore, C., Sprich, S., & Tsuang, M. T. (1992). Segregation analysis of attention deficit hyperactivity disorder. *Psychiatric Genetics, 2,* 257–275.

Faraone, S. V., Biederman, J., Lehman, B., Keenan, K., Norman, D., Seidman, L. J., Kolodny, P., Kraus, I., Perrin, J., & Chen, W. (1993). Evidence for the independent familial transmission of attention deficit hyperactivity disorder and learning disabilities: Results from a family genetic study. *American Journal of Psychiatry, 150,* 891–895.

Felton, R. H., Wood, F. B., Brown, I. S., Campbell, S. K., & Harter, M. R. (1987). Separate verbal memory and naming deficits in attention deficit disorder and reading disability. *Brain and Language, 31,* 171–184.

Ferguson, H. B., & Pappas, B. A. (1979). Evaluation of psychophysiological, neurochemical, and animal models of hyperactivity. In R. L. Trites (Eds.), *Hyperactivity in children*. Baltimore, MD: University Park Press.

Fergusson, D. M., Fergusson, I. E., Horwood, L. J., & Kinzett, N. G. (1988). A longitudinal study of dentine lead levels, intelligence, school performance, and behaviour. *Journal of Child Psychology and Psychiatry, 29,* 811–824.

Filipek, P. A., Semrud-Clikeman, M., Steingard, R. J., Renshaw, P. F., Kennedy, D. N., & Biederman, J. (1997). Volumetric MRI analysis comparing subjects having attention-deficit hyperactivity disorder with normal controls. *Neurology, 48,* 589–601.

Fingerman, K. L., & Perlmutter, M. (1994). Future time perspective and life events across adulthood. *Journal of General Psychology, 122,* 95–111.

Fischer, M. (1990). Parenting stress and the child with attention deficit hyperactivity disorder. *Journal of Clinical Child Psychology, 19,* 337–346.

Fischer, M., Barkley, R., Fletcher, K., & Smallish, L. (1990). The adolescent outcome of hyperactive children diagnosed by research criteria: II. Academic, attentional, and neuropsychological status. *Journal of Consulting and Clinical Psychology, 58,* 580–588.

Fischer, M., Barkley, R. A., Fletcher, K., & Smallish, L. (1993). The adolescent outcome of hyperactive children diagnosed by research criteria: V. Predictors of outcome. *Journal of the American Academy of Child and Adolescent Psychiatry, 32,* 324-332.

Flavell, J. H. (1970). Developmental studies of mediated memory. In H. W. Reese & L. P. Lipsett (Eds.), *Advances in child development and behavior* (pp. 181-211). New York: Academic Press.

Flavell, J. H., Green, F. L., Flavell, E. R., & Grossman, J. B. (1997). The development of children's knowledge about inner speech. *Child Development, 68,* 39–47.

Flavell, J. H., Miller, P. h., & Miller, S. A. (1993). *Cognitive development.* Englewood Cliffs, NJ: Prentice Hall.

Forisha, B. D. (1975). Mental imagery and verbal processes: A developmental study. *Developmental Psychology, 11,* 259–267.

Frank, Y., Lazar, J. W., & Seiden, J. A. (1992). Cognitive event-related potentials in learning-disabled children with or without attention-deficit hyperactivity disorder [Abstract]. *Annals of Neurology, 32,* 478.

Frauenglass, M. H., & Diaz, R. M. (1985). Self-regulatory functions of children's private speech: A critical analysis and recent challenges to Vygotsky's theory. *Developmental Psychology, 21,* 357–364.

Freibergs, V., & Douglas, V. I. (1969). Concept learning in hyperactive and normal children. *Journal of Abnormal Psychology, 74,* 388–395.

Frick, P. J., & Jackson, Y. K. (1993). Family functioning and childhood antisocial behavior: Yet another reinterpretation. *Journal of Clinical Child Psychology, 22,* 410–419.

Friedman, H. S., Tucker, J. S., Schwartz, J. E., Tomlinson-Keasey, C., Martin, L. R., Wingard, D. L., & Criqui, M. H. (1995). Psychosocial and behavioral predictors of longevity: The aging and death of the "Termites." *American Psychologist, 50,* 69–78.

Frijda, N. H. (1994). Emotions are functional, most of the time. In P. Ekman & R. J. Davidson (Eds.), *The nature of emotion: Fundamental questions* (pp. 112–122). New York: Oxford University Press.

Frisk, V., & Milner, B. (1990). The relationship of working memory to the immediate recall of stories following unilateral temporal or frontal lobectomy. *Neuropsychologia, 28,* 121–135.

Friston, K. J., Frith, C. D., Liddle, P. F., & Frackowiak, R. S. J. (1993). Functional connectivity: The principal component analysis of large (PET) data sets. *Journal of Cerebral Blood Flow and Metabolism, 13,* 5–14.

Frith, C. D., Friston, K. J., Liddle, P. F., & Frackowiak, R. S. (1991). Willed action and the prefrontal cortex in man: A study with PET. *Proceedings of the Royal Society of London, 244,* 241–246.

Frost, L. A., Moffitt, T. E., & McGee, R. (1989). Neuropsychological correlates of psychopathology in an unselected cohort of young adolescents. *Journal of Abnormal Psychology, 98,* 307–313.

Funder, D. C., Block, J. H., & Block, J. (1983). Delay of gratification: Some longitudinal personality correlates. *Journal of Personality and Social Psychology, 57,* 1041–1050.

Funk, J. B., Chessare, J. B., Weaver, W. T., & Exley, A. R. (1993). Attention deficit hyperactivity disorder, creativity, and the effects of methylphenidate. *Pediatrics, 91,* 816–819.

Fuster, J. M. (1989). *The prefrontal cortex.* New York: Raven Press.

Fuster, J. M. (1995). Memory and planning: Two temporal perspectives of frontal lobe function. In H. H. Jasper, S. Riggio, & P. S. Goldman-Rakic (Eds.), *Epilepsy and the functional anatomy of the frontal lobe* (pp. 9–18). New York: Raven Press.

Garber, J., & Dodge, K. A. (1991). (Eds.), *The development of emotional regulation and dysregulation.* Cambridge, England: Cambridge University Press.

Gelernter, J. O., O'Malley, S., Risch, N., Kranzler, H. R., Krystal, J., Merikangas, K., & Kennedy, J. L. (1991). No association between an allele at the D2 dopamine receptor gene (DRD2) and alcoholism. *Journal of the American Medical Association, 266,* 1801–1807.

Gerbing, D. W., Ahadi, S. A., & Patton, J. H. (1987). Toward a conceptualization of impulsivity: Components across the behavioral and self-report domains. *Multivariate Behavioral Research, 22,* 357–379.

Gershberg, F. B., & Shimamura, A. P. (1995). Impaired use of organizational strategies in free recall following frontal lobe damage. *Neuropsychologia, 33,* 1305–1333.

Giedd, J. N., Castellanos, F. X., Casey, B. J., Kozuch, P., King, A. C., Hamburger, S. D., & Rapoport, J. L. (1994). Quantitative morphology of the corpus callosum in attention deficit hyperactivity disorder. *American Journal of Psychiatry, 151,* 665–669.

Giedd, J. N., Snell, J. W., Lange, N., Rajapakse, J. C., Casey, B. J., Kozuch, P. L., Vaituzis, A. C., Vauss, Y. C., Hamburger, S. D., Kaysen, D., &

Rapoport, J. L. (1996). Quantitative magnetic resonance imaging of human brain development: Ages 4–18. *Cerebral Cortex, 6,* 551–560.

Gilger, J. W., Pennington, B. F., & DeFries, J. C. (1992). A twin study of the etiology of comorbidity: Attention-deficit hyperactivity disorder and dyslexia. *Journal of the American Academy of Child and Adolescent Psychiatry, 31,* 343–348.

Gillis, J. J., Gilger, J. W., Pennington, B. F., & DeFries, J. C. (1992). Attention deficit disorder in reading-disabled twins: Evidence for a genetic etiology. *Journal of Abnormal Child Psychology, 20,* 303–315.

Gittelman, R., & Eskinazi, B. (1983). Lead and hyperactivity revisited. *Archives of General Psychiatry, 40,* 827–833.

Gjone, H., Stevenson, J., & Sundet, J. M. (1996). Genetic influence on parent-reported attention-related problems in a Norwegian general population twin sample. *Journal of the American Academy of Child and Adolescent Psychiatry, 35,* 588–596.

Gjone, H., Stevenson, J., Sundet, J. M., & Eilertsen, D. E. (1996). Changes in heritability across increasing levels of behavior problems in young twins. *Behavior Genetics, 26,* 419–426.

Glosser, G., & Goodglass, H. (1990). Disorders of executive control functions among aphasic and other brain-damaged patients. *Journal of Clinical and Experimental Neuropsychology, 12,* 485–501.

Glow, P. H., & Glow, R. A. (1979). Hyperkinetic impulse disorder: A developmental defect of motivation. *Genetic Psychology Monographs, 100,* 159–231.

Godbout, L., & Doyon, J. (1995). Mental representation of knowledge following frontal-lobe or post-rolandic lesions. *Neuropsychologia, 33,* 1671–1696.

Goel, V., & Grafman, J. (1995). Are the frontal lobes implicated in "planning" functions? Interpreting data from the Tower of Hanoi. *Neuropsychologia, 33,* 623–642.

Gold, J. M., Berman, K. F., Randolph, C., Goldberg, T. E., & Weinberger, D. R. (1996). PET validation of a novel prefrontal task: Delayed response alternation. *Neuropsychology, 10,* 3–10.

Goldberg, E., & Podell, K. (1995). Lateralization in the frontal lobes. In H. H. Jasper, S. Riggio, & P. S. Goldman-Rakic (Eds.), *Epilepsy and the functional anatomy of the frontal lobe* (pp. 85–96). New York: Raven Press.

Golden, J. (1996). Are tests of working memory and inattention diagnostically useful in children with ADHD? *ADHD Report, 4* (5), 6–8.

Goldman-Rakic, P. S. (1995a). Anatomical and functional circuits in prefrontal cortex of nonhuman primates: Relevance to epilepsy. In H. H. Jasper, S. Riggio, & P. S. Goldman-Rakic (Eds.), *Epilepsy and the functional anatomy of the frontal lobe* (pp. 51–62). New York: Raven Press.

Goldman-Rakic, P. S. (1995b). Architecture of the prefrontal cortex and the central executive. In J. Grafman, K. J. Holyoak, & F. Boller (Eds.), *Structure and functions of the human prefrontal cortex: Vol. 769. Annals of the New York Academy of Sciences* (pp. 71–83). New York: New York Academy of Sciences.

Gomez, R., & Sanson, A. V. (1994a). Effects of experimenter and mother presence on the attentional performance and activity of hyperactive boys. *Journal of Abnormal Child Psychology, 22,* 517–529.

Gomez, R., & Sanson, A. V. (1994b). Mother–child interactions and noncompliance in hyperactive boys with and without conduct problems. *Journal of Child Psychology and Psychiatry, 35,* 477–490.

Goodman, J. R., & Stevenson, J. (1989). A twin study of hyperactivity: II. The aetiological role of genes, family relationships, and perinatal adversity. *Journal of Child Psychology and Psychiatry, 30,* 691–709.

Goodwin, S. H. (1981). The integration of verbal and motor behavior in preschool children. *Child Development, 52,* 280–289.

Goodyear, P., & Hynd, G. (1992). Attention deficit disorder with (ADD/H) and without (ADD/WO) hyperactivity: Behavioral and neuropsychological differentiation. *Journal of Clinical Child Psychology, 21,* 273–304.

Gordon, M. (1979). The assessment of impulsivity and mediating behaviors in hyperactive and nonhyperactive children. *Journal of Abnormal Child Psychology, 7,* 317–326.

Gottman, J. (1986). The world of coordinated play: Same- and cross-sex friendship in young children. In J. M. Gottman & J. G. Parker (Eds.), *Conversations of friends: Speculations on affective development* (pp. 139–191). Cambridge, England: Cambridge University Press.

Goyette, C. H., Conners, C. K., & Ulrich, R. F. (1978). Normative data on revised Conners Parent and Teacher Rating Scales. *Journal of Abnormal Child Psychology, 6,* 221–236.

Grattan, L. N., Bloomer, R. H., Archambault, F. X., & Eslinger, P. J. (1994). Cognitive flexibility and emphathy after frontal lobe lesion. *Neuropsychiatry, Neuropsychology, and Behavioral Neurology, 7,* 251–259.

Grattan, L. M., & Eslinger, P. J. (1991). Frontal lobe damage in children and adults: A comparative review. *Developmental Neuropsychology, 7,* 283–326.

Gray, J. A. (1982). *The neuropsychology of anxiety.* New York: Oxford University Press.

Gray, J. A. (1987). *The psychology of fear and stress.* New York: Cambridge University Press.

Gray, J. A. (1994). Three fundamental emotional systems. In P. Ekman & R. J. Davidson (Eds.), *The nature of emotion: Fundamental questions* (pp. 243–247). New York: Oxford University Press.

Green, L., Fry, A. F., & Myerson, J. (1994). Discounting of delayed rewards: A life-span comparison. *Psychological Science, 5,* 33–36.

Green, L., Myerson, J., Lichtman, D., Rosen, S., & Fry, A. (1996). Temporal discounting in choice between delayed rewards; The role of age and income. *Psychology and Aging, 11,* 79–84.

Greenburg, L., & Waldman, I. (1992). *The Test of Variables of Attention.* Minneapolis: Attention, Inc.

Gregory, R. L. (1987). *The Oxford companion to the mind.* Oxford, England: Oxford University Press.

Greve, K. W., Williams, M. C., & Dickens, T. J., Jr. (1996, February). *Concept formation in attention disordered children.* Poster presented at the annual meeting of the International Neuropsychological Society, Chicago.

Grodzinsky, G., & Barkley, R. A. (February, 1996). *The predictive power of executive function tests for the diagnosis of attention deficit hyperactivity disorder.* Paper presented at the annual meeting of the International Neuropsychological Society, Chicago.

Grodzinsky, G. M., & Diamond, R. (1992). Frontal lobe functioning in boys with attention-deficit hyperactivity disorder. *Developmental Neuropsychology, 8,* 427–445.

Gross-Tsur, V., Shalev, R. S., & Amir, N. (1991). Attention deficit disorder: Association with familial-genetic factors. *Pediatric Neurology, 7,* 258–261.

Grskovic, J. A., Zentall, S. S., & Stormont-Spurgin, M. (1995). Time estimation and planning abilities: Students with and without mild disabilities. *Behavioral Disorders, 20,* 197–203.

Gualtieri, C. T., & Hicks, R. E. (1985). Neuropharmacology of methylphenidate and a neural substrate for childhood hyperactivity. *Psychiatric Clinics of North America, 8,* 875–892.

Haenlein, M., & Caul, W. F. (1987). Attention deficit disorder with hyperactivity: A specific hypothesis of reward dysfunction. *Journal of the American Academy of Child and Adolescent Psychiatry, 26,* 356–362.

Hale, S., Bronik, M. D., & Fry, A. F. (1997). Verbal and spatial working memory in school-age children: Developmental differences in susceptibility to interference. *Developmental Psychology, 33,* 364–371.

Halperin, J. M., & Gittelman, R. (1982). Do hyperactive children and their siblings differ in IQ and academic achievement? *Psychiatry Research, 6,* 253–258.

Halperin, J. M., Matier, K., Bedi, G., Sharma, V., & Newcorn, J. H. (1992). Specificity of inattention, impulsivity, and hyperactivity to the diagnosis of attention-deficit hyperactivity disorder. *Journal of the American Academy of Child and Adolescent Psychiatry, 31,* 190–196.

Halverson, C. F., & Waldrop, M. F. (1976). Relations between preschool activity and aspects of intellectual and social behavior at age 7½. *Developmental Psychology, 12,* 107–112.

Hamlett, K. W., Pellegrini, D. S., & Conners, C. K. (1987). An investigation of executive processes in the problem-solving of attention deficit disorder-hyperactive children. *Journal of Pediatric Psychology, 12,* 227–240.

Hart, E. L., Lahey, B. B., Loeber, R., Applegate, B., & Frick, P. J. (1995). Developmental changes in attention-deficit hyperactivity disorder in boys: A four-year longitudinal study. *Journal of Abnormal Child Psychology, 23,* 729–750.

Hartsough, C. S., & Lambert, N. M. (1985). Medical factors in hyperactive and normal children: Prenatal, developmental, and health history findings. *American Journal of Orthopsychiatry, 55,* 190–210.

Hastings, J., & Barkley, R. A. (1978). A review of psychophysiological research with hyperactive children. *Journal of Abnormal Child Psychology, 7,* 413–337.

Hayes, S. (1989). *Rule-governed behavior.* New York: Plenum Press.

Hayes, S. C., Gifford, E. V., & Ruckstuhl, L. E. Jr. (1996). Relational frame theory and executive function: A behavioral analysis. In G. R. Lyon & N. A. Krasnegor (Eds.), *Attention, memory, and executive function* (pp. 279–306). Baltimore: Paul H. Brookes.

Heaton, R. K. (1981). *A manual for the Wisconsin Card Sort Test.* Odessa, FL: Psychological Assessment Resources.

Heffron, W. A., Martin, C. A., & Welsh, R. J. (1984). Attention defcit disorder in three pairs of monozygotic twins: A case report. *Journal of the American Academy of Child Psychiatry, 23,* 299–301.

Heilman, K. M., Voeller, K. K. S., & Nadeau, S. E. (1991). A possible pathophysiological substrate of attention deficit hyperactivity disorder. *Journal of Child Neurology, 6,* 74–79.

Higgins, A. T., & Turnue, J. E. (1984). Distractibility and concentration of attention in children's development. *Child Development, 55,* 1799–1810.

Hill, J. C., & Schoener, E. P. (1996). Age-dependent decline of attention deficit hyperactivity disorder. *American Journal of Psychiatry, 153,* 1143–1146.

Hinshaw, S. P. (1987). On the distinction between attentional deficits/hyperactivity and conduct problems/aggression in child psychopathology. *Psychological Bulletin, 101,* 443–447.

Hinshaw, S. P. (1992). Externalizing behavior problems and academic underachievement in childhood and adolescence: Causal relationships and underlying mechanisms. *Psychological Bulletin, 111,* 127–155.

Hinshaw, S. P. (1994). *Attention deficits and hyperactivity in children.* Thousand Oaks, CA: Sage.

Hinshaw, S. P., & Anderson, C. A. (1996). Conduct and oppositional defiant disorders. In E. J. Mash & R. A. Barkley (Eds.), *Child psychopathology* (pp. 113–152). New York: Guilford Press.

Hinshaw, S. P., Buhrmeister, D., & Heller, T. (1989). Anger control in response to verbal provocation: Effects of stimulant medication for boys with ADHD. *Journal of Abnormal Child Psychology, 17,* 393–408.

Hinshaw, S. P., Heller, T., & McHale, J. P. (1992). Covert antisocial behavior in boys with attention-deficit hyperactivity disorder: External validation and effects of methylphenidate. *Journal of Consulting and Clinical Psychology, 60,* 274–281.

Hinshaw, S. P., Henker, B., Whalen, C. K., Erhardt, D., & Dunnington, R. E., Jr. (1989). Aggressive, prosocial, and nonsocial behavior in hyperactive boys: Dose effects of methylphenidate in naturalistic settings. *Journal of Consulting and Clinical Psychology, 57,* 636–643.

Hinshaw, S. P., Herbsman, C., Melnick, S., Nigg, J., & Simmel, C. (1993, February). *Psychological and familial processes in ADHD: Continuous or discontinuous with those in normal comparison children?* Paper presented at the meeting of the International Society for Research in Child and Adolescent Psychopathology, Santa Fe, NM.

Hinshaw, S. P., & Melnick, S. M. (1995). Peer relationships in boys with attention-deficit hyperactivity disorder with and without comorbid aggression. *Development and Psychopathology, 7,* 627–647.

Hinshaw, S. P., Morrison, D. C., Carte, E. T., & Cornsweet, C. (1987). Factorial dimensions of the Revised Behavior Problem Checklist: Replication and validation within a kindergarten sample. *Journal of Abnormal Child Psychology, 15,* 309–327.

Hinshaw, S. P., Simmel, C., & Heller, T. L. (1995). Multimethod assessment of covert antisocial behavior in children: Laboratory observations, adult ratings, and child self-report. *Psychological Assessment, 7,* 209–219.

Hoffman, M. L. (1970). Moral development. In P. H. Mussen (Ed.), *Handbook of child psychology* (Vol. 2, pp. 261–293). New York: Wiley.

Hofstadter, M., & Reznick, J. S. (1996). Response modality affects human infant delayed-response performance. *Child Development, 67,* 646–658.

Holdnack, J. A., Moberg, P. J., Arnold, S. E., Gur, R. C., & Gur, R. E. (1995). Speed of processing and verbal learning deficits in adults diagnosed with attention deficit disorder. *Neuropsychiatry, Neuropsychology, and Behavioral Neurology, 8,* 282–292.

Homan, L. B. (1922). Post-encephalitic behavior disorders in children. *Johns Hopkins Hospital Bulletin, 33,* 372–375.

Houk, J. C., & Wise, S. P. (1995). Distributed modular architectures linking basal ganglia, cerebellum, and cerebral cortex: Their role in planning and controlling action. *Cerebral Cortex, 2,* 95–110.

Hoy, E., Weiss, G., Minde, K., & Cohen, N. (1978). The hyperactive child at adolescence: Cognitive, emotional, and social functioning. *Journal of Abnormal Child Psychology, 6,* 311–324.

Hudson, J. A., & Fivush, R. (1991). Planning in the preschool years: The emergence of plans from general event knowledge. *Cognitive Development, 6,* 393–415.

Hulme, C., & Roodenrys, S. (1995). Practitioner review: Verbal working memory development and its disorders. *Journal of Child Psychology and Psychiatry, 36,* 373–398.

Humphries, T., Swanson, J., Kinsbourne, M., & Yiu, L. (1979). Stimulant effects on persistence of motor performance of hyperactive children. *Journal of Pediatric Psychology, 4,* 55–66.

Humphrey, N. (1984). *Consciousness regained.* Oxford, England: Oxford University Press.

Hynd, G. W., Hern, K. L., Novey, E. S., Eliopulos, D., Marshall, R., Gonzalez, J. J., & Voeller, K. K. (1993). Attention-deficit hyperactivity disorder and asymmetry of the caudate nucleus. *Journal of Child Neurology, 8,* 339–347.

Hynd, G. W., Semrud-Clikeman, M., Lorys, A. R., Novey, E. S., & Eliopulos, D. (1990). Brain morphology in developmental dyslexia and attention deficit disorder/hyperactivity. *Archives of Neurology, 47,* 919–926.

Hynd, G. W., Semrud-Clikeman, M., Lorys, A. R., Novey, E. S., Eliopulos, D., & Lyytinen, H. (1991). Corpus callosum morphology in attention deficit-hyperactivity disorder: Morphometric analysis of MRI. *Journal of Learning Disabilities, 24,* 141–146.

Iaboni, F., Douglas, V. I., & Baker, A. G. (1995). Effects of reward and response costs on inhibition in ADHD children. *Journal of Abnormal Psychology, 104,* 232–240.

Ingersoll, B. D., & Goldstein, S. (1993). *Attention deficit disorder and learning disabilities: Realities, myths, and controversial treatments.* New York: Doubleday.

Ingvar, D. H. (1993). Language functions related to prefrontal cortical activity: Neurolinguistic implications. In P. Tallal, A. M. Galaburda, R. R. Llinas, & C. von Euler (Eds.), *Temporal information processing in the nervous system: Vol. 682. Annals of the New York Academy of Sciences* (pp. 240–247). New York: New York Academy of Sciences.

Iversen, S. D., & Dunnett, S. B. (1990). Functional organization of striatum as studied with neural grafts. *Neuropsychologia, 28,* 601–626.

Jackson, J. P. (1974). The relationship between the development of gestural imagery and the development of graphic imagery. *Child Development, 45,* 432–438.

Jacobvitz, D., & Sroufe, L. A. (1987). The early caregiver-child relationship and attention-deficit disorder with hyperactivity in kindergarten: A prospective study. *Child Development, 58,* 1488–1495.

James, W. (1992). *Principles of psychology.* Chicago: Encyclopedia Brittanica. (Original work published 1890)

Jennings, J. R., van der Molen, M. W., Pelham, W., Debski, K. B., & Hoza, B. (1997). Inhibition in boys with attention deficit hyperactivity disorder as indexed by heart rate change. *Developmental Psychology, 33,* 308–318.

Kagan, J. (1966). Reflection–impulsivity: The generality and dynamics of conceptual tempo. *Journal of Abnormal Psychology, 71,* 17–24.

Kagan, J., Reznick, S., & Snidman, N. (1988). Biological bases of childhood shyness. *Science, 240,* 167–171.

Kanfer, F. H., & Karoly, P. (1972). Self-control: A behavioristic excursion into the lion's den. *Behavior Therapy, 3,* 398–416.

Kaufman, A. S. (1975). Factor analysis of the WISC-R at eleven age levels betwen 6.5 and 16.5 years. *Journal of Consulting and Clinical Psychology, 43,* 135–147.

Kaufman, A. S. (1980). Issues in psychological assessment: Interpreting the WISC-R intelligently. In B. Lahey & A. Kazdin (Eds.), *Advances in clinical child psychology* (Vol. 3, pp. 177–214). New York: Plenum Press.

Kaufman, A. S., & Kaufman, N. L. (1983). *Kaufman Assessment Battery for Children.* Circle Pines, MN: American Guidance Services.

Kelsoe, J. R., Ginns, E. I., Egeland, J. A., Gerhard, D. S., Goldstein, A. M., Bale, S. J., & Pauls, D. L. (1989). Re-evaluation of the linkage relationship between chromosome 11p loci and the gene for bipolar affective disorder in the Old Order Amish. *Nature, 342,* 238–243.

Keltner, D., Moffitt, T. E., & Stouthamer-Loeber, M. (1995). Facial expressions of emotion and psychopathology in adolescent boys. *Journal of Abnormal Psychology, 104,* 644–652.

Keogh, B. K., & Margolis, J. S. (1976). A component analysis of attentional problems of educationally handicapped boys. *Journal of Abnormal Child Psychology, 4,* 349–359.

Kertesz, A., Nicholson, I., Cancelliere, A., Kassa, K., & Black, S. E. (1985). Motor impersistence: A right hemisphere syndrome. *Neurology, 35,* 662–666.

Kesner, R. P., Hopkins, R. O., & Fineman, B. (1994). Item and order dissociation in humans with prefrontal cortex damage. *Neuropsychologia, 32,* 881–891.

Kessler, J. W. (1980). History of minimal brain dysfunction. In H. Rie & E. Rie (Eds.), *Handbook of minimal brain dysfunctions: A critical view* (pp. 18–52). New York: Wiley.

Klorman, R. (1992). Cognitive event-related potentials in attention deficit disorder. In S. E. Shaywitz & B. A. Shaywitz (1992), *Attention deficit disorder comes of age: Toward the twenty-first century* (pp. 221–244). Austin, TX: Pro-ed.

Klorman, R., Brumaghim, J. T., Coons, H. W., Peloquin, L., Strauss, J., Lewine, J. D., Borgstedt, A. D., & Goldstein, M. G. (1988). The contributions of event-related potentials to understanding effects of stimulants on information processing in attention deficit disorder. In L. M. Bloomingdale & J. A. Sergeant (Eds.), *Attention deficit disorder: Criteria, cognition, intervention* (pp. 199–218). London: Pergamon Press.

Klorman, R., Salzman, L. F., & Borgstedt, A. D. (1988). Brain event-related potentials in evaluation of cognitive deficits in attention deficit disorder and outcome of stimulant therapy. In L. Bloomingdale (Ed.), *Attention deficit disorder. Vol. 3. New research in attention, treatment, and psychopharmacology* (pp. 49–80). New York: Pergamon.

Klorman, R., Brumaghim, J. T., Fitzpatrick, P. A., & Borgstedt, A. D. (1991). Methylphenidate speeds evaluation processes of attention deficit disorder adolescents during a continuous performance test. *Journal of Abnormal Child Psychology, 19,* 263–283.

Klorman, R., Salzman, L. F., & Borgstedt, A. D. (1988). Brain event-related potentials in evaluation of cognitive deficits in attention deficit disorder and outcome of stimulant therapy. In L. Bloomingdale (Ed.), *Attention deficit disorder* (Vol. 3, pp. 49–80). New York: Pergamon Press.

Knight, R. T., Grabowecky, & Scabini, D. (1995). Role of human prefrontal cortex in attention control. In H. H. Jasper, S. Riggio, & P. S. Goldman-Rakic (Eds.), *Epilepsy and the functional anatomy of the frontal lobe* (pp. 21–34). New York: Raven Press.

Knobel, M., Wolman, M. B., & Mason, E. (1959). Hyperkinesis and organicity in children. *Archives of General Psychiatry, 1,* 310–321.

Kochanska, G., Aksan, N., & Koenig, A. L. (1995). A longitudinal study of the roots of preschoolers conscience: Committed compliance and emerging internalization. *Child Development, 66,* 1752–1769.

Kochanska, G., DeVet, K., Goldman, M., Murray, K., & Putnam, S. P. (1994). Maternal reports of conscience development and temperament in young children. *Child Development, 65,* 852–868.

Kochanska, G., Murray, K., Jacques, T. Y., Koenig, A. L., & Vandegeest, K.

A. (1996). Inhibitory control in young children and its role in emerging internalization. *Child Development, 67,* 490–507.

Kohlberg, L. (1963). The development of children's orientations toward moral order: I. Sequence in the development of moral thought. *Vita Humanity, 6,* 11–33.

Kohlberg, L., Yaeger, J., & Hjertholm, E. (1968). Private speech: Four studies and a review of theories. *Child Development, 39,* 691–736.

Kopp, C. B. (1982). Antecedents of self-regulation: A developmental perspective. *Developmental Psychology, 18,* 199–214.

Kopp, C. B. (1989). Regulation of distress and negative emotions: A developmental view. *Developmental Psychology, 25,* 343–354.

Kosslyn, S. M. (1994). *Image and brain: The resolution of the imagery debate.* Cambridge, MA: MIT Press.

Krener, P., Carter, C., Chaderjian, M., Wolfe, V., & Northcutt, C. (1993, October). *Executive function in children with ADHD and controls.* Paper presented at the annual meeting of the American Academy of Child and Adolescent Psychiatry, San Antonio, TX.

Krueger, R. F., Caspi, A., Moffitt, T. E., White, J., & Stouthamer-Loeber, M. (in press). Delay of gratification, psychopathology, and personality: Is low self-control specific to externalizing problems? *Journal of Personality.*

Kuperman, S., Johnson, B., Arndt, S., Lindgren, S., & Wolraich, M. (1996). Quantitative EEG differences in a nonclinical sample of children with ADHD and undifferentiated ADD. *Journal of the American Academy of Child and Adolescent Psychiatry, 35,* 1009–1017.

Kupietz, S. S., Camp, J. A., & Weissman, A. D. (1976). Reaction time performance of behaviorally deviant children: Effects of prior preparatory interval and reinforcement. *Journal of Child Psychology and Psychiatry, 17,* 123–131.

Lahey, B. B., Applegate, B., McBurnett, K., Biederman, J., Greenhill, L., Hynd, G. W., Barkley, R. A., Newcorn, J., Jensen, P., Richters, J., Garfinkel, B., Kerdyk, L., Frick, P. J., Ollendick, T., Perez, D., Hart, E. L., Waldman, I., & Shaffer, D. (1994). DSM-IV field trials for attention deficit/hyperactivity disorder in children and adolescents. *American Journal of Psychiatry, 151,* 1673–1685.

Lahey, B. B., & Carlson, C. L. (1992). Validity of the diagnostic category of attention deficit disorder without hyperactivity: A review of the literature. In S. E. Shaywitz & B. A. Shaywitz (Eds.), *Attention deficit disorder comes of age: Toward the twenty-first century* (pp. 119–144). Austin, TX: Pro-ed.

Lahey, B. B., Pelham, W. E., Schaughency, E. A., Atkins, M. S., Murphy, H. A., Hynd, G. W., Russo, M., Hartdagen, S., & Lorys-Vernon, A. (1988). Dimensions and types of attention deficit disorder with hyperactivity in children: A factor and cluster-analytic approach. *Journal of the American Academy of Child and Adolescent Psychiatry, 27,* 330–335.

Lahoste, G. J., Swanson, J. M., Wigal, S. B., Glabe, C., Wigal, T., King, N., & Kennedy, J. L. (1996). Dopamine D4 receptor gene polymorphism is associated with attention deficit hyperactivity disorder. *Molecular Psychiatry, 1,* 121–124.

Lamminmaki, T., Ahonen, T., Narhi, V., Lyytinen, H., & de Barra, H. T. (1995). Attention deficit hyperactivity disorder subtypes: Are there differences in academic problems? *Developmental Neuropsychology, 11,* 297–310.

Landau, S., Berk, L. E., & Mangione, C. (1996, March). *Private speech as a problem-solving strategy in the face of academic challenge: The failure of impulsive children to get their act together.* Paper presented at the annual meeting of the National Association of School Psychologists, Atlanta.

Landau, S., Lorch, E. P., & Milich, R. (1992). Visual attention to and comprehension of television in attention deficit hyperactivity disordered and normal boys. *Child Development, 63,* 928–937.

Lang, P. J. (1995). The emotion probe: Studies of motivation and attention. *American Psychologist, 50,* 372–385.

Lapierre, D., Braun, C. M. J., & Hodgins, S. (1995). Ventral frontal deficits in psychopathy: Neuropsychological test findings. *Neuropsychologia, 33,* 139–151.

Laufer, M., Denhoff, E., & Solomons, G. (1957). Hyperkinetic impulse disorder in children's behavior problems. *Psychosomatic Medicine, 19,* 38–49.

Lazarus, R. (1994). Appraisal: The long and the short of it. In P. Ekman & R. J. Davidson (Eds.), *The nature of emotion: Fundamental questions* (pp. 208–215). New York: Oxford University Press.

Lee, G. P., Strauss, E., McCloskey, L., Loring, D., & Drane, D. L. (1996, February). *Localization of frontal lobe lesions using verbal and nonverbal fluency measures.* Paper presented at the annual meeting of the International Neuropsychological Society, Chicago.

Lee, M., Vaughn, B. E., & Kopp, C. B. (1983). The role of self-control in young children's performance on a delayed response memory for location task. *Developmental Psychology, 19,* 40–44.

Lerer, R. J., & Lerer, P. (1976). The effects of methyphnidate on the soft neurological signs of hyperactive children. *Pediatrics, 57,* 521–525.

Lerer, R. J., Lerer, P., & Artner, J. (1977). The effects of methylphenidate on the handwriting of children with minimal brain dysfunction. *Journal of Pediatrics, 91,* 127–132.

Leung, P. W. L., & Connolly, K. J. (1996). Distractibility in hyperactive and conduct-disordered children. *Journal of Child Psychology and Psychiatry, 37,* 305–312.

Levenson, R. W. (1994). Human emotions: A functional view. In P. Ekman & R. J. Davidson (Eds.), *The nature of emotion: Fundamental questions* (pp. 123–126). New York: Oxford University Press.

Levin, H. S., Culhane, K. A., Hartmann, J., Evankovich, K., Mattson, A. J., Harwood, H., Ringholz, G., Ewing-Cobbs, L., & Fletcher, J. M. (1991). Developmental changes in performance on tests of purported frontal lobe functions. *Developmental Neuropsychology, 7,* 377–396.

Levin, H. S., Fletcher, J. M., Kufera, J. A., Harward, H., Lilly, M. A., Mendelsohn, D., Bruce, D., & Eisenberg, H. M. (1996). Dimensions of cognition measured by the Tower of London and other cognitive tasks in head-injured children and adolescents. *Developmental Neuropsychology, 12,* 17–34.

Levin, H. S., Mendelsohn, D., Lilly, M. A., Fletcher, J. M., Culhane, K. A., Chapman, S. B., Harward, H., Kusnerik, L., Bruce, D., & Eisenberg, H. M. (1994). Tower of London performance in relation to magnetic resonance imaging following closed head injury in children. *Neuropsychology, 8,* 171–179.

Levin, I., Wilkening, F., & Dembo, Y. (1984). Development of time quantification: Integration and nonintegration of beginnings and endings in comparing durations. *Child Development, 55,* 2160–2172.

Levin, P. M. (1938). Restlessness in children. *Archives of Neurology and Psychiatry, 39,* 764–770.

Levy, F., & Hay, D. (1992, February). *ADHD in twins and their siblings.* Paper presented at the annual meeting of the International Society for Research in Child and Adolescent Psychopathology, Sarasota, FL.

Levy, F., Hay, D. A., McStephen, M., Wood, C., & Waldman, I. (1977). Attention-deficit hyperactivity disorder: A category or a continuum? Genetic analysis of a large-scale twin study. *Journal of the American Academy of Child and Adolescent Psychiatry, 36,* 737–744.

Levy, F., & Hobbes, G. (1989). Reading, spelling, and vigilance in attention deficit and conduct disorder. *Journal of Abnormal Child Psychology, 17,* 291–298.

Lhermitte, F. (1983). "Utilization behavior" and its relation to lesions of the frontal lobes. *Brain, 106,* 237–255.

Lhermitte, F., Pillion, B., & Sraru, M. (1985). Human autonomy and the frontal lobes: I. Imitation and utilization behavior: A neuropsychological study of 75 patients. *Annals of Neurology, 19,* 326–334.

Light, J. G., Pennington, B. F., Gilger, J. W., & DeFries, J. C. (1995). Reading disability and hyperactivity disorder: Evidence for a common genetic etiology. *Developmental Neuropsychology, 11,* 323–335.

Livesay, J., Liebke, A., Samaras, M., & Stanley, A. (1996). Covert speech behavior during a silent language recitation task. *Perceptual and Motor Skills, 83,* 1355–1362.

Loeber, R. (1990). Development and risk factors of juvenile antisocial behavior and delinquency. *Clinical Psychology Review, 10,* 1–42.

Loeber, R., Green, S. M., Lahey, B. B., Christ, M. A. G., & Frick, P. J. (1992). Developmental sequences in the age of onset of disruptive child behaviors. *Journal of Child and Family Studies, 1,* 21–41.

Logan, G. D., & Cowan, W. B. (1984). On the ability to inhibit thought and action: A model and a method. *Psychological Review, 91,* 295–327.

Loge, D. V., Staton, D., & Beatty, W. W. (1990). Performance of children with ADHD on tests sensitive to frontal lobe dysfunction. *Journal of the American Academy of Child and Adolescent Psychiatry, 29,* 540–545.

Loney, J., & Milich, R. (1982). Hyperactivity, inattention, and aggression in clinical practice. In D. Routh & S. Wolraich (Eds.), *Advances in developmental and behavioral pediatrics* (Vol. 3, pp. 113–147). Greenwich, CT: JAI Press.

Lopez, R. (1965). Hyperactivity in twins. *Canadian Psychiatric Association Journal, 10,* 421.

Losier, B. J., McGrath, P. J., & Klein, R. M. (1996). Error patterns on the continuous performance test in non-medication and medicated samples of children with and without ADHD: A meta-analysis. *Journal of Child Psychology and Psychiatry, 37,* 971–987.

Lou, H. C., Henriksen, L., & Bruhn, P. (1984). Focal cerebral hypoperfusion in children with dysphasia and/or attention deficit disorder. *Archives of Neurology, 41,* 825–829.

Lou, H. C., Henriksen, L., & Bruhn, P. (1990). Focal cerebral dysfunction in developmental learning disabilities. *Lancet, 335,* 8–11.

Lou, H. C., Henriksen, L., Bruhn, P., Borner, H., & Nielsen, J. B. (1989). Striatal dysfunction in attention deficit and hyperkinetic disorder. *Archives of Neurology, 46,* 48–52.

Loughton, K., & Daehler, M. (1973). The effects of distraction and added perceptual cues on the delayed reaction of very young children. *Child Development, 44,* 384–388.

Ludlow, C., Rapoport, J., Brown, G., & Mikkelson, E. (1979). The differential effects of dextroamphetamine on the language and communication skills of hyperactive and normal children. In R. Knights & D. Bakker (Eds.), *Rehabilitation, treatment, and management of learning disorders.* Baltimore: University Park Press.

Lufi, D., Cohen, A., & Parish-Plass, J. (1990). Identifying ADHD with the WISC-R and the Stroop Color–Word Test. *Psychology in the Schools, 27,* 28–34.

Luk, S. (1985). Direct observations studies of hyperactive behaviors. *Journal of the American Academy of Child and Adolescent Psychiatry, 24,* 338–344.

Luo, D., Petrill, S. A., & Thompson, L. A. (1994). An exploration of genetic g: Hierarchical factor analysis of cognitive data from the Western Reserve Twin Project. *Intelligence, 18,* 335–347.

Luria, A. R. (1961). *The role of speech in the regulation of normal and abnormal behavior* (J. Tizard, Ed.). New York: Liveright.

Lynam, D., Moffitt, T., & Stouthamer-Loeber, M. (1993). Explaining the relation between IQ and delinquency: Class, race, test motivation, school failure, or self-control? *Journal of Abnormal Psychology, 102,* 187–196.

Lyon, G. R., & Krasnegor, N. (1996). *Attention, memory, and executive function.* Baltimore, MD: Paul H. Brookes.

Maccoby, E. E., Dowley, E. M., Hagen, J. W., & Degerman, R. (1965). Activity level and intellectual functioning in normal preschool children. *Child Development, 36,* 761–770.

MacLeod, D., & Prior, M. (1996). Attention deficits in adolescents with ADHD and other clinical groups. *Child Neuropsychology, 2,* 1–10.

Mahon, N. E., & Yarcheski, T. J. (1994). Future time perspective and positive health practices in adolescents. *Perceptual and Motor Skills, 79,* 395–398.

Malone, M. A., & Swanson, J. M. (1993). Effects of methylphenidate on impulsive responding in children with attention deficit hyperactivity disorder. *Journal of Child Neurology, 8,* 157–163.

Mangels, J. A., Gershberg, F. B., Shimamura, A. P., & Knight, R. T. (1996). Impaired retrieval from remote memory in patients with frontal lobe damage. *Neuropsychology, 10,* 32–41.

Mangelsdorf, S. C., Shapiro, J. R., & Marzolf, D. (1995). Developmental and temperamental differences in emotion regulation in infancy. *Child Development, 66,* 1817–1828.

Marenco, S., Coppola, R., Daniel, D. G., Zigun, J. R., & Weinberger, D. R. (1993). Regional cerebral blood flow during the Wisconsin Card Sorting Test in normal subjects studied by Xenon-133 dynamic SPT: Comparison of absolute values, percent distribution values, and covariance analysis. *Psychiatry Research: Neuroimaging, 50,* 177–192.

Mariani, M., & Barkley, R. A. (1997). Neuropsychological and academic functioning in preschool children with attention deficit hyperactivity disorder. *Developmental Neuropsychology, 13,* 111–129.

Masters, J. C., & Binger, C. G. (1978). Interrupting the flow of behavior: The stability and development of children's initiation and maintenance of compliant response inhibition. *Merrill–Palmer Quarterly, 24,* 229–242.

Masters, J. C., & Santrock, J. W. (1976). Studies in the self-regulation of behavior: Effects of contingent cognitive and affective events. *Developmental Psychology, 12,* 334–348.

Matier-Sharma, K., Perachio, N., Newcorn, J. H., Sharma, V., & Halperin, J. M. (1995). Differential diagnosis of ADHD: Are objective measures of attention, impulsivity, and activity level helpful? *Child Neuropsychology, 1,* 118–127.

Matochik, J. A., Rumsey, J. M., Zametkin, A. J., Hamburger, S. D., & Cohen, R. M. (1996). Neuropsychological correlates of familial attention-deficit hyperactivity disorder in adults. *Neuropsychiatry, Neuropsychology, and Behavioral Neurology, 9,* 186–191.

Mattes, J. A. (1980). The role of frontal lobe dysfunction in childhood hyperkinesis. *Comprehensive Psychiatry, 21,* 358–369.

Mazur, J. E. (1993). Predicting the strength of a conditioned reinforcer: Effects of delay and uncertainty. *Current Directions in Psychological Science, 2,* 70–74.

McAndrews, M. P., & Milner, B. (1991). The frontal cortex and memory for temporal order. *Neuropsychologia, 29,* 849–859.

McBurnett, K., Harris, S. M., Swanson, J. M., Pfiffner, L. J., Tamm, L., & Freeland, D. (1993). Neuropsychological and psychophysiological differentiation of inattention/overactivity and aggression/defiance symptom groups. *Journal of Clinical Child Psychology, 22,* 165–171.

McCall, R. B. (1994). What process mediates predictions of childhood IQ from infant habituation and recognition memory? Speculations on the roles of inhibition and rate of information processing. *Intelligence, 18,* 107–125.

McCarthy, G., Puce, A., Constable, R. T., Krystal, J. H., Gore, J. C., & Goldman-Rakic, P. (1996). Activation of human prefrontal cortex during spatial and nonspatial working memory tasks measured by functional MRI. *Cerebral Cortex, 6,* 600–611.

McGee, R., Williams, S., & Feehan, M. (1992). Attention deficit disorder and age of onset of problem behaviors. *Journal of Abnormal Child Psychology, 20,* 487–502.

McGee, R., Williams, S., Moffitt, T., & Anderson, J. (1989). A comparison of 13-year old boys with attention deficit and/or reading disorder on neuropsychological measures. *Journal of Abnormal Child Psychology, 17,* 37–53.

McGee, R., Williams, S., & Silva, P. A. (1984). Behavioral and developmental characteristics of aggressive, hyperactive, and aggressive–hyperactive boys. *Journal of the American Academy of Child Psychiatry, 23,* 270–279.

McMahon, S. A., & Greenberg, L. M. (1977). Serial neurologic examination of hyperactive children. *Pediatrics, 59,* 584–587.

Mercugliano, M. (1995). Neurotransmitter alterations in attention-deficit/hyperactivity disorder. *Mental Retardation and Developmental Disabilities Research Reviews, 1,* 220–226.

Methany, A. P., Jr., & Fisher, J. E. (1984). Behavioral perspectives on children's accidents. In M. Wolraich & D. K. Routh (Eds.), *Advances in behavioral pediatrics* (Vol. 5, pp. 221–263). Greenwich, CT: JAI Press.

Michon, J. A. (1985). Introduction. In J. Michon, & T. Jackson (Eds.), *Time, mind, and behavior.* Berlin: Springer-Verlag.

Michon, J. A., & Jackson, J. L. (1984). Attentional effort and cognitive strategies in the processing of temporal information. In J. Gibbon & L. Allan (Eds.), *Timing and time perception: Vol. 423. Annals of the New York Academy of Sciences* (pp. 298–321). New York: New York Academy of Sciences.

Michon, J. A., Jackson, J. L., & Vermeeren, A. (1984). The processing of temporal information. In J. Gibbon & L. Allan (Eds.), *Timing and time perception: Vol. 423. Annals of the New York Academy of Sciences* (pp. 603–604). New York: New York Academy of Sciences.

Milberger, S., Biederman, J., Faraone, S. V., Chen, L., & Jones, J. (1996a). ADHD is associated with early initiation of cigarette smoking in children and adolescents. *Journal of the American Academy of Child and Adolescent Psychiatry, 36,* 37–44.

Milberger, S., Biederman, J., Faraone, S. V., Chen, L., & Jones, J. (1996b). Is maternal smoking during pregnancy a risk factor for attention deficit hyperactivity disorder in children? *American Journal of Psychiatry, 153,* 1138–1142.

Milich, R. (in press). The response of children with ADHD to failure: If at first you don't succeed, do you try, try again? *School Psychology Review.*

Milich, R., Carlson, C. L., Pelham, W. E., & Licht, B. G. (1991). Effects of methylphenidate on the persistence of ADHD boys following failure experiences. *Journal of Abnormal Child Psychology, 19,* 519–536.

Milich, R., Hartung, C. M., Martin, C. A., & Haigler, E. D. (1994). Behavioral disinhibition and underlying processes in adolescents with disruptive behavior disorders. In D. K. Routh (Ed.), *Disruptive behavior disorders in childhood* (pp. 109–138). New York: Plenum Press.

Milich, R., & Kramer, J. (1985). Reflections on impulsivity: An empirical investigation of impulsivity as a construct. In K. Gadow & I. Bialer (Eds.), *Advances in learning and behavioral disabilities,* (Vol. 3, pp. 57–94). Greenwich, CT: JAI Press.

Milich, R., & Loney, J. (1979). The factor composition of the WISC for hyperkinetic/MBD males. *Journal of Learning Disabilities, 12,* 67–70.

Milich, R., Loney, J., & Landau, S. (1982). The independent dimensions of hyperactivity and aggression: A validation with playroom observation data. *Journal of Abnormal Psychology, 91,* 183–198.

Milich, R., & Lorch, E. P. (1994). Television viewing methodology to understand cognitive processing of ADHD children. In T. H. Ollendick & R. J. Prinz (Eds.), *Advances in clinical child psychology* (Vol. 16, pp. 177–202). New York: Plenum Press.

Miller, L. T., & Vernon, P. A. (1996). Intelligence, reaction time, and working memory in 4- to 6-year-old children. *Intelligence, 22,* 155–190.

Milner, B. (1995). Aspects of human frontal lobe function. In H. H. Jasper, S. Riggio, & P. S. Goldman-Rakic (Eds.), *Epilepsy and the functional anatomy of the frontal lobe* (pp. 67–81). New York: Raven Press.

Mirsky, A. F. (1996). Disorders of attention: A neuropsychological perspective. In R. G. Lyon & N. A. Krasnegor (Eds.), *Attention, memory, and executive function* (pp. 71–96). Baltimore: Paul H. Brookes.

Mischel, W. (1983). Delay of gratification as process and as person variable in development. In D. Magnusson & U. L. Allen (Eds.), *Human development: An interactional perspective* (pp. 149–166). New York: Academic Press.

Mischel, W., Shoda, Y., & Peake, P. K. (1988). The nature of adolescent competencies predicted by preschool delay of gratification. *Journal of Personality and Social Psychology, 54,* 687–696.

Mischel, W., Shoda, Y., & Rodriguez, M. I. (1989). Delay of gratification in children. *Science, 244,* 933–938.

Mitchell, E. A., Aman, M. G., Turbott, S. H., & Manku, M. (1987). Clinical characteristics and serum essential fatty acid levels in hyperactive children. *Clinical Pediatrics, 26,* 406–411.

Moffitt, T. E. (1990). Juvenile delinquency and attention deficit disorder: Boys' developmental trajectories from age 3 to 15. *Child Development, 61,* 893–910.

Moffitt, T. E., & Silva, P. A. (1988). Self-reported delinquency, neuropsychological deficit, and history of attention deficit disorder. *Journal of Abnormal Child Psychology, 16,* 553–569.

Morgan, A. E., Hynd, G. W., Riccio, C. A., & Hall, J. (1996). Validity of DSM-IV ADHD predominantly inattentive and combined types: Relationship to previous DSM diagnoses/subtype differences. *Journal of the American Academy of Child and Adolescent Psychiatry, 35,* 325–333.

Mori, L., & Peterson, L. (1995). Knowledge of safety of high and low active-impulsive boys: Implications for child injury prevention. *Journal of Clinical Child Psychology, 24,* 370–376.

Morris, R. G., Ahmed, S., Syed, G. M., & Toone, B. K. (1993). Neural correlates of planning ability: Frontal lobe activation during the Tower of London test. *Neuropsychologia, 31,* 1367–1378.

Morrison, J., & Stewart, M. (1973). The psychiatric status of the legal families of adopted hyperactive children. *Archives of General Psychiatry, 28,* 888–891.

Munir, K., Biederman, J., & Knee, D. (1987). Psychiatric comorbidity in patients with attention deficit disorder: A controlled study. *Journal of the American Academy of Child and Adolescent Psychiatry, 26,* 844–848.

Murphy, D. A., Pelham, W. E., & Lang, A. R. (1992). Aggression in boys with attention deficit-hyperactivity disorder: Methylphenidate effects on naturalistically observed aggression, response to provocation, and social information processing. *Journal of Abnormal Child Psychology, 20,* 451–465.

Murphy, K., & Barkley, R. A. (1996a). Attention deficit hyperactivity disorder in adults. *Comprehensive Psychiatry, 37,* 393–401.

Murphy, K., & Barkley, R. A. (1996b). Prevalence of DSM-IV symptoms of ADHD in adult licensed drivers: Implications for clinical diagnosis. *Journal of Attention Disorders, 1,* 147–161.

Narhi, V., & Ahonen, T. (1995). Reading disability with or without attention deficit hyperactivity disorder: Do attentional problems make a difference? *Developmental Neuropsychology, 11,* 337–349.

Nasrallah, H. A., Loney, J., Olson, S. C., McCalley-Whitters, M., Kramer, J., & Jacoby, C. G. (1986). Cortical atrophy in young adults with a history of hyperactivity in childhood. *Psychiatry Research, 17,* 241–246.

Needleman, H. L., Gunnoe, C., Leviton, A., Reed, R., Peresie, H., Maher, C., & Barrett, P. (1979). Deficits in psychologic and classroom performance of children with elevated dentine lead levels. *New England Journal of Medicine, 300,* 689–695.

Newman, J. P., & Wallace, J. F. (1993). Diverse pathways to deficient self-regulation: Implications for disinhibitory psychopathology in children. *Clinical Psychology Review, 13,* 699–720.

Nichols, P. L., & Chen, T. C. (1981). *Minimal brain dysfunction: A prospective study.* Hillsdale, NJ: Erlbaum.

Nucci, L. P., & Herman, S. (1982). Behavioral disordered children's conceptions of moral, conventional, and personal issues. *Journal of Abnormal Child Psychology, 10,* 411–426.

O'Connor, M., Foch, T., Sherry, T., & Plomin, R. (1980). A twin study of specific behavioral problems of socialization as viewed by parents. *Journal of Abnormal Child Psychology, 8,* 189–199.

Olson, R., Forsberg, H., Wise, B., & Rack, J. (1994). Measurement of word recognition, orthographic, and phonological skills. In G. R. Lyon (Ed.), *Frames of reference for the assessment of learning disabilities: New views on measurement issues* (pp. 243–268). Baltimore: Paul H. Brookes.

Olson, S. L. (1989). Assessment of impulsivity in preschoolers: Cross-measure convergences, longitudinal stability, and relevance to social competence. *Journal of Clinical Child Psychology, 18,* 176–183.

Olson, S. L., Bates, J. E., & Bayles, K. (1990). Early antecedents of childhood impulsivity: The role of parent–child interaction, cognitive competence, and temperament. *Journal of Abnormal Child Psychology, 18,* 317–334.

Oosterlaan, J., & Sergeant, J. A. (1995). Response choice and inhibition in ADHD, anxious, and aggressive children: The relationship between S-R compatibility and stop signal task. In J. A. Sergeant (Ed.), *Eunethydis: European approaches to hyperkinetic disorder* (pp. 225–240). Amsterdam: J. A. Sergeant.

Oosterlaan, J., & Sergeant, J. A. (1996a). Inhibition in ADHD, aggressive and anxious children: A biologically based model of child psychopathology. *Journal of Abnormal Child Psychology, 24,* 19–36.

Oosterlaan, J., & Sergeant, J. A. (1996b). *Response inhibition and response engagement in ADHD, disruptive, anxious, and normal children.* Manuscript submitted for publication.

Oosterlaan, J., & Sergeant, J. A. (in press). The effects of reward and response cost on response inhibition in ADHD, disruptive, anxious, and normal children. *Journal of Abnormal Child Psychology.*

Osmon, D. C., Zigun, J. R., Suchy, Y., & Blint, A. (1996). Whole brain MRI activation on Wisconsin-like card sorting measures: Clues to test specificity.

Ott, D. A., & Lyman, R. D. (1993). Automatic and effortful memory in children exhibiting attention deficit hyperactivity disorder. *Journal of Clinical Child Psychology, 22,* 420–427.

Owen, A. M., Evans, A. C., Petrides, M. (1996). Evidence for a two-stage model of spatial working memory processing within the lateral frontal cortex: A positron emission tomography study. *Cerebral Cortex, 6,* 31–38.

Ownby, R. L., & Matthews, C. G. (1985). On the meaning of the WISC-R third factor: Relations to selected neuropsychological measures. *Journal of Consulting and Clinical Psychology, 53,* 531- 534.

Pardo, J. V., Fox, P. T., & Raichle, M. E. (1991). Localization of a human system for sustained attention by positron emission tomography. *Nature, 349,* 61–64.

Parker, H. (1992). *ADAPT: Accomodations help students with attention deficit disorders.* Plantation, FL: Impact Publications.

Parry, P. A., & Douglas, V. I. (1983). Effects of reinforcement on concept identification in hyperactive children. *Journal of Abnormal Child Psychology, 11,* 327–340.

Partiot, A., Verin, M., Pillon, B., Teixeira-Ferreira, C., Agid, Y., & Dubois, B. (1996). Delayed response tasks in basal gnaglia lesions in man: Further evidence for a striato-frontal cooperation in behavioral adaptation. *Neuropsychologia, 34,* 709–721.

Passler, M. A., Isaac, W., & Hynd, G. W. (1985). Neuropsychological development of behavior attributed to frontal lobe functioning in children. *Developmental Neuropsychology, 1,* 349–370.

Patterson, G. R. (1982). *Coercive family process.* Eugene, OR: Castalia.

Patterson, G. R. (1986). Performance models for antisocial boys. *American Psychologist, 41,* 432–444.

Patterson, G. R., Dishion, T., & Reid, J. (1992). *Antisocial boys.* Eugene, OR: Castalia.

Pauls, D. L. (1991). Genetic factors in the expression of attention-deficit hyperactivity disorder. *Journal of Child and Adolescent Psychopharmacology, 1,* 353–360.

Pearson, D. A., Yaffee, L. S., Loveland, K. A., & Norton, A. M. (1995). Covert visual attention in children with attention deficit hyperactivity disorder: Evidence for developmental immaturity? *Development and Psychopathology, 7,* 351–367.

Pedersen, N. L., Plomin, R., & McClearn, G. E. (1994). Is there G beyond *g*? (Is there genetic influence on specific cognitive abilities independent of genetic influence on general cognitive ability?). *Intelligence, 18,* 133–143.

Pelham, W. E., Milich, R., & Walker, J. L. (1986). Effects of continuous and partial reinforcement and methylphenidate on learning in children with attention deficit disorder. *Journal of Abnormal Psychology, 95,* 319–325.

Pennington, B. F., Bennetto, L., McAleer, O., Roberts, R. J., Jr. (1996). Executive functions and working memory: Theoretical and measurement issues. In G. R. Lyon & N. Krasnegor (Eds.), *Attention, memory, and executive function* (pp. 327–348). Baltimore: Paul H. Brookes.

Pennington, B. F., Grossier, D., & Welsh, M. C. (1993). Contrasting cognitive deficits in attention deficit disorder versus reading disability. *Developmental Psychology, 29,* 511–523.

Pennington, B. F., & Ozonoff, S. (1996). Executive functions and developmental psychopathology. *Journal of Child Psychology and Psychiatry, 37,* 51–87.

Peterson, L. (1982). Altruism and the development of internal control: An integrative model. *Merrill–Palmer Quarterly, 28,* 197–222.

Petrides, M. (1994). Frontal lobes and working memory: Evidence from investigations of the effects of cortical excisions in nonhuman primates. In F. Boller & J. Grafman (Eds.), *Handbook of neuropsychology* (Vol. 9, pp. 59–82). New York: Elsevier.

Pike, A., & Plomin, R. (1996). Importance of nonshared environmental factors for childhood and adolescent psychopathology. *Journal of the American Academy of Child and Adolescent Psychiatry, 35,* 560–570.

Pinker, S. (1995). *The language instinct.* New York: Harper.

Pless, I. B., Taylor, H. G., & Arsenault, L. (1995). The relationship between vigilance deficits and traffic injuries involving children. *Pediatrics, 95,* 219–224.

Plomin, R. (1995). Genetics and children's experiences in the family. *Journal of Child Psychology and Psychiatry, 36,* 33–68.

Pontius, A. A. (1973). Dysfunction patterns analogous to frontal lobe system and caudate nucleus sundromes in some groups of minimal brain dysfunction. *Journal of the American Medical Women's Association, 26,* 285–292.

Popper, K., & Eccles, J. (1977). *The self and its brain.* Berlin/London: Springer-Verlag.

Porrino, L. J., Rapoport, J. L., Behar, D., Sceery, W., Ismond, D. R., & Bunney, W. E., Jr. (1983). A naturalistic assessment of the motor activity of hyperactive boys. *Archives of General Psychiatry, 40,* 681–687.

Quay, H. C. (1997). Inhibition and attention deficit hyperactivity disorder. *Journal of Abnormal Child Psychology, 25,* 7–13.

Quay, H. C. (1988a). Attention deficit disorder and the behavioral inhibition system: The relevance of the neuropsychological theory of Jeffrey A. Gray. In L. M. Bloomingdale & J. Sergeant (Eds.), *Attention deficit disorder: Criteria, cognition, intervention* (pp. 117–126). New York: Pergamon Press.

Quay, H. C. (1988b). The behavioral reward and inhibition systems in childhood behavior disorder. In L. M. Bloomingdale (Ed.), *Attention deficit disorder: III. New research in treatment, psychopharmacology, and attention* (pp. 176–186). New York: Pergamon Press.

Quay, H. C. (1996, January). *Gray's behavioral inhibition in ADHD: An update.* Paper presented at the annual meeting of the International Society for Research in Child and Adolescent Psychopathology, Los Angeles.

Rapoport, J. L., Donnelly, M., Zametkin, A., & Carrougher, J. (1986). "Situational hyperactivity" in a U.S. clinical setting. *Journal of Child Psychology and Psychiatry, 27,* 639–646.

Rapport, M. D., & Kelly, K. L. (1993). Psychostimulant effects on learning and cognitive function. In J. L. Matson (Ed.), *Handbook of hyperactivity in children* (pp. 97–135). Boston: Allyn & Bacon.

Rapport, M. D., Tucker, S. B., DuPaul, G. J., Merlo, M., & Stoner, G. (1986). Hyperactivity and frustration: The influence of control over and size of rewards in delaying gratification. *Journal of Abnormal Child Psychology, 14,* 181–204.

Rasile, D. A., Burg, J. S., Burright, B. G., & Donovick, P. J. (1995). The relationship between performance on the Gordon Diagnostic System and other measures of attention. *International Journal of Psychology, 30,* 35–45.

Raver, C. C. (1996). Relations between social contingency in mother–child interaction and 2-year-olds' social competence. *Developmental Psychology, 32,* 850–859.

Reader, M. J., Harris, E. L., Schuerholz, L. J., & Denckla, M. B. (1994). Attention deficit hyperactivity disorder and executive dysfunction. *Developmental Neuropsychology, 10,* 493–512.

Rezai, K., Andreason, N. C., Alliger, R., Cohen, G., Swayze, V., & O'Leary, D. S. (1993). The neuropsychology of the prefrontal cortex. *Archives of Neurology, 50,* 636–642.

Rhee, S. H., Waldman, I. D., Hay, D. A., & Levy, F. (1995). Sex differences in genetic and environmental influences on DSM-III-R attention-deficit hyperactivity disorder (ADHD). *Behavior Genetics, 25,* 285.

Riccio, C. A., Hall, J., Morgan, A., Hynd, G. W., & Gonzalez, R. M. (1994). Executive function and the Wisconsin Card Sort Test: Relationship with behavioral ratings and cognitive ability. *Developmental Neuropsychology, 10,* 215–229.

Roberts, M. A. (1990). A behavioral observation method for differentiating hyperactive and aggressive boys. *Journal of Abnormal Child Psychology, 18,* 131–142.

Roberts, R. J., & Pennington, B. F. (1996). An integrative framework for examining prefrontal cognitive processes. *Developmental Neuropschology, 12,* 105–126.

Robertson, I. H., Ward, T., Ridgeway, V., & Nimmo-Smith, I. (1996). The structure of normal human attention: The test of everyday attention. *Journal of the International Neuropsychological Society, 2,* 525–534.

Robins, P. M. (1992). A comparison of behavioral and attentional functioning in children diagnosed as hyperactive or learning-disabled. *Journal of Abnormal Child Psychology, 20,* 65–82.

Robins, R. W., John, O. P., Caspi, A., Moffitt, T. E., & Stouthamer-Loeber, M. (1996). Resilient, overcontrolled, and undercontrolled boys: Three replicable personality types. *Journal of Personality and Social Psychology, 70,* 151–171.

Rolls, E. T., Hornak, J., Wade, D., & McGrath, J. (1994). Emotion–related learning in patients with social and emotional changes associated with frontal lobe damage. *Journal of Neurology, Neurosurgery, and Psychiatry, 57,* 1518–1524.

Rosen, B. N., & Peterson, L. (1990). Gender differences in children's outdoor play injuries: A review and an integration. *Clinical Psychology Review, 10,* 187–205.

Rosenbaum, M., & Baker, E. (1984). Self-control behavior in hyperactive and nonhyperactive children. *Journal of Abnormal Child Psychology, 12,* 303–318.

Rosenthal, R. H., & Allen, T. W. (1978). An examination of attention, arousal, and learning dysfunctions of hyperkinetic children. *Psychological Bulletin, 85,* 689–715.

Rosenthal, R. H., & Allen, T. W. (1980). Intratask distractibility in hyperkinetic and nonhyperkinetic children. *Journal of Abnormal Child Psychology, 8,* 175–187.

Ross, D. M., & Ross, S. A. (1982). *Hyperactivity: Research, theory and action.* New York: Wiley.

Ross, R. G., Hommer, D., Brieger, D., Varley, C., & Radant, A. (1994). Eye movement task related to frontal lobe functioning in children with attention deficit disorder. *Journal of the American Academy of Child and Adolescent Psychiatry, 33,* 869–874.

Rothenberger, A. (1995). Electrical brain activity in children with hyperkinetic syndrome: Evidence of a frontal cortical dysfunction. In J. A. Sergeant (Ed.), *Eunethydis: European approaches to hyperkinetic disorder* (pp. 255–270). Amsterdam: J. A. Sergeant.

Routh, D. K., & Schroeder, C. S. (1976). Standardized playroom measures as indices of hyperactivity. *Journal of Abnormal Child Psychology, 4,* 199–207.

Rubin, P., Holm, S., Friberg, L., Videbech, P., Andersen, H. S., Bjerg-Bendsen, B., Stromsp, N., Larsen, J. K., Lassen, N. A., & Hemmingsen, R. (1991). Altered modulation of prefrontal and subcortical brain activity in newly diagnosed schizophrenia and schizophreniform disorder: A regional cerebral blood flow study. *Archives of General Psychiatry, 48,* 987–995.

Rueckert, L., & Grafman, J. (1996). Sustained attention deficits in patients with right frontal lesions. *Neuropsychologia, 34,* 953–963.

Rutter, M. (1977). Brain damage syndromes in childhood: Concepts and findings. *Journal of Child Psychology and Psychiatry, 18,* 1–21.

Rutter, M. (1983). Introduction: Concepts of brain dysfunction syndromes. In M. Rutter (Ed.), *Developmental neuropsychiatry* (pp. 1–14). New York: Guilford Press.

Ryding, E., Bradvik, B., & Ingvar, D. H. (1996). Silent speech activates prefrontal cortical regions asymmetrically, as well as speech-related areas in the dominant hemisphere. *Brain and Language, 52,* 435–451.

Sadeh, M., Ariel, R., & Inbar, D. (1996). Rey-Osterrieth and Taylor Complex Figures: Equivalent measures of visual organization and visual memory in ADHD and normal children. *Child Neuropsychology, 2,* 63–71.

Sagvolden, T., Wultz, B., Moser, E. I., Moser, M., & Morkrid, L. (1989). Results from a comparative neuropsychological research program indicate altered reinforcement mechanisms in children with ADD. In T. Sagvolden & T. Archer (Eds.), *Attention deficit disorder: Clinical and basic research* (pp. 261–286). Hillsdale, NJ: Erlbaum.

Sandberg, S. (1996). Hyperkinetic or attention deficit disorder. *British Journal of Psychiatry, 169,* 19–17.

Satterfield, J. H., Hoppe, C. M., & Schell, A. M. (1982). A prospective study of delinquency in 110 adolescent boys with attention deficit disorder and 88 normal adolescent boys. *American Journal of Psychiatry, 139,* 795–798.

Scarr, S., & McCartney, K. (19893). How people make their own environments: A theory of genotype–environment effeects. *Child Development, 54,* 424–435.

Schachar, R. J., & Logan, G. D. (1990). Impulsivity and inhibitory control in normal development and childhood psychopathology. *Developmental Psychology, 26,* 710–720.

Schachar, R. J., Tannock, R., & Logan, G. (1993). Inhibitory control, impulsiveness, and attention deficit hyperactivity disorder. *Clinical Psychology Review, 13,* 721–739.

Schachar, R. J., Tannock, R., Marriott, M., & Logan, G. (1995). Deficient inhibitory control in attention deficit hyperactivity disorder. *Journal of Abnormal Child Psychology, 23,* 411–438.

Schaughency, E., McGee, R., Raja, S. N., Feehan, M., & Silva, P. A. (1994). Self-reported inattention, impulsivity, and hyperactivity at ages 15 and 18 years in the general population. *Journal of the American Academy of Child and Adolescent Psychiatry, 33,* 173–184.

Scherer, K. R. (1994). Emotion serves to decouple stimulus and response. In P. Ekman & R. J. Davidson (Eds.), *The nature of emotion: Fundamental questions* (pp. 127–130). New York: Oxford University Press.

Schleifer, M., Weiss, G., Cohen, N. J., Elman, M., Cvejic, H., & Kruger, E. (1975). Hyperactivity in preschoolers and the effect of methylphenidate. *American Journal of Orthopsychiatry, 45,* 38–50.

Scholnick, E. K., & Friedman, S. L. (1993). Planning in context: Developmental and situational considerations. *International Journal of Behavioral Development, 16,* 145–167.

Schonfeld, I. S., Shaffer, D., & Barmack, J. E. (1989). Neurological soft signs and school achievement: The mediating effects of sustained attention. *Journal of Abnormal Child Psychology, 17,* 575–596.

Schothorst, P. F., & van Engeland, H. (1996). Long-term behavioral sequelae of prematurity. *Journal of the American Academy of Child and Adolescent Psychiatry, 35,* 175–183.

Schweitzer, J. B., & Sulzer-Azaroff, B. (1995). Self-control in boys with attention-deficit hyperactivity disorder: Effects of added stimulation and time. *Journal of Child Psychology and Psychiatry, 36,* 671–686.

Seidman, L. J., Benedict, K. B., Biederman, J., Bernstein, J. H., Seiverd, K., Milberger, S., Norman, D., Mick, E., & Faraone, S. V. (1995). Performance of children with ADHD on the Rey–Osterrieth Complex Figure: A pilot neuropsychological study. *Journal of Child Psychology and Psychiatry, 36,* 1459–1473.

Seidman, L. J., Biederman, J., Faraone, S. V., Milberger, S., Norman, D., Seiverd, K., Benedict, K., Guite, J., Mick, E., & Kiely, K. (1995). Effects of family history and comorbidity on the neuropsychological performance of children with ADHD: Preliminary findings. *Journal of the American Academy of Child and Adolescent Psychiatry, 34,* 1015–1024.

Seidman, L. J., Biederman, J., Faraone, S. V., Milberger, S., Seiverd, K., Benedict, K., Bernstein, J. H., Weber, W., & Ouellette, C. (1996). Toward defining a neuropsychology of ADHD: Performance of children and adolescents from a large clinically referred sample. *Journal of Consulting and Clinical Psychology, 65,* 150–160.

Semrud-Clikeman, M., Filipek, P. A., Biederman, J., Steingard, R., Kennedy, D., Renshaw, P., & Bekken, K. (1994). Attention-deficit hyperactivity disorder: Magnetic resonance imaging morphometric analysis of the corpus callosum. *Journal of the American Academy of Child and Adolescent Psychiatry, 33,* 875–881.

Senior, N., Towne, D., & Huessy, D. (1979). Time estimation and hyperactivity, a replication. *Perceptual and Motor Skills, 49,* 289–290.

Sergeant, J. (1988). From DSM-III attentional deficit disorder to functional defects. In L. Bloomingdale & J. Sergeant (Eds.), *Attention deficit disorder: Criteria, cognition, and intervention* (pp. 183–198). New York: Pergamon Press.

Sergeant, J. A. (1995a). Hyperkinetic disorder revisited. In J. A. Sergeant (Ed.), *Eunethydis: European approaches to hyperkinetic disorder* (pp. 7–17). Amsterdam: J. A. Sergeant.

Sergeant, J. A. (1996, January). *The cognitive-energetic model of ADHD.* Paper presented at the annual meeting of the International Society for Research in Child and Adolescent Psychopathology, Los Angeles.

Sergeant, J., & Scholten, C. A. (1985). On resource strategy limitations in hyperactivity: Cognitive impulsivity reconsidered. *Journal of Child Psychology and Psychiatry, 26,* 97–109.

Sergeant, J. A., & van der Meere, J. J. (1988). What happens when the hyperactive child commits an error? *Psychiatry Research, 24,* 157–164.

Sergeant, J., & van der Meere, J. J. (1989). The diagnostic significance of attentional processing: Its significance for ADDH classification—A future DSM. In T. Sagvolden & T. Archer (Eds.), *Attention deficit disorder: Clinical and basic research* (pp. 151–166). Hillsdale, NJ: Erlbaum.

Sergeant, J., & van der Meere, J. J. (1990). Convergence of approaches in localizing the hyperactivity deficit. In B. B. Lahey & A. E. Kazdin (Eds.), *Advances in clinical child psychology* (Vol. 13, pp. 207–245). New York: Plenum Press.

Shapiro, E. G., Hughes, S. J., August, G. J., & Bloomquist, M. L. (1993). Processing emotional information in children with attention deficit hyperactivity disorder. *Developmental Neuropsychology, 9,* 207–224.

Shaw, G. A., & Brown, G. (1990). Laterality and creativity concomitants of attention problems. *Developmental Neuropsychology, 6,* 39–57.

Shaw, G. A., & Giambra, L. (1993). Task-unrelated thoughts of college students diagnosed as hyperactive in childhood. *Developmental Neuropsychology, 9,* 17–30.

Shaywitz, S. E., Cohen, D. J., & Shaywitz, B. E. (1980). Behavior and learning difficulties in children of normal intelligence born to alcoholic mothers. *Journal of Pediatrics, 96,* 978–982.

Shaywitz, B. A., Shaywitz, S. E., Byrne, T., Cohen, D. J., & Rothman, S. (1983). Attention deficit disorder: Quantitative analysis of CT. *Neurology, 33,* 1500–1503.

Shaywitz, S. E., & Shaywitz, B. A. (1984). Diagnosis and management of attention deficit disorder: A pediatric perspective. *Pediatric Clinics of North America, 31,* 429–457.

Sherman, D. K., Iacono, W. G., & McGue, M. K. (1997). Attention-deficit hyperactivity disorder dimensions: A twin study of inattention and impulsivity–hyperactivity. *Journal of the American Academy of Child and Adolescent Psychiatry, 36,* 745–753.

Sherman, D. K., McGue, M. K., & Iacono, W. G. (1997). Twin concordance for attention deficit hyperactivity disorder: A comparison of teachers' and mothers' reports. *American Journal of Psychiatry, 154,* 532–535.

Shoda, Y., Mischel, W., & Peake, P. K. (1990). Predicting adolescent cognitive and self-regulatory competencies from preschool delay of gratification: Identifying diagnostic conditions. *Developmental Psychology, 26,* 978–986.

Shue, K., & Douglas, V. I. (1989). Attention deficit hyperactivity disorder, normal development, and frontal lobe syndrome. *Canadian Psychology, 30,* 498 (Abstract).

Shute, G. E., & Huertas, V. (1990). Developmental variability in frontal lobe function. *Developmental Neuropsychology, 6,* 1–11.

Sieg, K. G., Gaffney, G. R., Preston, D. F., & Hellings, J. A. (1995). SPECT brain imaging abnormalities in attention deficit hyperactivity disorder. *Clinical Nuclear Medicine, 20,* 55–60.

Siegel, L. S., & Ryan, E. B. (1989). The development of working memory in normally achieving and subtypes of learning disabled children. *Child Development, 60,* 973–980.

Silberg, J., Rutter, M., Meyer, J., Maes, H., Hewitt, J., Simonoff, E.,

Pickles, A., Loeber, R., & Eaves, L. (1996). Genetic and environmental influences on the covariation between hyperactivity and conduct disturbance in juvenile twins. *Journal of Child Psychology and Psychiatry, 37,* 803–816.

Silva, P. A., Hughes, P., Williams, S., & Faed, J. M. (1988). Blood lead, intelligence, reading attainment, and behaviour in eleven year old children in Dunedin, New Zealand. *Journal of Child Psychology and Psychiatry, 29,* 43–52.

Silverman, I. W., & Ragusa, D. M. (1991). Child and maternal correlates of impulse control in 24-month-old children. *Genetic, Social, and General Psychology Monographs, 116,* 435–473.

Silverman, I. W., & Ragusa, D. M. (1992). A short-term longitudinal study of the early development of self-regulation. *Journal of Abnormal Child Psychology, 20,* 415–435.

Simmell, C., & Hinshaw, S. P. (1993, March). *Moral reasoning and antisocial behavior in boys with ADHD.* Poster presented at the binennial meeting of the Society for Research in Child Development, New Orleans.

Sirigu, A., Zalla, T., Pillon, B., Grafman, J., Bubois, B., & Agid, Y. (1995). Planning and script analysis following prefrontal lobe lesions. In J. Grafman, K. J. Holyoak, & F. Boller (Eds.), *Structure and functions of the human prefrontal cortex: Vol. 769. Annals of the New York Academy of Sciences* (pp. 277–288). New York: New York Acdaemy of Sciences.

Skinner, B. F. (1953). *Science and human behavior.* New York: Macmillan.

Skinner, B. F. (1969). *Contingencies of reinforcement: A theoretical analysis.* New York: Appleton-Century-Crofts.

Skotko, D. J. (1992). Structural properties of verbal commands and their effects on the regulation of motor behavior. In R. Diaz & L. E. Berk (Eds.), *Private speech: From social interaction to self-regulation* (pp. 225–243). Mahwah, NJ: Erlbaum.

Sleator, E. K., & Pelham, W. E. (1986). *Attention deficit disorder.* Norwalk, CT: Appleton-Century-Crofts.

Sleator, E. K., & Ullmann, R. L. (1981). Can the physician diagnose hyperactivity in the office? *Pediatrics, 67,* 13–17.

Smith, E. E., Jonides, J., & Koeppe, R. A. (1996). Dissociating verbal and spatial working memory using PET. *Cerebral Cortex, 11,* 11–20.

Solanto, M. V. (1990). The effects of reinforcement and response-cost on a delayed response task in children with attention deficit hyperactivity disorder: A research note. *Journal of Child Psychology and Psychiatry, 31,* 803–808.

Solanto, M. V. (1991). Dosage effects of Ritalin on cognition. In L. Greenhill & B. B. Osman (Eds.), *Ritalin: Theory and patient management* (pp. 233–246). New York: Mary Ann Liebert.

Solanto, M. V., & Wender, E. H. (1989). Does methylphenidate constrict cognitive functioning? *Journal of the American Academy of Child and Adolescent Psychiatry, 28,* 897–902.

Sonneville, L. M. J., Njiokiktjien, C., & Bos, H. (1994). Methylphenidate and information processing: Part 1. Differentiation between responders and nonresponders. Part 2: Efficacy in responders. *Journal of Clinical and Experimental Neuropsychology, 16,* 877–897.

Sonuga-Barke, E. J. S. (1995). Disambiguating inhibitory dysfunction in childhood hyperactivity. In J. A. Sergeant (Ed.), *Eunethydis: European approaches to hyperkinetic disorder* (pp. 209–223). Amsterdam: J. A. Sergeant.

Sonuga-Barke, E. J. S., Houlberg, K., & Hall, M. (1994). When is "impulsiveness" not impulsive? The case of hyperactive children's cognitive style. *Journal of Child Psychology and Psychiatry, 35,* 1247–1255.

Sonuga-Barke, E. J. S., Lamparelli, M., Stevenson, J., Thompson, M., & Henry, A. (1994). Behaviour problems and pre-school intellectual attainment: The associations of hyperactivity and conduct problems. *Journal of Child Psychology and Psychiatry, 35,* 949–960.

Sonuga-Barke, E. J. S., Taylor, E., & Hepinstall, E. (1992). Hyperactivity and delay aversion: II. The effect of self versus externally imposed stimulus presentation periods on memory. *Journal of Child Psychology and Psychiatry, 33,* 399–409.

Sonuga-Barke, E. J. S., Taylor, E., Sembi, S., & Smith, J. (1992). Hyperactivity and delay aversion: I. The effect of delay on choice. *Journal of Child Psychology and Psychiatry, 33,* 387–398.

Sonuga-Barke, E. J. S., Williams, E., Hall, M., & Saxton, T. (1996). Hyperactivity and delay aversion: III. The effect on cognitive style of imposing delay after errors. *Journal of Child Psychology and Psychiatry, 37,* 189–194.

Sparrow, S. S., Baila, D. A., & Cicchetti, D. V. (1984). *Vineland Adaptive Behavior Scales.* Circle Pines, MN: American Guidance Service.

Speece, M. W., & Brent, S. B. (1984). Children's understanding of death: A review of three components of a death concept. *Child Development, 55,* 1671–1686.

Sprick-Buckminster, S., Biederman, J., Milberger, S., Faraone, S. V., & Lehman, B. (1993). Are perinatal complications relevant to the manifestation of ADD? Issues of comorbidity and familiality. *Journal of the American Academy of Child and Adolescent Psychiatry, 32,* 1032–1037.

Stein, M. A., Szumowski, E., Blondis, T. A., & Roizen, N. J. (1995). Adaptive skills dysfunction in ADD and ADHD children. *Journal of Child Psychology and Psychiatry, 36,* 663–670.

Steinkamp, M. W. (1980). Relationships between environmental distractions and task performance of hyperactive and normal children. *Journal of Learning Disabilities, 13,* 40–45.

Sternberg, R. J., & Lubart, T. I. (1996). Investing in creativity. *American Psychologist, 51,* 677–688.

Stevenson, J. (1994, June). *Genetics of ADHD.* Paper presented at the annual meeting of the Professional Group for ADD and Related Disorders, London.

Stewart, K. J., & Moely, B. E. (1983). The WISC-R third factor: What does it mean? *Journal of Consulting and Clinical Psychology, 51,* 940-941.

Stewart, M. A. (1970). Hyperactive children. *Scientific American, 222,* 94–98.

Stewart, M. A., Pitts, F. N., Craig, A. G., & Dieruf, W. (1966). The hyperactive child syndrome. *American Journal of Orthopsychiatry, 36,* 861–867.

Stewart, M. A., Thach, B. T., & Friedin, M. R. (1970). Accidental poisoning and the hyperactive child syndrome. *Disease of the Nervous System, 31,* 403–407.

Stifter, C. A., & Braungart, J. M. (1995). The regulation of negative reactivity in infancy: Function and development. *Developmental Psychology, 31,* 448–455.

Still, G. F. (1902). Some abnormal psychical conditions in children. *Lancet, 1,* 1008–1012, 1077–1082, 1163–1168.

Strauss, A. A., & Kephart, N. C. (1955). *Psychopathology and education of the brain-injured child: Vol II. Progress in theory and clinic.* New York: Grune & Stratton.

Strauss, A. A., & Lehtinen, L. E. (1947). *Psychopathology and education of the brain-injured child.* New York: Grune & Stratton.

Streissguth, A. P., Bookstein, F. L., Sampson, P. D., & Barr, H. M. (1995). Attention: Prenatal alcohol and continuities of vigilance and attentional problems from 4 through 14 years. *Development and Psychopathology, 7,* 419–446.

Streissguth, A. P., Martin, D. C., Barr, H. M., Sandman, B. M., Kirchner, G. L., & Darby, B. L. (1984). Intrauterine alcohol and nicotine exposure: Attention and reaction time in 4-year-old children. *Developmental Psychology, 20,* 533–541.

Stroop, J. P. (1935). Studies of interference in serial verbal reactions. *Journal of Experimental Psychology, 18,* 643–662.

Stryker, S. (1925). Encephalitis lethargica—The behavior residuals. *Training School Bulletin, 22,* 152–157.

Stuss, D. T., & Benson, D. F. (1986). *The frontal lobes.* New York: Raven.

Stuss, D. T., Gow, C. A., & Hetherington, C. R. (1992). "No longer Gage": Frontal lobe dysfunction and emotional changes. *Journal of Consulting and Clinical Psychology, 60,* 349–359.

Swanson, H. L., & Berninger, V. (1995). The role of working memory in skilled and less skilled readers' comprehension. *Intelligence, 21,* 83–108.

Swanson, J. M., McBurnett, K., Christian, D. L., & Wigal, T. (1995). Stimulant medications and the treatment of children with ADHD. In T. H. Ollendick & R. J. Prinz (Eds.), *Advances in clinical child psychology* (Vol. 17, pp. 265–322). New York: Plenum Press.

Swanson, J. M., Posner, M. I., Potkin, S., Bonforte, S., Youpa, D., Cantwell, D., & Crinella, F. (1991). Activating tasks for the study of visual–spatial attention in ADHD children: A cognitive anatomical approach. *Journal of Child Neurology, 6*(Suppl.), S119–S127.

Szatmari, P. (1992). The epidemiology of attention-deficit hyperactivity disorders. In G. Weiss (Ed.), *Child and adolescent Psychiatry Clinics of North America: Attention deficit hyperactivity disorder* (pp. 361–372). Philadelphia: Saunders.

Szatmari, P., Offord, D. R., & Boyle, M. H. (1989). Correlates, associated

impairments, and patterns of service utilization of children with attention deficit disorders: Findings from the Ontario Child Health Study.
Journal of Child Psychology and Psychiatry, 30, 205–217.

Szatmari, P., Saigal, S., Rosenbaum, P., & Campbell, D. (1993). Psychopathology and adaptive functioning among extremely low birthweight children
at eight years of age. *Development and Psychopathology, 5,* 345–357.

Tannock, R. (1996, January). *Discourse deficits in ADHD: Executive dysfunction
as an underlying mechanism?* Paper presented at the annual meeting of the
International Society for Research in Child and Adolescent Psychopathology, Santa Monica, CA.

Tannock, R. (in press). Attention deficit disorders with anxiety disorders. In
T. E. Brown (Ed.), *Subtypes of attention deficit disorders in children, adolescents,
and adults.* Washington, DC: American Psychiatric Press.

Tannock, R., Ickowicz, A., & Schachar, R. (1995). Differential effects of
methylphenidate on working memory in ADHD children with and
without comorbid anxiety. *Journal of the American Academy of Child and
Adolescent Psychiatry, 34,* 886–896.

Tannock, R., Purvis, K. L., & Schachar, R. J. (1992). Narrative abilities in
children with attention deficit hyperactivity disorder and normal peers.
Journal of Abnormal Child Psychology, 21, 103–117.

Tannock, R., Schachar, R. J., Carr, R. P., Chajczyk, D., & Logan, G. D. (1989).
Effects of methylphenidate on inhibitory control in hyperactive children.
Journal of Abnormal Child Psychology, 17, 473–491.

Tant, J. L., & Douglas, V. I. (1982). Problem-solving in hyperactive, normal,
and reading-disabled boys. *Journal of Abnormal Child Psychology, 10,*
285–306.

Tarver-Behring, S., Barkley, R. A., & Karlsson, J. (1985). The mother-child
interactions of hyperactive boys and their normal siblings. *American
Journal of Orthopsychiatry, 55,* 202–209.

Taylor, E. (1986). *The overactive child.* Philadelphia: Lippincott.

Taylor, E., Sandberg, S., Thorley, G., & Giles, S. (1991). *The epidemiology of
childhood hyperactivity.* London: Oxford University Press.

Taylor, H. G., Schatschneider, C., Petrill, S., Barry, C. T., & Owens, C. (1996).
Executive dysfunction in children with early brain disease: Outcomes
post *Haemophilus influenzae* meningitis. *Developmental Neuropsychology, 12,*
35–51.

Teicher, M. H., Ito, Y, Glod, C. A., & Barber, N. I. (1996). Objective
measurement of hyperactivity and attentional problems in ADHD.
Journal of the American Academy of Child and Adolescent Psychiatry, 35,
334–342.

Terman, L. M. (1954). Scientists and nonscientists in a group of 800 gifted
men. *Psychological Monographs: Genereal and Applied, 68,* 1–44.

Thapar, A., Hervas, A., & McGuffin, P. (1995). Childhood hyperactivity
scores are highly heritable and show sibling competition effects: Twin
study evidence. *Behavior Genetics, 25,* 537–544.

Thomson, G. O. B., Raab, G. M., Hepburn, W. S., Hunter, R., Fulton, M.,
& Laxen, D. P. H. (1989). Blood-lead levels and children's behavior—

Results from the Edinburgh lead study. *Journal of Child Psychology and Psychiatry, 30,* 515–528.

Thoresen, C. E., & Mahoney, M. J. (1974). *Behavioral self-control.* New York: Holt, Rinehart & Winston.

Torgesen, J. K. (1994). Issues in the assessment of of executive function: An information-processing perspective. In G. R. Lyon (Ed.), *Frames of reference for the assessment of learning disabilities: New views on measurement issues* (pp. 143–162). Baltimore: Paul H. Brookes.

Trommer, B. L., Hoeppner, J., & Zecker, S. G. (1991). The Go-No Go Test in attention deficit disorder is sensitive to methylphenidate. *Journal of Child Neurology, 6,* 126–129.

Trommer, B. L., Hoeppner, J. B., Lorber, R., & Armstrong, K. (1988). Pitfalls in the use of a continuous performance test as a diagnostic tool in attention deficit disorder. *Developmental and Behavioral Pediatrics, 9,* 339–346.

Truelle, J. L., Le Gall, D., Joseph, P. A., Aubin, G., Derouesne, C., & Lezak, M. D. (1995). Movement disturbances following frontal lobe lesions: Qualitative analysis of gesture and motor programming. *Neuropsychiatry, Neuropsychology, and Behavioral Neurology, 8,* 14–19.

Tucker, D. M., Luu, P., & Pribram, K. H. (1995). Social and emotional self-regulation. In J. Grafman, K. J. Holyoak, & F. Boller (Eds.), *Structure and functions of the human prefrontal cortex: Vol. 769. Annals of the New York Academy of Sciences* (pp. 213–239). New York: New York Academy of Sciencs.

Ullman, D. G., Barkley, R. A., & Brown, H. W. (1978). The behavioral symptoms of hyperkinetic children who successfully responded to stimulant drug treatment. *American Journal of Orthopsychiatry, 48,* 425–437.

van den Oord, E. J. C. G., & Rowe, D. C. (1997). Continuity and change in children's social maladjustment: A developmental behavior genetic study. *Developmental Psychology, 33,* 319–332.

van den Oord, E. J. C. G., Boomsma, D. I., & Verhulst, F. C. (1994). A study of problem behaviors in 10- to 15-year-old biololgically related and unrelated international adoptees. *Behavior Genetics, 24,* 193–205.

van den Oord, E. J. C. G. Verhulst, F. C., & Boomsma, D. I. (1996). A genetic study of maternal and paternal ratings of problem behaviors in 3 year-old twins. *Journal of Abnormal Psychology, 105,* 349–357.

van der Meere, J. (in press). The role of attention. In S. Sandberg (Ed.), *Mongraphs on child and adolesent psychiatry: Hyperactivity disorders* (pp. 109–146). Cambridge, England: Cambridge University Press.

van der Meere, J., Gunning, W. B., & Stemerdink, N. (1996). Changing response set in normal development and in ADHD children with and without tics. *Journal of Abnormal Child Psychology, 24,* 767–786.

van der Meere, J., Hughes, K. A., Borger, N., & Sallee, F. R. (1995). The effect of reward on sustained attention in ADHD children with and without CD. In J. A. Sergeant (Ed.), *Eunethydis: European approaches to hyperkinetic disorder* (pp. 241–253). Amsterdam: J. A. Sergeant.

van der Meere, J., & Sergeant, J. (1988a). Controlled processing and vigilance in hyperctivity: Time will tell. *Journal of Abnormal Child Psychology, 16,* 641–656.

van der Meere, J., & Sergeant, J. (1988b). Focused attention in pervasively hyperactive children. *Journal of Abnormal Child Psychology, 16,* 627–640.

van der Meere, J., Shalev, R., Borger, N., & Gross-Tsur, V. (1995). Sustained attention, activation and MPH in ADHD: A research note. *Journal of Child Psychology and Psychiatry, 36,* 697–703.

van der Meere, J., van Baal, M., & Sergeant, J. (1989). The additive factor method: A differential diagnostic tool in hyperactivity and learning disability. *Journal of Abnormal Child Psychology, 17,* 409–422.

van der Meere, J., Vreeling, H. J., & Sergeant, J. (1992). A motor presetting study in hyperactive, learning disabled and control children. *Journal of Child Psychology and Psychiatry, 33,* 1347–1354.

van der Meere, J., Wekking, E., & Sergeant, J. (1991). Sustained attention and pervasive hyperactivity. *Journal of Child Psychology and Psychiatry, 32,* 275–284.

Vaughn, B. E., Kopp, C. B., & Krakow, J. B. (1984). The emergence and consolidation of self-control from eighteen to thirty months of age: Normative trends and individual differences. *Child Development, 55,* 990–1004.

Vendrell, P., Junque, C., Pujol, J., Jurado, M. A., Molet, J., & Grafman, J. (1995). The role of prefrontal regions in the Stroop task. *Neuropsychologia, 33,* 341–352.

Verin, M., Pillon, P. B., Malapani, C., Agid, Y., & Dubois, B. (1993). Delayed response tasks and prefrontal lesions in man—Evidence for self generated patterns of behaviour with poor environmental modulation. *Neuropsychologia, 31,* 1379–1396.

Voelker, S. L., Carter, R. A., Sprague, D. J., Gdowski, C. L., & Lachar, D. (1989). Developmental trends in memory and metamemory in children with attention deficit disorder. *Journal of Pediatric Psychology, 14,* 75–88.

Voeller, K. K. S., & Heilman, K. M. (1988). Motor impersistence in children with attention deficit hyperactivity disorder: Evidence for right hemisphere dysfunction, abstract. *Annals of Neurology, 24,* 323.

Vygotsky, L. S. (1962). *Thought and language* (E. Hanfmann & G. Vakar, Eds. & Trans.). Cambridge, MA: MIT Press.

Vygotsky, L. S. (1978). *Mind in society.* Cambridge, MA: Harvard University Press.

Vygotsky, L. S. (1987). Thinking and speech. In *The collected works of L. S. Vygotsky: Vol. 1. Problems in general psychology* (N. Minick, Trans., pp. 37–285). New York: Plenum Press.

Wadsworth, S. J., DeFries, J. C., Fulker, D. W., Olson, R. K., & Pennington, B. F. (1995). Reading performance and verbal short-term memory: A twin study of reciprocal causation. *Intelligence, 20,* 145–167.

Walker, N. W. (1982). Comparison of cognitive tempo and time estimation by young boys. *Perceptual and Motor Skills, 54,* 715–722.

Weiss, G., & Hechtman, L. T. (1993). *Hyperactive children grown up* (2nd ed.): *ADHD in children adolescents, and adults.* New York: Guilford Press.

Weithorn, C. J., & Kagen, E. (1984). Verbal mediation in high-active and cognitively impulsive second graders. *Journal of Learning Disabilities, 17,* 87–96.

Welner, Z., Welner, A., Stewart, M., Palkes, H., & Wish, E. (1977). A controlled study of siblings of hyperactive children. *Journal of Nervous and Mental Disease, 165,* 110–117.

Welsh, M. C., & Pennington, B. F. (1988). Assessing frontal lobe functioning in children: Views from developmental psychology. *Developmental Neuropsychology, 4,* 199–230.

Welsh, M. C., Pennington, B. F., & Grossier, D. B. (1991). A normative-developmental study of executive function: A window on prefrontal function in children. *Developmental Neuropsychology, 7,* 131–149.

Werry, J. S. (1988). Differential diagnosis of attention deficits and conduct disorders. In L. M. Bloomingdale & J. A. Sergeant (Eds.), *Attention deficit disorder: Criteria, cognition, intervention* (pp. 83–96). London: Pergamon Press.

Werry, J. S., Elkind, G. S., & Reeves, J. S. (1987). Attention deficit, conduct, oppositional, and anxiety disorders in children: III. Laboratory differences. *Journal of Abnormal Child Psychology, 15,* 409–428.

Werry, J. S., Minde, K., Guzman, A., Weiss, G., Dogan, K., & Hoy, E. (1972). Studies on the hyperactive child: VII. Neurological status compared with neurotic and normal children. *American Journal of Orthopsychiatry, 42,* 441–451.

Weyandt, L. L., & Willis, W. G. (1994). Executive functions in school-aged children: Potential efficacy of tasks in discriminating clinical groups. *Developmental Neuropsychology, 19,* 27–38.

Whalen, C. K., Henker, B., Collins, B. E., McAuliffe, S., & Vaux, A. (1979). Peer interaction in structured communication task: Comparisons of normal and hyperactive boys and of methylphenidate (Ritalin) and placebo effects. *Child Development, 50,* 388-401.

Whalen, C. K., Henker, B., & Dotemoto, S. (1980). Methylphenidate and hyperactivity: Effects on teacher behaviors. *Science, 208,* 1280–1282.

White, J., Barratt, E., & Adams, P. (1979). The hyperactive child in adolescence: A comparative study of physiological and behavioral patterns. *Journal of the American Academy of Child Psychiatry, 18,* 154–169.

White, J. L., Moffitt, T. E., Caspi, A., Bartusch, D. J., Needles, D. J., & Stouthamer-Loeber, M. (1994). Measuring impulsivity and examining its relationship to delinquency. *Journal of Abnormal Psychology, 103,* 192–205.

Wigal, T., Swanson, J. M., Douglas, V. I., Wigal, S. B., Stoiber, C. M., & Fulbright, K. K. (1993). *Reinforcement effects on frustration and persistence in children with attention-deficit hyperactivity disorder.* Manuscript submitted for publication.

Wilkison, P. C., Kircher, J. C., McMahon, W. M., & Sloane, H. N. (1995). Effects of methylphenidate on reward strength in boys with attention-deficit hyperactivity disorder. *Journal of the American Academy of Child and Adolescent Psychiatry, 34,* 877–885.

Willerman, L. (1973). Activity level and hyperactivity in twins. *Child Development, 44,* 288–293.

Williams, G. V., & Goldman-Rakic, P. S. (1995). Modulation of memory fields by dopamine D1 receptors in prefrontal cortex. *Nature, 376,* 572–575.

Willis, T. J., & Lovaas, I. (1977). A behavioral approach to treating hyperactive children: The parent's role. In J. B. Millichap (Ed.), *Learning disabilities and related disorders* (pp. 119–140). Chicago: Yearbook Medical Publications.

Wolraich, M. L., Wilson, D. B., & White, J. W. (1995). The effect of sugar on behavior or cognition in children; A meta-analysis. *Journal of the American Medical Association, 274,* 1617–1621.

Zagar, R., & Bowers, N. D. (1983). The effect of time of day on problem-solving and classroom behavior. *Psychology in the Schools, 20,* 337–345.

Zahn, T. P., Krusei, M. J. P., & Rapoport, J. L. (1991). Reaction time indices of attention deficits in boys with disruptive behavior disorders. *Journal of Abnormal Child Psychology, 19,* 233–252.

Zakay, D. (1990). The evasive art of subjective time measurement: Some methodological dilemmas. In R. A. Block (Ed.), *Cognitive models of psychological time* (pp. 59–84). Hillsdale, NJ: Erlbaum.

Zakay, D. (1992). The role of attention in children's time perception. *Journal of Experimental Child Psychology, 54,* 355–371.

Zametkin, A. J., Liebenauer, L. L., Fitzgerald, G. A., King, A. C., Minkunas, D. V., Herscovitch, P., Yamada, E. M., & Cohen, R. M. (1993). Brain metabolism in teenagers with attention-deficit hyperactivity disorder. *Archives of General Psychiatry, 50,* 333–340.

Zametkin, A. J., Nordahl, T. E., Gross, M., King, A. C., Semple, W. E. , Rumsey, J., Hamburger, S., & Cohen, R. M. (1990). Cerebral glucose metabolism in adults with hyperactivity of childhood onset. *New England Journal of Medicine, 323,* 1361–1366.

Zelazo, P. D., & Resnick, J. S. (1991). Age-related asynchrony of knowledge and action. *Child Development, 62,* 719–735.

Zelazo, P. R., Kearsley, R. B., & Stack, D. M. (1995). Mental representations for visual sequences: Increased speed of central processing from 22 to 32 months. *Intelligence, 20,* 41–63.

Zelazo, P. R., Reznick, J. S., & Pinon, D. E. (1995). Response control and the execution of verbal rules. *Developmental Psychology, 31,* 508–517.

Zentall, S. S. (1985). A context for hyperactivity. In K. D. Gadow & I. Bialer (Eds.), *Advances in learning and behavioral disabilities* (Vol. 4, pp. 273–343). Greenwich, CT: JAI Press.

Zentall, S. S. (1988). Production deficiencies in elicited language but not in the spontaneous verbalizations of hyperactive children. *Journal of Abnormal Child Psychology, 16,* 657–673.

Zentall, S. S., & Smith, Y. S. (1993). Mathematical performance and behavior of children with hyperactivity with and without coexisting aggression. *Behavior Research and Therapy, 31,* 701–710.

Zentall, S. S., Smith, Y. N., Lee, Y. B., & Wieczorek, C. (1994). Mathematical outcomes of attention-deficit hyperactivity disorder. *Journal of Learning Disabilities, 27,* 510–519.

Index